W9-BVL-293

Praise for Teaching Yoga

"*Teaching Yoga* is an urgently needed manual that will be a valuable tool in the arsenal of aspiring yoga teachers to add perspective and to hone their skills. It provides a wealth of foundational information, advice, tips, guidance, and grist for the mill."

  –Ganga White, founder, White Lotus Yoga Foundation, Santa Barbara, California, and author of *Yoga Beyond Belief: Insights to Awaken and Deepen Your Practice*

"*Teaching Yoga* is friendly, well-thought-out, helpful, clear, and tremendously thorough. Many people will benefit from this gift, it being exactly what is needed to help a growing teacher teach at his or her best. I'm glad it is finally in print and it is coming out just in time for my next teacher training!"

  –Erich Schiffmann, author of *Yoga: The Spirit and Practice of Moving into Stillness*

"Mark Stephens is making a real offering to yoga teachers, providing practical tools and inspiration for the path that embraces all forms of embodied yoga. There are hard-to-find gems that make this a great resource, from the section on the mythological meaning behind the *asanas* to teaching cues for the core *asanas* and sequencing tools from *vinyasa krama.* Enjoy this great resource and dive deeply into your own transformational process of teaching yoga."

  –Shiva Rea, leading instructor of Transformational Prana Flow Yoga and Yoga Trance Dance

"Yoga luminary Mark Stephens has written a book that embodies Hatha yoga itself, offering a highly informative guide for all yoga teachers. *Teaching Yoga* answers our questions and addresses our controversies. This comprehensive and scholarly guide is now required reading for our teaching staff."

  –Mary Lynn Fitton, founder and director of programs, The Art of Yoga Project

"Dedicated yoga students and their teachers will find Mark Stephens's comprehensive book an essential and timeless resource. Filled with profound insights presented with clarity and intelligence, *Teaching Yoga* is a wonderful resource that beautifully models the practice of yoga itself; it unites many diverse threads of truth into a cohesive, vibrant whole. It has quickly become an indispensable part of my teaching library."

  –Daniel Stewart, cofounder and director, Rising Lotus Yoga, Los Angeles, California

"Fifteen years after starting a successful movement to bring yoga into inner city schools, prisons, treatment centers, and veterans' facilities, Mark Stephens is back with a treasure trove of wisdom and insight drawn from years of training teachers for success in those settings as well as more traditional yoga spaces such as studios, retreats, and conferences. *Teaching Yoga* is destined to be a classic that every yoga teacher and student will consult for years to come."

  –James Wvinner, yogi and cofounder of Yoga, Tribe, and Culture

ALSO BY MARK STEPHENS

Yoga Sequencing: Designing Transformative Yoga Classes

TEACHING YOGA

Essential Foundations and Techniques

MARK STEPHENS

North Atlantic Books
Berkeley, California

Copyright © 2010 by Mark Stephens. All rights reserved. No portion of this book, except for brief review, may be reproduced, stored in a retrieval system, or transmitted in any form or by any means—electronic, mechanical, photocopying, recording, or otherwise—without the written permission of the publisher. For information contact North Atlantic Books.

Published by
North Atlantic Books
P.O. Box 12327
Berkeley, California 94712

Front and back cover photographs © James Wvinner
Cover and book design © Ayelet Maida, A/M Studios
Printed in the United States of America

Teaching Yoga: Essential Foundations and Techniques is sponsored by the Society for the Study of Native Arts and Sciences, a nonprofit educational corporation whose goals are to develop an educational and cross-cultural perspective linking various scientific, social, and artistic fields; to nurture a holistic view of arts, sciences, humanities, and healing; and to publish and distribute literature on the relationship of mind, body, and nature.

North Atlantic Books' publications are available through most bookstores. For further information, visit our website at www.northatlanticbooks.com or call 800-733-3000.

Library of Congress Cataloging-in-Publication Data
Stephens, Mark, 1958–
  Teaching yoga : essential foundations and techniques / Mark Stephens.
      p. ; cm.
  Includes bibliographical references and index.
  ISBN 978-1-55643-885-1
  1. Yoga—Study and teaching. I. Title.
  [DNLM: 1. Yoga. 2. Teaching—methods. QT 18 S829t 2009]
  RA781.7.S7277 2009
  613.7'04607—dc22
                2009041082

6 7 8 9 10 11 12 SHERIDAN 17 16 15 14 13 12

To the best teacher
you'll ever have—
the one singing and dancing
in your heart.

ACKNOWLEDGMENTS

This book would not have been conceivable without the students I've been honored to teach over the past fifteen years in yoga studios, shelters, prisons, treatment centers, and public schools, along with hundreds of participants in my teacher-training courses over the years. Together they remain my most influential source of inspiration and insight as a yoga teacher and teacher trainer, giving concrete expression and meaning to the more formal yoga teacher training and instruction I received at Yoga Works in the early to mid-1990s.

The formative voices of my first teachers—Erich Schiffmann, Chuck Miller, Steve Ross, Lisa Walford, and Maty Ezraty—still echo in my approach to the practice. In-depth apprenticeships with Jasmine Lieb and Shiva Rea gave me the opportunity to hone my ability to see and relate to students in a more meaningful way, amplified by assisting Shiva on several yoga retreats from 1995 to 1997. In-depth workshops over the years with Ramanand Patel, Richard Freeman, Dona Holleman, Kofi Busia, Patricia Walden, Rodney Yee, Tias Little, John Schumacher, Tim Miller, John Friend, and Judith Lasater influenced my approach to teaching in often quite different ways.

Conversations with several friends and colleagues helped me to refine my presentation of every topic covered here. Sally Kempton, Joel Kramer, Diana Alstad, Shiva Rea, Kofi Busia, Mariel Hemingway, James Bailey, Ganga White, James Wvinner, Jennifer Stanley, Ralph Quinn, and Sarah Powers led me to refine the text in ways they might not recognize but that are nonetheless expressed in these pages. Scores of participants in my Yoga Teacher Training and In-Depth Studies Program in Santa Cruz, California, read and shared in discussions of early drafts of every chapter; Jody Greene, Lynda Lewitt, Karen Parrish, Jim Frandeen, and Jenna Jeantet offered thorough readings and critiques.

My research assistant, yoga teacher Cindy Cheung, was helpful in finding and organizing a variety of resources; she also read and critiqued each chapter. Melinda Stephens-Bukey read and critiqued several early drafts and assisted with the appendices. Laurie Gibson read and edited the initial draft of the manuscript, offering questions and suggestions conceivable only by a thoughtful professional editor from outside the yoga community. Many other friends, students, and fellow teachers read portions of the manuscript and offered invaluable suggestions.

Bryce Florian, Maya Gil-Cantu, Jody Greene, Debbie Jordan, JuJu Kim, Jeanette Lehouillier, Joanna Saxby, Jennifer Stanley, and Dana Wingfield graciously modeled the asanas shown in Chapter Seven. Photographs appearing in all other chapters are courtesy of James Wvinner. Chris MacIvor provided the anatomy illustrations that appear in Chapter Four, all which he originally drew for Ray Long, MD's Bandha Yoga series of yoga anatomy books.

The folks at North Atlantic Books were delightful to work with, starting with copublisher Lindy Hough pulling the needle of my original manuscript from a haystack of book proposals and embracing my vision of the book. My wonderful project editor at North Atlantic, Jessica Sevey, expertly guided me through all the phases of translating a draft manuscript into a complete book, providing a wide array of insights on every element of the book. Christopher Church masterfully edited the entire manuscript, bringing much greater clarity and consistency to the overall narrative. Ayelet Maida's beautiful design speaks for itself.

Any errors are entirely my responsibility.

None of this would have been possible without the loving support of Michael, Melinda, Reatha, John, Jennifer, Jo, and DiAnna.

CONTENTS

Appendices

FOREWORD

by Mariel Hemingway

Yoga has been such an amazing teacher in my life. What was at first a "work-out" and a challenge from a friend who thought it would "kick my butt" became a ritual that led me to a path of understanding more about myself. It guided me to honor my body and my soul in a way that I had never done before. I learned what it meant to listen to my movement in concert with my breath. It would bring up things that led me to become aware of myself at a profound level. Before yoga I was always moving too fast and feeling pushed to achieve, reach a goal, and win (I was a downhill racer as a kid). Then came yoga, and I was led into a place where breath and movement informed who I became every day. It was not a physical movement that invoked self-judgment and criticism; to the contrary, it was a gentle lover of self. I learned through yoga *asana* that the body is a map to the soul and that my own body speaks a language that is designed for me to hear and learn from. Everyone's body and practice are different in the sense that the language that the body speaks is entirely different from one person to the next, but the template is the same.

When I met Mark Stephens I had been a practicing yogini for nearly twenty years, and yet I knew that Mark would be a significant teacher in my life. He was and still is an inspiration to me because of his grounded understanding of the principles of yoga and the relationship of the body to asana. But what really moves me about Mark is his relationship to the spirit of yoga and his depth of understanding of the science behind yogic tradition. He understands the template of what is needed to become the best you can be as a practitioner and especially as a teacher.

Mark helped me to put together my first book, *Finding My Balance,* and through that experience we became close friends. He helped me with the yoga sequencing in my book as well as the photos, and he provided space for me to take gorgeous yoga pictures in his new yoga studio he was opening in LA at that time. We laughed a lot and had fun. I helped him choose colors for the walls and the best place for a bookshelf or a Natarajasana statue while he guided me to understand that what I spoke in the sequence of my book had a deeper impression than I might have thought. The depth of what I was doing by sharing yoga in my book was bigger than just showing postures for a yoga routine. It was a gift of sharing who I was as a person at that time. Mark was conscious of the power of what I was sharing with others—maybe more than even I realized. I am sure today we would come up with different sequencing as I am a different person than I was in 2003. Still, Mark helped me find the teacher in me and how to share her through asana in concert with who I was at that time.

Between brainstorming the studio look and my own personal requirements for my book, we also took time to do yoga. We often remained quiet for hours in order to let the experience of our own individual practice do what needed to be done for the body and soul. Mark understands the dance of the physical with the spirit in relationship with yoga. He is a scientist and a spiritual man who is guided by his passion for yoga and teaching. He is a teacher's teacher. He gives the student the empowering feeling that they know more than they do while making sure they get what they need to from the science, the history, and the mystery of yoga. I am so excited that Mark has been guided to share his profound knowledge of this ancient tradition. He is bringing it to us in a modern, tangible, and practical way so that we as practitioners and teachers can be more efficient and qualified as we grow into this magical experience we call our yoga practice for ourselves and in service of others.

INTRODUCTION

Teaching yoga will change your life. It will continually bring you back to your earliest motivations to practice and add abundant clarity to the first questions you asked yourself about yoga. These questions are almost invariably philosophical and personal, the answers shifting amid the currents of our lives. Who am I? What makes me feel happy and balanced? How can I make things easier and steadier in my life? Even after years or decades of practice, most teachers' motives are still evolving. Jim Frandeen, sixty-five, a yoga teacher for many years and a student since his early forties, just completed his fourth teacher-training program in part because, as he puts it, "the more I practice and teach, the more I realize there is to learn about myself and life—so here I am, feeling like it's all just beginning."

Students come to yoga for a variety of reasons. For many it is a way to relax and reduce stress from living in a world of cell phones, high-pressure jobs, relationship challenges, and the fast pace of modern life. Yoga's widely proclaimed health benefits bring many people to the practice. Some are looking for the "hot workout" and perfectly sculpted body highlighted in the media courtesy of yoga-practicing stars like Madonna and Sting. Others, however, are interested in inner harmony, balance, and a sense of overall well-being. Some are motivated by pain or suffering, looking to yoga as a way to heal and feel whole. Still others consciously gravitate to yoga seeking a sense of spiritual connection or growth. For most it is a combination of these and other goals.

The role of the teacher is to provide inspired support and informed guidance to students pursuing these varied and changing aims. When teachers create safe and nurturing yoga classes where students can explore and experience anew the body, mind, and spirit, amazing things start to happen. New sensations arise in the body. Just breathing becomes a profound tool of awareness. The mind becomes clearer and stronger. Emotions even out, the heart opens, and the spirit soars. You simply feel better—more vibrant, more alive.

Our ability as teachers to help students develop and sustain their yoga practice in keeping with their personal intentions rests upon three basic foundations. First, continually cultivating our own personal practice keeps us strong, clear, and connected to the evolution of yoga. It also refreshes the well from which we draw new insight and inspiration. In his autobiographical introduction to his book *Yoga: The Spirit and Practice of Moving into Stillness*, Erich Schiffmann (1996, xxiii) tells the story of how he first fully awakened as a teacher. In learning from Joel Kramer to be "guided from within," Schiffmann tapped into an endless well of experience in which "each session is a learning event." The lessons we learn on the mat as well as from our teachers and students are invaluable when giving guidance to others on their mats.

Second, deepening our understanding of how bodies work—biomechanically, physiologically, and as the embodiment of spirit and life experience—gives us an essential set of tools for offering appropriate instruction. While our experience on the mat is essential, the marvelous diversity of people and the different needs and conditions they uniquely bring to the mat requires ongoing learning about functional anatomy, common injuries, alignment principles, physical and emotional risks, pregnancy, the respiratory process, and many other aspects of our being. Equipped with more knowledge and greater understanding, we can teach more safely. As yoga continues to grow in popularity, many teachers are entering the profession unprepared for working with the diverse array of students in their classes. Popular news articles on yoga teaching with titles like "In Over Their Heads" (*Los Angeles Times,* August 13, 2001) and "When Yoga Hurts" (*Time,* October 4, 2007) are an unfortunate reflection of a growing trend of students getting hurt in classes. This is the last thing a teacher wants written about his or her own heartfelt work.

Third, drawing intelligently from the wide variety of styles and sources available to us from the historical evolution of yoga provides an essential foundation for effective teaching. For just about every intention one finds in a yoga class, there is a tradition and style of yoga to inform and fulfill it. Within the various traditions and styles, a teacher's approach to the craft gives further nuance to students' experience. Most of the styles and approaches are, wittingly or not, rooted in a vast and rich web of ancient to contemporary writings on the nature of being, the physical body and mind, healing, and spirit. Tapping into these sources, teachers find greater ease in navigating the shifting tides of interest, need, and motivation arising from students and their own lives. Exploring the vastness of yoga philosophy and literature creates a richer, deeper palette from which to draw in the art of teaching yoga. This is the focus of Chapters One and Two, exploring the received wisdom of ancient yoga traditions and the development of modern Hatha yoga, respectively.

A marvelous quality of human beings is our natural dynamism. Even when choosing stillness we are still moving, our hearts beating, breath flowing, all our systems at work. When we choose to move, it is often with unconscious actions as our neuromuscular and skeletal systems interact. In the body-mind-spirit practice of Hatha yoga, we are becoming more and more aware of how we move, how we position our bodies, how we breathe, where we are in our minds, how we feel throughout our being, how we might move into a sense of stillness. In this way, all Hatha yoga is Vinyasa Flow—*vinyasa* meaning simply "to place in a special way" and *flow* denoting the conscious dynamism of movement within and between poses. While some classes flow more than others, even in a Restorative or Iyengar-oriented practice with long holds, there is always dynamic movement that involves consciously placing the body-breath-mind in a special way. To flow we need form and a stabilizing structure. Like a river flowing from the mountains, the riverbank, riverbed, and objects along the way channel the flow just as the flow changes the shape and conditions of that which holds it. Sometimes a powerful flow will break the banks, creating a new relationship along a different path in a way that could be a disaster or a blessing, depending on what happens. Sometimes the structure is so rigid, like the concrete walls of the Los Angeles River, that the flow is constricted to a point of seeming lifelessness. With time, with evolution, a new balance is always emerging, the flow expressed in new and wondrous ways. "The interplay of structure, rigidity, and form with formlessness," says Ganga White (2007, 114), "makes up the movement of life."

In consciously flowing in Hatha yoga practice, there are two sources of guidance: the outer teacher and the inner teacher. Their roles are similar even while their experiences of what is happening in the moment are different. Both are listening, watching, using what they feel and know to adjust and refine in ways that create a more beautiful experience. The inner teacher is ultimately the best guide, using physical sensations, emotional states, and knowledge to find what feels right. The outer teacher—being trained and well practiced in sensing how subtle energy flows in the body, how muscles and joints work and possible risks of injury, how to modify *asanas* to cultivate ease and stability, how to work with the breath—guides the student in deepening his or her relationship with that student's own inner teacher and thereby his or her practice.

Understanding how the body works is a key part of being a yoga teacher. Part of the challenge is that the human being is described with a completely different language and set of concepts in traditional yogic and Western scientific models. One has *prana, koshas, nadis,* and *chakras;* the other has systems made up of bones, tissues, nerves, organs, and fluids. Each makes sense only when understood as a whole comprised of its interrelated elements. Prana makes no sense without the concept of nadis, just as bones are largely devoid of practical meaning when viewed separately from tendons, ligaments, and muscles. Furthermore, each perspective has a view of the other. The traditional yogic perspective sees the physical body as an expression of cosmic and subtle elements, while the Western scientific model tends to dismiss any notion of nonmaterial or nonphysiological forces as religious mysticism or creative imagination. Some who believe in the traditional perspective suggest that technology is simply not yet capable of detecting the reality of subtle energy, while some who are committed to the Western scientific perspective acknowledge the possible material effect of mystical or spiritual forces. In the dance-like interplay of these two views, we are treated to a rich array of insights to guide us in our teaching.

Chapters Three and Four explore the elements of energetic flow, form, and structure that expand the scientific foundations of our teaching palette. We first review concepts of subtle energy and anatomy, recognizing the formative stream of *tantra*—a conception of human beings and the universe as an integrated whole—as a key element in *hatha,* or physical, yoga. Then we look at basic functional anatomy and biomechanics through the lens of the yoga teacher, paying close attention to the spine, pelvic and shoulder girdles, feet, ankles, knees, elbows, wrists, and hands. Here we will lay the foundation for what to watch for, how to see not merely bodies but people in their bodies dynamically doing yoga.

We expand this part of the teaching palette in Chapters Five and Six, exploring how to create favorable space for students to deepen their practice (Chapter Five) and fundamental principles and techniques for guiding that practice (Chapter Six). These general principles are given practical application as we look closely at teaching 108 asanas (Chapter Seven), several *pranayama* techniques (Chapter Eight), various approaches to meditation (Chapter Nine), sequencing asanas and planning classes (Chapter Ten), and working with diverse student conditions and intentions (Chapter Eleven). And in Chapter Twelve, we look at yoga as a profession, offering guidance on navigating the business aspect of yoga in a way that allows you to sustain yourself as a teacher.

Print media such as this book offer a potentially timeless resource that we can continually return to in our teaching. But some teaching skills, in particular the art and science of looking at, seeing, understanding, and appropriately relating to different students in their asana practices, are more effectively conveyed by observing teaching in action. Applying the foundational material offered throughout this book (especially in chapters 6 and 7), we have created short video vignettes showing methods of asana demonstration, modification, hands-on adjustments, and use of props for all of the 108 asanas presented in Chapter Seven. These clips are available online at www.markstephensyoga.com/teaching.html.

Yoga originated in India, where much of its development was expressed through the ancient Sanskrit language. The meaning of many yoga concepts is still best stated in Sanskrit, and wherever there is translation there is concern about accuracy. This might not be an issue for teachers whose approach eschews all reference to yoga's ancient roots. Many other teachers (as well as books, periodicals, and electronic media) do draw from the ancient teachings and also employ the Sanskrit terms for concepts and asanas (which means "to take one seat"). The most commonly accepted and used terms for asanas and other aspects of yoga are drawn from the Krishnamacharya lineage, reflecting the widespread influence of teachers such as B. K. S. Iyengar, Pattabhi Jois, and T. V. K. Desikachar. *Yoga Journal* magazine has further popularized this terminology (and the related spelling forms). Throughout this book we use these terms and forms, providing English translation with each first instance of the term. All Sanskrit terms can be found in the glossary, and all asanas are additionally listed in Appendix C with their English and Sanskrit names.

The ultimate language of yoga is expressed in doing yoga, a practice that transcends words as we open our lives to living more consciously through the infinite wisdom of the heart. It is in this wisdom that we take the seat of the teacher, sharing yoga with all who cross our path. In my own experience as a yoga teacher, nothing has so changed my life as the commitment to sharing yoga in a way that helps students to develop their own personal and sustainable practice. From my earliest days as a teacher in Los Angeles to the present—and whether teaching public or private classes, beginners workshops or teacher trainings, working with famous celebrities or convicted felons—every one of my students has been my teacher, each in his or her way bringing new light to my practice and teaching. May this book similarly inspire and guide you along your path as teacher.

CHAPTER ONE

ANCIENT ROOTS OF MODERN YOGA

There is a light that shines beyond all things
on earth, beyond us all, beyond the heavens,
beyond the highest, the very highest heavens.
This is the light that shines in our heart.
—*Chandogya Upanishad*

Yoga comes from a wide and deep river of ancient tradition. Its many currents flow from a complex history of spiritual exploration, philosophical reflection, scientific experimentation, and spontaneous creative expression. Arising from the diverse and evolving cultures of India, often moored to and conditioned by Hinduism, Buddhism, Jainism, and other religions, the philosophies, teachings, and practices of yoga are as richly varied as the innumerable tributaries of the vastness of yoga in all its manifestations. What we know of the origins and development of yoga comes to us from a variety of sources, including ancient texts, oral transmission through certain yogic or spiritual lineages, iconography, dances, and songs. While for some yoga students and teachers the history matters little, for others full appreciation of the practice is richer and clearer when informed by a deeper understanding of where it all came from.

Here we will use broad brushstrokes to paint a canvas depicting the received wisdom of tradition that still informs the practices we explore and share today. We will look at the foundational literature of yoga to identify the traditional practices, pausing along the way to consider the relevance and practical application of these practices in doing and teaching yoga in the twenty-first century.

THE VEDAS

While the history of yoga may be several thousand years old, the earliest known writings on yoga are found in ancient Hindu spiritual texts known as the Vedas

1

(meaning "knowledge"), the oldest being the Rig Veda. Though scholars debate the exact date and origins of the Vedas (1700–1100 BCE), most agree that the 1,028 hymns that make up the Rig Veda, considered by many to be of divine origin, are the original written source on yoga (Witzel 1997). Composed as poems by spiritual leaders (seers) in a culture where most spiritual practices connected directly and immediately with nature in the quest for meaning and well-being, these hymns reflect the mystical exploration of consciousness, being, and connection with the divine. It is here that yoga, meaning "to yoke" or "to make one," is first mentioned. The intended yoking is that of one's mind and the divine, a self-transcendent quality creating a pure state of consciousness in which the awareness of "I" disappears into a sense of divine essence.

The ancient Rig Veda

Meditation is the principal tool the Vedic seers describe in the Rig Veda for attaining this state of consciousness and oneness. The primary form of meditation is through *mantra,* the repetitive singing of certain sounds found to create an inner resonance with divine essence. The sounds themselves are put forth by the seers in what is considered a pure form of divine expression, undiluted by thought. The meditative state is deepened by visualizing a deity and fully absorbing a sense of the deity within one's heart. These interrelated practices anticipate qualities of meditation found much later in the Yoga Sutras: withdrawal of the senses from their external distractions, concentration on a single point, release of the mind into a heart-centered awareness of being, and opening to oneness with the divine. Many of the Vedic hymns are shared today in *kirtan*—or call-and-response singing—led by practitioners of *bhakti* (devotional) yoga. While the Hare Krishnas might have first popularized the chanting of mantras in the West, popular singers like Jai Uttal, Deva Premal, and Krishna Das have integrated this practice into mainstream yoga studios throughout the West. It is now more and more common to hear the chanting of ancient Hindu hymns in Western yoga classes, whether as part of the background music or with full student participation.

Many students find that this practice deepens their sense of spiritual connection while extending a feeling of community. Whether the effect is from the specific vibrations created in the tonality of certain Sanskrit words as claimed in

The Gayatri Mantra, taken from the Rig Veda, is one of the most highly revered mantras in Hinduism. The most popular translation and recording in the West are from Deva Premal:

Om bhur bhuvah svah
Tat savitur varenyam
Bhargo devasya dhimahi
Dhiyo yonah prachodayat

Translation:
Through the coming, going, and the balance of life
The essential nature illuminating existence is the adorable one
May all perceive through subtle intellect
The brilliance of enlightenment

the Rig Veda, or arises from simply being in the joy of singing and breathing, is the subject of some lively discussion. Despite the pleasant and affirming experiences many students report, some studios discourage chanting (including *"aum"*) because there are many other students, especially those new to yoga, who feel that chanting is a weird and esoteric religious ritual, possibly one at odds with their belief system or sense of spirituality. Cultivating and tapping into your authentic spiritual sensibilities while being attuned to the openness of your students will help guide you in whether or when to bring chanting into your classes.

THE UPANISHADS

At the later end of the Vedic period, another set of ancient writings on yoga appeared in India. Considered by some to be part of the Vedas, the earliest Upanishads were written in the first millennium BCE as part of a spiritual movement in which reliance on elaborate and secretive rituals gave way to more purely internal practices. Here we first find thorough explanations of yoga practice, although they are still focused on meditation, particularly in the later Upanishads in the first millennium CE. There are various estimates of the number of Upanishads, ranging between fifty and three hundred, each presented in the form of philosophical dialogue on the nature of being and the fate of the soul (Easwaran 1987). Considered the essence and final word of the Vedas, they became known as the philosophy of Vedanta ("the end of the Vedas") (Michaels 2004).

As an expression of Hindu religious philosophy, the Upanishads hold forth the belief in a universal spirit, *brahman,* and an individual soul, *atman.* Brahman is the absolute infinite, all that ever was and all that will ever be. Atman, or the inner self, is the self we experience in our limited awareness, in which we are said to experience ourselves as alienated from the true self: the absolute, or brahman. The ritualistic and contemplative practices described in the Upanishads aim to unite—yoke—atman and brahman by attaining release from the worldly constraints and limited consciousness that keep us from realizing the true state of oneness. As Georg Feuerstein (2001, 127) notes, "The transcendental ground of the world is identical with the ultimate core of the human being. That supreme Reality, which is pure, formless Consciousness, cannot be adequately described or defined. It must simply be *realized.*" The pathway to this self-realization includes inner reflection on the mind that brings one to a place of pure wisdom (Manchester 2002).

While the practices described in the Upanishads bear very little resemblance to what we find in most yoga classes in the Western world today, they do shape the language and experience of teaching in powerful ways. *Upanishad* means "sitting down beside," referring to the practice of sitting near the feet of one's guru as a means of enlightenment. The practice of *satsang* (from *sat,* meaning "true," and

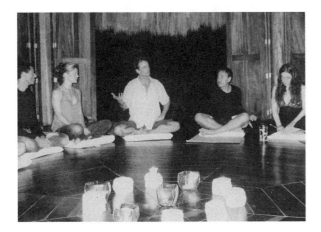

sangha, meaning "company"), which involves sitting with a teacher, guru, or an assembly of others with the aim of learning and experiencing spiritual awakening through assimilation of the teacher's thoughts, is found in some yoga studios in the West.

The Upanishads are also the earliest written source describing what is referred to today as the traditional yogic anatomy of the subtle body. The concept of the three-part body (causal, subtle, and physical) and koshas (or "five sheaths," discussed in detail in Chapter Three) are found in one of the oldest Upanishads, the Taittiriya Upanishad (2.1–9). Prana, or "life force," is found in several Upanishads. A passage in the Kaushitaki Upanishad (3.2) gives one of the most familiar descriptions of prana today: "Life is prana, prana is life. So long as prana remains in the body, so long is there life. Through prana, one obtains, even in this world, immortality."

In the later Upanishads, written through the fifteenth century, we begin to see evidence of experimentation in various yogic practices utilizing breath and sound as tools of physical transformation. As we see later in this chapter, much of this exploration was associated with the rise of tantra and created the groundwork for the future development of Hatha yoga. This culminates in the fifteenth century

Darshana Upanishad's description of specific asanas, all but one of which are sitting positions in which the essential practice is pranayama (Aiyar 1914).

THE BHAGAVAD GITA

Some of the Upanishads describe in detail the meditative and contemplative practices for finding oneness. Thought to be part of the Upanishadic movement, the Bhagavad Gita, or Song of God, explores the mystery of the mind, providing a set of guiding principles for a life of conscious action. Though it may be based on a historical event, the symbolism of the Bhagavad Gita is a guide to spiritual liberation. The flame of desire and manifestations of ego create inner conflicts that keep us from enlightenment or self-realization. The practices described in the Bhagavad Gita offer a pathway to "inner peace" through connection with the divine. Inner peace resides within us, but the constant rambling noise of the mind—the "I"—keeps us from this awareness.

The story unfolds in the middle of the epic Mahabharata as a conversation between the warrior-prince Arjuna and his charioteer, Krishna. Peering across the battlefield, Arjuna sees those he knows and loves. They have sought to destroy him and have made his life miserable, yet he thinks it wrong to fight the war and kill them to win back the kingdom. He turns to Krishna for advice. Krishna expounds on the idea of *dharma*, or destined duty. By coming to identify with the immortal self, with brahman, the one, the ultimate divine consciousness, we can transcend our mortality, our attachment to the material world, and live in the love of the infinite. With Arjuna wanting to abstain from action, Krishna warns that it is through action that one's destined duty and divine nature are manifested. To clarify his point, Krishna explains the three yogic paths corresponding to the dharmas associated with the varied natures of people (Prabhavananda and Isherwood 1944).

1. *Karma yoga*—the yoga of service. Literally translated as the path of "union through action," karma yoga involves acting without consideration of desire or selfish need. This, says Krishna, purifies the mind and makes clearer the divine nature of one's existence: "Freedom from activity is never achieved by abstaining from action. Nobody can be perfect by merely ceasing to act.... The world is imprisoned in its own activity, except when actions are performed as worship of God.... The reward of all action is to be found in enlightenment."

2. *Jnana yoga*—the yoga of knowledge. Exercising the faculties of discrimination and detachment, it is possible to transcend the temporal limitations that occupy the "I" mind. Krishna explains that jnana yoga brings about an intellect that has rid itself of delusions and created an awareness of the difference

between the body and soul. In this awareness, one becomes indifferent to the results of all action through knowledge of the absolute.

3. *Bhakti yoga*—the yoga of devotion. Staying constantly in touch with God, the bhakti yogi, in Krishna's words, is guided by love and pure innocence in spiritual life: "Engage your mind in always thinking of Me, become my devotee, offer obeisances to Me and worship Me. Being completely absorbed in Me, surely you will come to be Me." The primary activities of this practice are chanting God's names and stories from scripture, meditating on God, providing selfless service, offering prayer and other means of always being in a state of purely devoted, loving being.

To the modern yoga teacher, relating these three paths of yoga to teaching classes at a studio or gym can seem like quite a stretch. Yet we can make some meaningful connections between these paths and how we live, which does have an immediate and vital relationship to the qualities we bring to our teaching. The act of committing yourself completely to teaching yoga can be a form of karma yoga, making the needs and intentions of your students the focus of your efforts as you expand and refine your skills and knowledge. Jnana yoga is a more difficult path: engaging yourself in a deep, rigorous, yet compassionate process of self-examination lends clarity to your mind and heart, which in turn lends greater clarity in giving guidance to your students. If your path is one of bhakti yoga, staying immersed in a sense of connection with the sounds and sensations of your spiritual guides will manifest in the voice and love you share in your classes. Taking these paths even further, it is important to remember that yoga is far more than the practice done in class, that the life of yoga extends well off the mat and into the world each and every day. In this integration and expression of yoga in life, the path of the teacher is most fully expressed.

THE YOGA SUTRAS OF PATANJALI

Most yoga students and teachers who study yoga philosophy have read excerpts from Patanjali's Yoga Sutras. Composed around 200 CE, many of the central themes in the Bhagavad Gita are given more focused and elaborate attention in this set of 196 aphorisms. This is the classical presentation of *raja yoga,* the "royal" yoga of the mind, and contains one of the earliest references to a practice involving both asanas and pranayama. Composing in the dialogue format found in many of the Vedas and Upanishads (many of which were composed after the Sutras), Patanjali begins with a simple question: "What is yoga?" His answer makes clear that the practice described here is centered around mental experience: *"chitta vritti nirodaha,"* he writes, meaning, "to calm the fluctuations of the mind" or "to steady the mind" (Bouanchaud 1999).

Considered by many to be the basic text on yoga, the Yoga Sutras explain how to cultivate one's path to *samadhi,* a blissful state where the practitioner is absorbed into oneness with the divine by releasing the ego. With the constant ego-centered activity of the mind always at work, our prejudices, desires, and passions bring us into the abyss of confusion, pain, and suffering. Yoga offers liberation from this suffering. Patanjali gives nuanced guidance on practices for stilling the mind and eradicating the mental afflictions that cause suffering in the world.

Many students and teachers of yoga are surprised that the Yoga Sutras do not discuss or describe a single asana or pose. A central point of the Sutras—and as we shall see later, what most distinguishes raja yoga from Hatha yoga is that one must begin with ethical and spiritual observations, moving steadily along an eight-limbed path to finally experience the full fruits of yoga. As B. K. S. Iyengar (2001, 29) emphasizes, "there are sequential stages in an individual's life journey through yoga." The eight-limbed path, or *ashtanga* yoga, is: *yama, niyama, asana, pranayama, pratyahara, dharana, dhyana, and samadhi.* With later chapters devoted to teaching asana, pranayama, and the meditative and transcendent practices of pratyahara, dharana, and dhyana, here we will look most closely at yama and niyama while briefly introducing the other limbs as described in the Yoga Sutras.

Yama

Yama explains the principles of ethical behavior one should follow in everyday life, in our relationships with others and with ourselves. The literal definition of *yama* is "to contain" or "to control." The yamas provide a source of guidance on teacher-student and life relationships. There are five yamas:

1. *Ahimsa:* Meaning "nonhurting," ahimsa is often interpreted as "nonviolence." It begins with respecting one's own body and extending this respect to all other beings in the world. In teaching yoga, this wisdom applies directly by creating a safe space for students to learn and practice, approaching students with compassion and understanding, and offering qualities of guidance that do not hurt or injure students or ourselves.

2. *Satya:* This means being honest with ourselves and others. A question sometimes arises over the possible conflict between this second principle and ahimsa. What if the truth hurts? In the ancient epic Mahabharata, this apparent conundrum is carefully navigated. "Truth should be told when agreeable,

should be said agreeably, and truth should not be said that does harm; how-ever, never lie to give pleasure."

3. *Asteya:* The essence of asteya, "not stealing," is freeing oneself from the desire to have something that one has not earned or paid for. Listing greed as one of the "seven spiritual sins," Gandhi emphasized that "wealth without work" is wrong. Some teachers extend this to their yoga classes, encouraging students to "pay their dues" on the yoga mat before expecting the fruits of the practice. Creating ways for students to experience a sense of abundance in their practice while honoring what is not readily there for them is one way of expressing this principle when teaching, while respecting that there are greater possibilities on the path beyond one's immediate experience.

4. *Brahmacharya:* The essence of this sutra is honoring yourself and others in intimate relationships. It is typically given loose interpretation as the "right use of energy." While Iyengar (2001, 35) points out that the literal definition means "a life of celibacy, religious study, and self-restraint," he goes on to underline that "without experiencing human love and happiness it is not possible to know divine love." The concept originates in the Bhagavad Gita, which stresses that living in the truth of brahman "a man's heart . . . is never again moved by the things of the senses." The Bhagavad Gita goes on to say that "The yogi should retire to a solitary place and live alone." (Prabhavananda and Isherwood 1944, 64–65). If one does have sexual relations, the strict interpretation of brahmacharya tells us that "the capacity to perceive the soul or realize the true Self become impossible."[1] Others emphasize "the correct balancing of actions, thoughts, and feelings, and channeling them first toward the quest for the absolute or higher realization" (Bouanchaud 1999, 111).

5. *Aparigraha:* Aparigraha means "noncovetousness"—not being greedy, or being free of desire, is how this is traditionally interpreted. It is about living with generosity of spirit and action, giving without expecting something in return. Applied to asana and pranayama, this principle can help students approach their practice with an attitude of patience in which steadiness and ease is more important than getting into a pose.

AHIMSA VERSUS SATYA: HOW TO NAVIGATE THE POTENTIAL CONFLICT WHEN TEACHING YOGA

Teaching Urdhva Dhanurasana, the Upward Bow Pose, sometimes called the Wheel Pose, in an intermediate class, a student named Christina, age thirty-one, with unstable shoulders, recent complaints of lower-back pain, and a go-for-it attitude, is struggling to straighten her arms. There is no evidence of *sthira* or *sukham,* steadiness or ease. She describes herself as a strong student and seems to have an attitude of accomplished practice. Telling her the truth—I think she is not ready for this asana—is almost certain to offend her sense of self, to hurt her feelings. So I approach her in a different way. Asking her to come down for a moment, I ask her if I can help her prepare to do the pose in a more stable and easier way as part of her "advancing practice." She likes the idea. We look closely at her strengths and limitations in setting up for the asana. I show her several preparatory stretches, prop supports, and energetic actions that will lead her into a happier, more graceful, and fuller expression of the pose. She smiles and gets to work. In Buddhism, this is called "skillful means," wherein the teacher draws from a variety of practices and teachings to lead a student along an appropriate path toward awakening. Redirecting the student's effort is not lying if the purpose and effect is to help her in deepening her practice.

Niyama

The niyamas are personal observances, a means of well-being that brings our attention from relationships with others to the intimacy of our relationship with ourselves. Living the niyamas leads to deeper authenticity in our teaching practice. While there are ten or more niyamas discussed in the Upanishads, the Yoga Sutras focus on five:

1. *Saucha:* In cultivating purity of body and mind, saucha suggests treating your body like a temple. Asana practice detoxifies the body, removing impurities caused by the environment and diet. Keeping yourself clean with regular bathing helps purify the external body while eating fresh and healthy food lends to more cleanliness inside. But even more important is cleansing the mind, keeping your mental state as clear as possible. When we cleanse the body and mind we are more attentive to the higher aspects of living consciously, staying grounded and centered in daily life. Modeling radiant health and vibrant well-being inspires your students to do the same in their lives.

2. *Santosa:* From a place of purity, we become humble and content in the modesty of how things are, as well as with the past and our sense of the future. Santosa opens us to happiness with who we are and what we presently have. When we recognize and accept that life is an ongoing process for learning, growing, and evolving, we are more inclined to self-acceptance. Being happy with what we have is also contagious, especially when manifested as a teacher. Being content with your students and classes just as they are liberates you from expectations and helps to make you the best teacher you can be.

3. *Tapas:* Being as present as we can to our contentment without apathy or self-satisfaction involves disciplined commitment. This is tapas, the burning fire of daily practice that creates an austerity of being, the forging of our character, which opens us more and more to our true nature. This burning fire of enthusiasm allows us to treat every experience as a tool for self-realization. Tapas helps us to direct our energy toward our innermost truth and intentions, being attentive to how we are in our body, breath, heart, and mind.

4. *Svadhyaya:* Dwelling in the yamas and niyamas requires a practice of self-study that deepens our sense of spiritual being. It involves intentional self-awareness in all we do in the world, welcoming and accepting our limitations while staying centered in our truth. Here we cultivate a more authentic way of being in the world, as human beings and as teachers. Pausing from time to time to ask basic questions about your teaching will deepen this authenticity.

5. *Ishvarapranidhana:* Letting go of the ego, our lives come to express all the qualities of the yamas and niyamas. For some this is surrender to God, to a sense of the divine; to others a feeling of being an expression of the whole of the natural universe. When grounded in a sense of being that is greater than the individual self, our *raison d'être*—reason for being—is clearer, and so is our teaching.

Asana

The third limb of yoga presented in the Yoga Sutras is asana. While the Yoga Sutras do not discuss any specific asanas, there is one sutra that addresses asana specifically, saying simply *"sthira sukham asanam"* (Bouanchaud 1997, 130–131). This ancient aphorism offers essential insight for the instruction of asana. The term *asana* is commonly translated as "pose," but contains within it a far richer meaning. Bernard Bouanchaud, in *The Essence of Yoga: Reflections on the Yoga Sutras of Patanjali,* notes that the verbal root *as* conveys the sense of "being present in one's body—inhabiting, existing, living in it." The literal translation of *asana* is "to take one seat," which can be interpreted to mean being just here, just now, in the present moment, thus

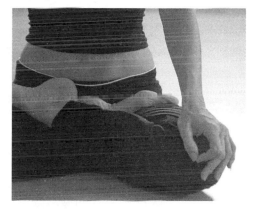

embodying the meditation practices found in earlier writings on yoga in the Vedas and Upanishads (Bouanchaud 1997, 130–131). *Sthira* means "to be stable or firm," while *sukham* means "to be soft, at ease, relaxed." Taken together and put into the context of a dynamic practice, we find a blended quality in which one is cultivating steadiness, ease, and presence of mind, breath by breath, within and between the asanas. This is the meaning of *asana* when expressed and embodied in an integrated practice.

Pranayama

Patanjali tells us that pranayama is the "controlled intake and outflow of breath in a firmly established posture" (Bouanchaud 1997, 135–136). When we observe the flow of the breath through its natural phases of inhale-pause-exhale-pause, the breath becomes smoother and its effects more subtle. Through delicate observation, the breath is refined. Gradually, more refined and difficult techniques are introduced. At each stage in this developing practice, one is always cultivating a feeling of steadiness and ease. Eventually, one moves beyond the technique, coming into a state of bliss. In preparation for this practice, Patanjali reminds us that the eight limbs are to be done in sequence. If one were to attempt pranayama prior to properly preparing the body and mind, tension would increase and cause harm. Mastering the asanas brings about the basic physical and mental health that allows pranayama to be done safely. As we will see, many modern-day gurus and teachers embrace this sequential approach. We will return to this later when looking at the rise of Hatha yoga as well as when looking in detail at guiding asana and pranayama practices, further examining these ancient views and considering them in light of teaching yoga today.

Pratyahara, Dharana, Dhyana

The practice of pratyahara is to draw the senses inward, relieving them of their external distractions. Here Patanjali is addressing the tendency of the mind to go toward whatever is stimulating the senses and thoughts (Yoga Sutras II.51). As we sense, so we think, and as we think, so we tend to act. By internalizing consciousness, pratyahara allows us to leave external circumstances in abeyance. What might otherwise be an annoying sound or smell is now just there. Without pratyahara, a bead of sweat gathering on your brow or the sound of someone entering class late might distract you from your breath or concentrated awareness. Now those sounds or sensations are simply there, while your awareness is turned more inside. This opens us to a state of focused concentration, or dharana (Bouanchaud 1997, 141). Staying with this state of concentration, dharana becomes dhyana as you become one in body-breath-mind, a state of awareness in which the sense of knower and known, subject and object, thought and thinker dissolve into one, leading to samadhi, or bliss (Bouanchaud 1997, 150).

Samadhi

The eight limbs of ashtanga yoga are often likened to a tree. B. K. S. Iyengar offers such a metaphor in his *Light on the Yoga Sutras of Patanjali.* Yama creates the roots for living clearly and honorably through ethical being. Niyama is the trunk of the tree, establishing a base of purity in one's body and mind. Asana creates the branches, extending strongly yet flexibly to move with the breezes of life. Pranayama is symbolized by the leaves on the tree, drawing in the life force through the exchange of breath. Pratyahara is the bark protecting the tree from outer elements and preventing its essence from flowing outward. Dharana is the sap running through the veins of the tree and its leaves, keeping the body-mind firm. Dhyana is the flower of whole consciousness, slowly ripening into the fullest fruit of the practice, samadhi, pure bliss.

Although the historical origins and philosophical foundations of Hatha yoga mark a departure from many of the tenets of Patanjali's raja yoga, many of today's yoga styles (or lineages) pay considerable homage to the Sutras. The Krishnamacharya lineage, which includes Iyengar, Ashtanga Vinyasa, and the basic foundations of Vinyasa Flow, Anusara, and other approaches, is tied quite strongly to Patanjali's philosophy. These roots will become clearer as we look at the major styles of yoga in the next chapter. A curious irony is that B. K. S. Iyengar, Pattabhi Jois, and others in the Krishnamacharya lineage immediately start their students with asana and *ujjayi* pranayama, the third and fourth limbs, while asserting that their approaches fully embody the Yoga Sutras. Regardless of whether or not one considers this inconsistency significant, the pure raja yoga path is very difficult, and as we will soon see, the tantric and hatha practices that emerged a few centuries later are a practical response to that difficulty. In practice and teaching we can find a variety of ways to look on the eight-limbed path as a whole tree of yoga, each limb inseparable from and offering insight, support, and guidance to the others, a mixing that later yogis found effective in their practice and teaching.

Teaching with integrity involves being clear about the sources of our instruction. The Yoga Sutras were written about two thousand years ago in a time and culture far removed from the modern West. When we draw from such a source, it is helpful to have thought through what we think about what is being put forth. What are you saying to your class? Do you believe it? Embrace it? We will continue to explore these questions as we look at the further evolution of yoga.

TANTRA

The paths from the Vedas, Upanishads, and Yoga Sutras to the modern and well-known contemporary practices of Hatha yoga are typically described as a series of straight evolutionary lines. But this is not correct. Rather, Hatha yoga arises from the formative influence of tantra, a fact shrouded in veils of illusion cast by many Hatha adherents who passionately reject tantra as being antithetical to their spiritual and social worldview. The tantra movement in India, arising from the influence of Mahayana Buddhism in the opening centuries of the first millennium, was in part a reaction against the dualistic and renunciate practices taught in the Vedas and Upanishads and further codified in the Yoga Sutras. The essential idea of tantra—that everything in the universe is an expression of the divine and thus can be tapped as a source of divine consciousness and being—is a marked departure from traditional Vedic and Upanishadic teachings that would put the devoted yogi in an isolated cave and insist that normal human experiences such as desire or sexuality prevent or at least limit true happiness or enlightened being. In some of the Upanishads—particularly the nondual Svetasvatara Upanishad—we can find an opening to the idea of fully living here and now in a state of self-realization and liberation—*jivan mukti*—but it is still largely situated within a dualistic perspective that separates the individual and his or her experiences from the whole of the natural order and spiritual being (Feuerstein 2001, 341).

From the root word *tan,* meaning "expansive" or "whole," tantra recognizes the entire fabric of existence as an expression of the divine feminine, or Shakti energy. The idea is to open up to a sense of the divine within *any* experience. The philosophy of tantra identifies the path of freedom not through renunciation of human desire and experience, but indeed largely through it:

> Tantra is that Asian body of beliefs and practices which, working from the principle that the universe we experience is nothing other than the concrete manifestation of the divine energy of the Godhead that creates and maintains that universe, seeks to ritually appropriate and channel that energy, within the human microcosm, in creative and emancipatory ways (D.G. White 2000).

Tantra offers an integrative approach to yoga in which we tap into every aspect of internal and external experience as a source of conscious awakening to divine energy, the omnipotent, omniscient, and omnipresent primordial creative force of the universe. This has a profound impact on how we think about the body and yoga practice. Since everything is a manifestation of the divine, yet different in its energetic expression, there are infinite possibilities for being in a sense of the divine, even amid what might seem entirely mundane. Tantric practitioners will go to what may seem the extremes of human experience, seeking energetic intensity in order to experience the purest awareness of being.

There are three traditional forms of tantric practice, sometimes referred to as initiations and usually said to require the intimate guidance of a guru (Tigunait 1999, 6).

- *Mantra:* This practice takes the practitioner into the divine vibrating energy of sound through repeated chanting of hymns or words, many found in the Vedas (such as the Gayatri Mantra), in concert with a rich set of rituals involving meditation, sacred space purification, and imagination of a protective wall of fire.

- *Yantra:* As the intimacy between practitioner and mantric energy grows, the practice extends into meditation on a yantra, a visible vibratory expression of the divine feminine represented in geometrical form. As a map of the mantric world, this embodies the forces of Shakti energy—intensity, radiance, delight, pleasure, desire, yantra speed, illumination, being, and *vighna vinashini,* the power that destroys resistance. Yantra practice involves an array of rituals, visualization, meditation, chanting, and offerings.

- *Puja:* In contrast to the "right-hand" tantric path of mantra and yantra, the "left-hand" path moves from esoteric internal practices to fully living in the world, embracing with intense concentration the most powerful expression of Shakti energy in the strongest sensual experiences. In puja practice, one is cultivating self-mastery, the union of sensuous pleasure and divine ecstasy, in the most intense of acts, aiming to "bring spirituality into day-to-day existence, and vice versa" (Tigunait 1999, 104–105).

At the heart of tantra is the idea, born of experience rather than grand philosophical speculation, that there is a continuity between what seems the ordinary realm of human life and the infinite. Instead of transcending the material reality of human experience, going more intensely into it is the path to enlightenment and happiness. Arising from ordinary people among the lower castes of India's highly stratified society, this approach opened up the fullness of spiritual practice to anyone (Davidson 2003). As Georg Feuerstein (2001, 343) emphasizes, these people "were responding to a widely felt need for a more practical orientation that would integrate the lofty metaphysical ideals of nondualism with down-to-earth procedures for living a sanctified life without necessarily abandoning one's belief in the local deities and the age-old rituals for worshipping them."

As tantra grew in influence, its essence was distorted by the reactions to some of its rituals, particularly those involving sex. Speaking of tantra in the West usually evokes notions of "sacred sex," thus rendering tantra as little more than "spiritual sexuality." While sexual relationship is part of tantra, the spiritual philosophy and practices of tantra are deeper and more subtle. This is perhaps most richly expressed in the form of tantra that took root in Kashmir in the ninth century, known as Kashmir Shaivism, poetically expressed in the Spanda Karika (Odier 2004). The main idea of the Spanda Karika is to take all of existence as one and not divide it into pure or impure. This is the central idea of tantra, the kernels of which were found in the most ancient Vedas and Upanishads, but largely lost or discarded in the Bhagavad Gita and in raja yoga as described by Patanjali. The idea of yoga in the tantric perspective is to be without separation, to reconcile the body, breath, mind, and emotion as one, without distinction, without anything considered impure or profane. Most of the tantric texts state that Shiva and Shakti, or divine masculine and feminine energy, are one—one in the body, one in the mind, one in the heart of emotional being (Davidson 2005). In this expression of being we are embracing the fullness of all of our energy, to be this one thing, not to be in distinction, not to be anything but the space where everything is alive. As we go into this practice, we find liberation from the ego, from dualistic thinking, experiencing and viscerally comprehending that we are this beautiful space, this amazing wholeness.

In the ninth century CE, the Vijnana Bhairava offered a rich array of simple-to-complex practices for tapping into this quality of awareness.[2] More recently, tantric yogis have expanded this to offer what Daniel Odier refers to as "micro-practices." The micro-practices are based on the fact that the mind is very fast, likes to be fast, and is good at it. The ancient yogis had a wonderful idea: to invent a practice that goes just as fast as the mind. Rather than trying to counteract the mind, one goes with it for a brief moment in which one tries to be completely present to something very simple. Sitting with your morning coffee, you pass the cup beneath your

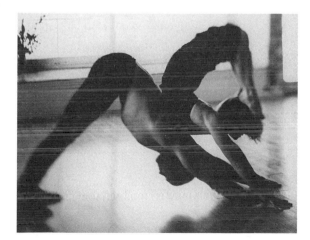

nose, and for a moment you are fully absorbed in all the sensations you are experiencing. Walking in the woods, your foot crosses over a dry leaf while a light breeze caresses your skin and damp forest aromas flow into your olfactory senses. There you are, in those few seconds, completely present to your senses of sound, light, aroma, your skin, your heart, and a sense of something far greater that is in it all, you and nature and spirit as one. The aim is to be fully present in just that moment, just that one breath, finding there a sense of being in a state of bliss or oneness. Bringing this into yoga asana and pranayama practices, a far more refined and subtle quality of awareness arises, lending a more nuanced body-breath-mind connection, a more expansive consciousness of the wholeness. At the heart of this practice is being present when you breathe in and out, bringing consciousness to the breath and feeling that you are breathing completely, letting go of the breath completely, and in that space feeling the body-mind going to a place of spontaneous awareness of spirit or bliss.

HATHA YOGA: THE HATHA PRADIPIKA, GHERANDA SAMHITA, AND SHIVA SAMHITA

All of the best-known styles of yoga practiced in the West today are a form of Hatha yoga: Vinyasa Flow, Iyengar, Anusara, Ashtanga Vinyasa, Power yoga, and dozens of others that offer only slight variations on a tradition or style but with a branded name. It may come as a surprise that the first in-depth writings on Hatha yoga and related explanations of asana practice are just a few hundred years old, not thousands as is often claimed or intimated in the popular yoga media and literature. Think of how many times you have read an article on Hatha yoga that begins, "In this ancient practice that dates back over five thousand years . . ."

The first substantial writing on Hatha yoga, the well-known Hatha Yoga Pradipika, was written in the fourteenth century by the Indian sage Swami Swatmarama. A fairly encyclopedic text, the Pradipika looks in detail at asana, *shatkarma,* pranayama, *mudra, bandha,* and samadhi, giving very specific guidance on each of these interrelated practices. (We will look at these elements below.) The Shiva Samhita, written sometime between the fifteenth and seventeenth centuries, shows more clearly than the Pradipika the influence of Buddhism and tantra in the development of Hatha yoga (Vasu 2004). While only four asanas are described in detail, the Shiva Samhita provides an elaborate explanation of nadis (the energy channels through which prana flows), the nature of prana or "life force," and the many obstacles faced in practice and how to overcome them through a variety of techniques. These techniques include *dristana* (conscious gazing), silent mantra and tantric practices for awakening and moving *kundalini* energy. The Gheranda Samhita, written in the late seventeenth century, reflects the diminishing influence of tantra, particularly anything involving sexual interaction (Mallinson 2004) Seven chapters describe the seven means to perfecting oneself on the yogic path: shatkarmas for purification, asanas for strength, mudras for steadiness, pratyahara for calmness, pranayama for lightness, dhyana for realization, and samadhi for bliss.

According to the original texts, there are three purposes of Hatha yoga: (1) the total purification of the body, (2) the complete balancing of the physical, mental, and energetic fields, and (3) the awakening of purer consciousness through which one ultimately connects with the divine by engaging in practices rooted in the physical body. Today we find most Hatha yoga traditions attributing their roots to the raja yoga philosophy of Patanjali. Raja yoga, greatly influenced by the Buddhist philosophy of yama and niyama, can be seen as having more to do with religion than a person's spiritual life. Living in the real world of relationships, work, adventure, culture, and society, you can drive yourself crazy trying to control the mind as a pure raja yogi is instructed to do. Hatha yoga, in its origins, is very much more tied to tantra, seeking spiritual development in the ordinary experiences of life and using the sensuous experience of the body to cultivate the balanced integration of body, mind, and spirit. Ultimately you may find the path of Hatha yoga brings you to a place where all the other paths converge, in simple bliss. This at least is what those who first wrote about Hatha yoga expected to happen.

Hatha yoga uses all of who we are—physically, mentally, emotionally, our most subtle and elusive inner nature—as the raw material for learning, seeing, and integrating our entire being, opening us to our fullest imagination, intelligence, enthusiasm, energy, and awareness of spiritual life. The term *hatha* derives from *ha,* meaning "sun," and *tha,* meaning "moon," symbolizing life force and consciousness. (The prism varies by tradition and perspective, with an emphasis in tantra on Shiva-Shakti, in Taoism on yin-yang, in physics on matter-energy.) To experience being fully alive and conscious, these oppositions come into one, a seamless harmony of being. The problem is that we tend to get stuck in our mind, our body, our heart. Hatha yoga offers a way to experience this integration along a path involving very specific practices that purify the body, calm the mind, and open the heart.

Shatkarma—Purification Practices

Shatkarma, from *shat,* meaning "six," and *karma,* meaning "action," are set forth as the initial stage of Hatha yoga practices. They are designed to bring the body's three doshas or energetic qualities—*kapha, pitta,* and *vata*—into balance, creating harmony in the body and mind that prepares one for asana, pranayama, and other Hatha practices. By cultivating energetic balance, we improve overall body function, allowing asana and pranayama practices to proceed with the greatest ease and effect. As with many other seemingly esoteric yoga practices, the ancient texts describe these as secret techniques to be learned only from an experienced and qualified teacher. Each of the six cleansing techniques—*dhauti* (internal cleansing), *basti* (yogic enema), *neti* (nasal cleansing), *trataka* (concentrated gazing), *nauli* (abdominal massage), *kapalabhati* (brain cleansing)—has a variety of practices, described most fully in the Gheranda Samhita and the Hatha Yoga Pradipika (Mallinson 1994, 1–15; Muktibodhananda 1993, 190–227).

Asana and Pranayama—Energetic Balancing Practices

At the beginning of most yoga classes, there is often a moment of sitting, getting an initial sense of calm, and typically a greeting of *"namaste"* followed by a brief bow. We find the roots of this ritual in the Pradipika, with Swami Swatmarama offering just such salutations and prostrations to his guru, Adinath. It is an act of humility, symbolizing the release of the ego and the opening to something far greater, to a higher force. The Pradipika then departs from raja yoga by prescribing a practice that begins with shatkarmas and asanas, with asana now involving a variety of specific bodily positions that help to open the nadis (energy channels) and chakras (psychic centers) of the subtle body. The ultimate aim is the same as in raja yoga: to come into a state of samadhi. So why start with asansas?

The Hatha yogis discovered that through the practice of asanas, one attains a delicate balance of body, mind, and spirit. Following the shatkarma purification practices, asanas further cleanse the body by creating the inner fire to burn out impurities. They stimulate increased circulation, revitalize all the organs of the body, tone the muscles and ligaments, stabilize the joints, create ease in the nerves, and promote the improved functioning of all the body's systems. In the Pradipika's first verse on asana, it is said, "having done asana one gets steadiness of body and mind, diseaselessness and lightness of the limbs" (Muktibodhananda 1993, verse 17). By deeply purifying the body and cultivating steadiness, prana moves more freely, nourishing, healing, and integrating the body and mind. As in the Yoga Sutras, the Pradipika instructs opening and steadying the body through asana practice before commencing with pranayama. This is echoed by B. K. S. Iyengar (1985, 10), who says, "if a novice attends to the perfection of the postures, he cannot concentrate on breathing. He loses balance and the depth of the asanas. Attain steadiness and stillness in asanas before introducing rhythmic breathing techniques."

In verse 33 of the Pradipika, Swatmarama tells us "eighty-four asanas were taught by Lord Shiva." Only fifteen asanas are described in the Pradipika. The

Gheranda Samhita tells us that Shiva taught 8,400,000 asanas, "as many asanas as there are species of living beings." The point is that asana is infinite, underlining a practice that is about process rather than the attainment of some preconceived perfect form. The Gheranda Samhita describes seventeen asanas, in addition to the fifteen found in the Pradipika. Several of these are very slight variations on one another (such as a change in hand position or gaze). Even though asanas have the same names as some found in the Pradipika, several have slight variations in the Gheranda Samhita. Throughout the continued development of Hatha yoga, the specific description and form of the asanas would change, with the same name often given to very different physical positions.

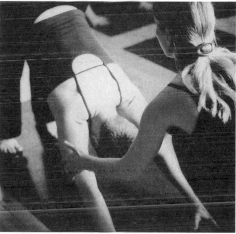

Neither of these writings offers detailed instruction on asana techniques. Four asanas are mentioned in the Pradipika as the "important ones." Of these, Padmasana (Lotus Pose) receives by far the most detailed explanation, which by today's standards is surprisingly brief: "Place the right foot on the left thigh and the left foot on the right thigh, cross the hands behind the back and firmly hold the toes. Press the chin against the chest and look at the tip of the nose." A few verses later we are told that "ordinary people cannot achieve this posture, only the few wise ones on this earth can" (Muktibodhananda 1993, verse 44). While wisdom is probably not what most determines who can or cannot do particular asanas, the intricacy of asana technique and clarity of instruction in the more recent development of Hatha yoga has certainly made this pose and others accessible to a constantly expanding world of practitioners, wise or not. Still, it would not be until the mid-twentieth century that the process of practicing asanas would be described in any greater detail than during the fifteenth century.

In contrast to their sparse discussion of asana, both the Gheranda Samhita and the Pradipika provide very detailed guidance on pranayama practice, beginning with statements on how prana and the mind are inextricably linked: "When prana moves, *chitta* (the mental faculty) moves. When prana is without movement, chitta is without movement. By this the yogi attains steadiness and should thus restrain the *vayu* (air)" (Muktibodhananda 1993, 150). Specific techniques are explained, including setting, season, location, pace, rhythm, retention, various alternate nostril methods, use of bandhas and mudras. We explore these practices Chapter Eight, offering safe and effective methods for teaching pranayama in different yoga class environments and to different levels of students.

Mudra and Bandha—Conscious Awakening Practices

As the serpent upholds the earth and its mountains, so *kundalini*
is the support of all the yoga practices. By guru's grace, this sleeping kundalini is awakened, then all the lotuses (chakras) and knots
(nadis) are opened. Then *sushumna* (the central energetic channel
through the spine) becomes the pathway of prana, mind is free of
all connections, and death is averted.

Thus begins the Pradipika's explanation of mudra and bandha. The energy that was
unleashed in creation, kundalini, lies coiled and sleeping at the base of the spine.
With the help of tantric practices described hundreds of years earlier in the Kanka-
malinitantra and other sources, it is the purpose of Hatha yoga to arouse this cosmic energy, causing it to rise back up through the increasingly subtler chakras until
union with God is achieved in the *sahasrara* chakra at the crown of the head. Mudras are the specific body positions, including precise placement of the fingers and
gaze, that direct the pranic energy generated in asana and pranayama practice to
flow in balance through the subtle body. Bandhas are "energy locks" that further
generate and accumulate prana in the physical and subtle bodies. Mudras and bandhas are explored in Chapter Three in conjunction with other elements of subtle
energy.

TOWARD MODERN HATHA YOGA

In these early writings on yoga, we begin to see two clearly divergent and often
conflicting pathways of practice: one renunciate and firmly rooted in Patanjali's
raja yoga, and the other influenced by the tantric movement. The development of
Hatha yoga in the centuries after the appearance of the Hatha Yoga Pradipika would
reflect these polarities of philosophical, practical, and spiritual orientation. The
distinctions between these tendencies would often come to blur as lineages, schools,
and teachers of yoga brought their own creative expression to the evolution of
yoga philosophy and practice. Yet as with all forms of evolution, even in those
instances of great leaps, the colorful ancient threads of wisdom and practice can
still be seen in the modern fabric of yoga, rooting even the most innovative contemporary teachings in the wisdom first articulated by yogis in India more than
five thousand years ago.

CHAPTER TWO

MODERN HATHA YOGA

I want to unfold.
Let no place in me hold itself closed,
for where I am closed, I am false.
—*Ranier Maria Rilke*

In the last twenty-five years there has been a dizzying yoga explosion in the West.[1] The styles and approaches are widely varied—Ananda, Anusara, Ashtanga, Bikram, Integral, Iyengar, Kundalini, Power, Sivananda, Viniyoga, Vinyasa Flow—and the list goes on. Some are "pure" forms with a direct and uninterrupted lineage connected to India, while others show only a faint resemblance to traditional forms of Hatha yoga. Navigating through the different schools and styles can be challenging, especially if you are just beginning to teach and you feel uncertain about the right fit for you.

While dating back more than five thousand years, yoga has changed more in the past thirty years than in all its history. It took until around the fourteenth century for Hatha yoga, the predominant form of practice throughout the Western world, to be given written form in texts like Hatha Yoga Pradipika. From then until the mid-twentieth century, Hatha and the many other strands of yoga were like proverbial ships in the night: even when their paths crossed, they rarely cross-fertilized. Where they did mix—not only among themselves but also with other practices such as Buddhism, Taoism, martial arts, dance, New Age philosophy, and modern science—it can sometimes take an acrobatic stretching of the imagination to recognize ancient teachings. The result is the predominance of asana practice, with most pranayama and meditation techniques largely missing in yoga classes in the West.

Reaction to this among teachers ranges from concern over losing the essence of yoga to a sense of relief in being freed from what can seem like esoteric authoritarian dogmas that may compromise health and freedom rather than lead to greater well-being and authentic spiritual awakening. In looking at the recent history of Hatha yoga we can see elements of truth at both ends of this continuum of thought, as well as many forms of integration reflecting the ongoing creative development of yoga. As a teacher, you might ask yourself: *What is the yoga that I'm teaching? How do I respond to a student asking about the deeper roots of my teaching? What is the received wisdom of tradition expressed in my classes, and what is from other sources? Where can I refer students whose interests in yoga are different from mine?* Gaining perspective on these questions helps to clarify the basis of our teaching while offering inspiration for the further creative development of yoga as a healing and empowering practice.

In reviewing the development of Hatha yoga, we will look at the major currents of the practice and how they came to be as they are today. We will look at what distinguishes the approaches of the best known and most widely practiced forms of yoga in the West today, looking for the kernels of wisdom and insight unique to each and relevant to the practical realities of teaching safe and effective classes in diverse settings and with a wide variety of students. With this background, we expand the palette that you as a yoga teacher can draw from in your own creative expression and sharing of the practice.

YOGA'S JOURNEY TO THE WEST

Much attention has been given to the gurus and ashrams that brought yoga to the West. These are commonly dated to Swami Vivekenanda's address to the World Parliament of Religions held in conjunction with the 1893 Chicago World's Fair,[2] though teachers from the East journeyed to the West a century prior to that. Well before Queen Victoria was anointed Empress of India in 1877, British imperialism began exposing Westerners to India and yoga. While British colonialists attempted to supplant Eastern traditions and impose their language and traditions on the people of India, the agents of colonial domination—military personnel, businesspeople, missionaries, and colonial authorities—were immersed in those traditions. The ancient literature of yoga began seeping into the West. These largely untold influences on the early transmission of yoga to the West and especially the United States are still evident in the way yoga is taught outside India.

Almost a century before Mahatma Gandhi, imprisoned in South Africa for protesting discrimination, read Henry David Thoreau's *Civil Disobedience,* Thoreau, on retreat at Walden Pond, read Charles Wilkin's 1785 translation of the Bhagavad Gita as well as the Vedas and the Upanishads (B. S. Miller 1986, 58–63). In a letter to his friend H. G. O. Blake in 1849, Thoreau wrote: "Free in this world as the birds in the air, disengaged from every kind of chains, those who practice the yoga gather in Brahma the certain fruits of their works. Depend upon it that, rude and careless as I am, I would fain the practice of yoga." He went on to say, "to some extent . . . even I am a yogi" (B. S. Miller 1986, 63). The writings of Ralph Waldo Emerson, Thoreau, and others in the early American transcendentalist movement spread knowledge of yoga in the West in a language that resonated with the non-Hindu culture in which they lived. Like contemporary yoga teachers and writers, they were interested in making the often-esoteric concepts and practices of yoga more accessible to the West. There were no yoga teachers, no yoga studios, no classes. Instead, early American yoga practices were based almost entirely on what these contemplative explorers gathered from the ancient literature, with recognizable asana practice nearly a century in the future.

The view from Thoreau's cabin

Soon spiritual seekers were traveling to India in hopes of finding the gurus the classical literature described as essential in learning yoga. These seekers included Helena Petrovna Blavatsky, founder of the Theosophical Society, and Annie Besant, under whose leadership the society later embraced a blending of Hinduism, Buddhism, and yoga as part of a belief that all religions contain portions of a larger truth. Besant played a key role, along with C. W. Leadbeater, in identifying a young boy named Jiddu Krishnamurti as the anticipated "world teacher," taking custody of him, training him in a variety of disciplines that included yoga, and eventually bringing him to the West. In young adulthood, Krishnamurti, who greatly influenced the development of yoga and other spiritual disciplines around the world, abandoned theosophy and declared, in a statement that continues to reverberate in the world of yoga teaching,

> I maintain that truth is a pathless land, and you cannot approach it by any path whatsoever, by any religion, by any sect. That is my point of view, and I adhere to that absolutely and unconditionally. Truth, being limitless, unconditioned, unapproachable by any path whatsoever, cannot be organized; nor should any organization be formed to lead or coerce people along a particular path (Lutyens 1975).

This tension between hierarchical, authority-based approaches to teaching yoga and the creative impulses within the practice had existed across the landscape of the American yoga scene in the early twentieth century. Indeed, as the early Americanization of yoga blended the received wisdom of tradition with the cultural and physical sensibilities of the United States and the larger Western world, innovative approaches to yoga were appearing across the country. Before the turn of the century, a native of Lincoln, Nebraska, Pierre Baker (a.k.a. "Oom the Omnipotent" or "Pierre Arnold Bernard") joined with the tantric yogi Sylvais Hamati to crisscross the United States giving quite original and creative yoga demonstrations. Years later, Baker founded New York Sanskrit College in midtown Manhattan, where wealthy celebrities such as Gloria Vanderbilt generously supported a yoga center, a countryside retreat facility, and a world-class spiritual research facility. In 1943, Baker's son, Theos, while teaching classes on the Upper East Side of Manhattan that reached out to elites in the cultural mainstream, wrote a Master's thesis on tantra and later a dissertation at Columbia University titled *Hatha Yoga: The Report of a Personal Experience.* The younger Bernard traveled extensively in

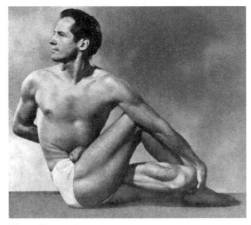

Theos Bernard

India and Tibet, generating significant media coverage of yoga and other Eastern spiritual practices.

Yoga teaching flourished in early to mid-twentieth century America with the rising influence of teachers from outside the United States. Yogendra Mastamani arrived from India in 1919, taught Hatha yoga for several years, and established one of the first yoga studio chains. A year later, Paramahansa Yogananda, whose *Autobiography of a Yogi* (1946) would become one of the best-selling yoga books of all time, arrived in Boston for the International Congress of Religious Liberals after founding a "how to live" school for boys in India in 1917 offering yoga classes and spiritual philosophy. He too soon joined the cross-continental lecture circuit, eventually settling in Los Angeles, where he established the Self-Realization Fellowship as the leading center for yoga in the West. His model is said to have inspired others such as B. K. S. Iyengar to bring their approach to the West.[3] Creating the first American yoga brand, called Yogoda, Yogananda's teaching—primarily bhakti and raja and very little Hatha—spread quickly as the media celebrated numerous Hollywood movie stars doing yoga. Yogananda's teachings would eventually create the foundation for Ananda yoga, while his younger brother, Bishnu Ghosh, would later teach Hatha yoga to a four-year-old boy named Bikram Choudhury.

Decades before Bikram and others would appropriate the title of "yoga teacher to the stars," others could legitimately claim the appellation. In the 1940s and 1950s, a young Latvian-born teacher who took the name Indra Devi popularized a form of Hatha yoga in Hollywood and across the country. At age twenty-eight, Devi, the daughter of a Swedish banker and Russian noblewoman and trained as a dancer and actress, set sail for India, where she acted in Indian films and married a Czechoslovakian diplomat. Cardiac problems led her to study yoga with a noted teacher named Tirumalai Krishnamacharya, who at the time was instructing young Brahman caste boys such as B. K. S. Iyengar and Pattabhi Jois at the Mysore Palace. Krishnamacharya asked Devi to teach yoga, and when she and her husband moved to Shanghai, she opened China's first yoga school. In 1947, she moved to California and set up a studio in Hollywood where Elizabeth Arden, whose line of beauty products and spas was well known, became a student, followed by some of Hollywood's biggest stars: Greta Garbo, Gloria Swanson, Ramon Navarro, Linda Christian, and Robert Ryan. Devi's book, *Forever Young, Forever Healthy,* became an instant classic among yoga teachers and students (Aboy 2002).

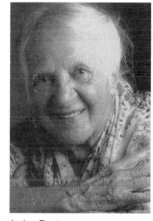

Indra Devi

Often overlooked in current times, Devi was the first well-known teacher to embody the eclectic creativity that characterizes most yoga teaching in the West today. With her background in dance and the influence of spiritual maverick Krishnamurti, she created a space in her classes for exploration beyond the structures and strictures inherited from the past. Others would soon join in this more playful and spiritually eclectic Americanization of yoga, breaking down barriers and opening up new possibilities for freedom in how yoga is taught, creating a liberalness that is often taken for granted in today's somewhat more forgiving yoga culture.

Soon yoga classes appeared across the American cultural landscape in a variety of forms and applications. Around the turn of the twenty-first century the media were highlighting yoga in sports clubs and Baron Baptiste's classes at the Philadelphia Eagle's football training camp, but in 1953, Selvarajan Yesudian published *Yoga and Sport,* which sold more than a hundred thousand copies and led many athletes and athletic training programs to begin integrating yoga into their training regimens. In Hartford, Connecticut, a journalist named Jack Zaiman wrote a regular column on yoga that helped get the practice into YMCAs and gyms across the country. Walt Baptiste, Baron's father and a popular San Francisco yoga teacher in the 1950s, promoted the benefits of yoga for bodybuilders in California. When word spread of Gary Cooper and Marilyn Monroe studying yoga, classes appeared everywhere. In the 1960s and 1970s, television shows on yoga, starring Richard Hittleman and later Lilias Folan, were hugely successful. When the Beatles began singing songs inspired by India, then embraced Maharishi Mahesh Yogi, yoga became almost the household word that it is today. With millions of viewers tuning in to Hittleman's *Twenty-Eight Day Yoga Plan* or Folan's *Lilias, Yoga and You,* the groundwork was set for future yoga teachers offering instruction through videos, CDs, DVDs, podcasts, and other media. With the rise of the human potential movement in centers such as Esalen Institute in Big Sur, California, where Joel Kramer profoundly influenced the future course of Hatha yoga, an Americanized approach to practice and teaching gained more attention.

More traditional forms of Hatha yoga based on claimed lineages continue to flourish. Teachers across the span of the yoga community have drawn from these more defined styles or systems of yoga. Most offer yoga teacher-training programs or other resources for learning their approach. Some continue to evolve, while others are committed to a strict maintenance of traditional teachings, said to be passed down through a lineage of gurus and students, and sometimes presented as the only correct system or method of teaching and practicing yoga. When traditional teaching methods and techniques appear to be unsupported or contradicted by Western medical or scientific research, teachers enter a fertile ground for exploration of ancient and contemporary perspectives, often on their own yoga mats, discovering anew and refining how yoga works in ways that can inform the practice and its sharing.

We can look at these traditional schools as spanning a continuum from relative insistence on teaching and practicing in a prescribed way to more open and eclectic approaches in which teachers feel a sense of creative freedom. Many observers have characterized the one extreme as fostering dependence on authority, diminishing spirit and humanity in the practice, and the latter as drifting into body sculpting or other practices that are more exercise than yoga, where traditional ideas of yoga virtually disappear.[4] Beautiful and authentic teachings can be found throughout the spectrum, as can sloppiness and practices that result in a high incidence of injury. We will look at the most popular styles of yoga taught in the West today, and consider these tendencies and ways that teachers' creative palettes are evolving.

CONTEMPORARY HATHA YOGA STYLES

The Hatha yoga styles discussed here represent the vast preponderance of approaches found in the West today. Our focus is on the development and distinct methods of each style. One of the challenges in describing some yoga traditions is evaluating the veracity of claims—the verifiable truthfulness about the origins and evolution of their practices. Many famous yogis claim to have received a yoga teaching directly from a divine source or from ancient writings that have since been lost. The belief that we are teaching or practicing in a tradition that was divinely inspired or passed down largely intact across thousands of years can be a powerful motivation to accept that tradition and create a sense of superior ordination. Yet whether or not the many fascinating stories about the creation or evolution of a style are true, what matters is whether the substance of the teachings has integrity. As a teacher, it is important to teach from a place of truth as you best feel it, know it, and understand it; ultimately this derives from intensive study and open-minded exposure to different traditions as well as experience on your mat and practice in the art of teaching. There is no question that much of the received wisdom of tradition was transmitted orally, often through memorization of songs or *slokas.* It may well be that every claim is true, although many stretch even the most tolerant imaginations, especially when considered in the context of other claims made by the guru that test credulity. A few things we do know can be applied in thinking about this and navigating our way through the traditions.

First, many early writings on yoga dating back thousands of years are well preserved and give extremely fine and richly detailed instruction on yoga practices, yet *none* of these give any details about asanas until the fourteenth century (although some tantric texts from the sixth to ninth centuries do discuss a few seated poses). This casts some doubt on the veracity of claims in many lineages that their system of asana practice was directly transmitted from the ancient past, when not a trace of that system (nor of any asana practice beyond sitting) can be found in the ancient writings and artifacts. Second, notions about property and responsibility in Indian and Hindu culture discourage a person taking credit for any divine practice, thus giving impetus to the assertion of the teachings being channeled or otherwise transmitted from ancient sources. This leads to a third consideration, that the legitimacy of teachings is bolstered if seen as received through an ancient lineage or from a divine source. Simply telling the complete truth—for instance, affirming that one synthesized a practice that draws from ancient and contemporary sources—should confer all the legitimacy one needs so long as the practice provides benefits such as physical well-being, emotional healing, or spiritual awakening to the practitioner. But when you believe that you are practicing something that was passed down largely intact for thousands of years, as we shall see is often claimed, that is compelling motivation to accept what the guru says and glow in the feeling of that connection, whether it is verifiable or not. What we find in the various teachings themselves is a beautiful tapestry of possibilities in the exploration and expression of yoga, tapping into the human body as a source of healing, wholeness, vitality, and spiritual awakening. This physical yoga described long ago thus can become in practice metaphysical, spanning the fullest range of human feeling, sensation, and awareness. As these practices evolve, drawing from developments in psychology, philosophy, science, and spirituality, our own creative contributions can extend, widen, and deepen them.

Ananda

Ananda yoga is based on the teachings of Paramahansa Yogananda, founder of the Self-Realization Fellowship and author of *Autobiography of a Yogi*. Yogananda's emphasis on opening to a direct inner experience of the divine—"self-realization"—is at the core of Ananda teachings, which were fully developed in 1968 by J. Donald Walters, a student of Yogananda's known as Swami Kriyananda (Kriyananda 1967). As a classical style of Hatha yoga that includes asana, pranayama, and meditation, Ananda is distinguished in part by a gentle form of asana practice.

As with most forms of Hatha yoga, the purpose of asana and pranayama in Ananda yoga is to awaken, experience, and ultimately control the flow of life-force energies within oneself, with the goal of increasing awareness and uplifting consciousness. What makes Ananda yoga unique are its "energization exercises" and asana affirmations. Ananda offers thirty-nine energy regulation techniques developed by Yogananda to help expand, direct, and control the life force. The affirmations are practiced silently while in a pose, "helping to reinforce the asana's natural effect on one's state of consciousness, bringing the mind actively and directly into one's practice" (Kriyananda 1967, 23). With a strong emphasis on safety and correct alignment, Ananda's teaching of yoga asana places considerably more attention than most other approaches on maintaining relaxation amid the effort required to do the asanas. The asana affirmations are said to foster an expanding awareness of the inner aspects of the practice, deepening awareness of how energy is moving in the body, including mental energy, giving rise to different states of mind. Rather than trying to force students into an idealized form of a pose, Ananda teachers encourage students to adapt their expression of the asanas to fit with their needs and abilities.

Anusara Yoga

John Friend founded Anusara yoga in 1997, integrating his largely Iyengar background with the tantric approach of *siddha* yoga. Friend (2006) describes Anusara as "a compelling Hatha yoga system that unifies a life-affirming tantric philosophy of intrinsic Goodness with remarkably elegant Universal Principles of Alignment," creating a system that was, he says, "immediately acknowledged by the greater yoga community in North America as a uniquely integrated style of Hatha yoga in which the artistic glory of the human heart blends seamlessly with the scientific principles of biomechanics." The central philosophy of Anusara begins with the belief that "God . . . is supreme consciousness and divine bliss. . . . As He thinks and feels, so He becomes the world." This belief, with clear roots in the Vedas and Kashmir Shaivist doctrines of tantra, holds that God is concealing his divine nature, creating the illusion of the self as a separate being and thus the source of our suffering. Yoga is a tool for realigning our awareness with the divine, creating a state of oneness that is our true nature.

In practicing and teaching Anusara yoga, the intention is to "align with the flow of Grace, to awaken to the truth that our essential nature is part of this divine flow, and to lovingly and joyfully serve this flow" (Friend 2006, 20); it is a "heart-oriented" practice in which asanas are expressed from the inside out as patterned by the "Optimal Blueprint," the master design for the body's potential. The center of this approach is the spiritual and emotional heart. For example, in describing the "three main directions of flow" of "Muscular Energy," the muscular hugging action is said to have "the qualities of firmness, love, security, and sensitivity. It is like how two loving family members hug each other when they are reunited after a long separation" (Friend 2006, 32–33). It is this heart-oriented emphasis that most differentiates the technical aspects of Anusara from Friend's roots in the Iyengar method. Many teachers gravitate to Anusara both for its heart-centered approach and for the feeling of belonging to a conscious community of like-minded teachers and students who are deeply immersed in a practice of aligning with the divine in yoga and daily life.

Ashtanga Vinyasa Yoga

There is often confusion about the meaning of *ashtanga*. The term means "eight limbs," as in Patanjali's eightfold path outlined in the Yoga Sutras, but it is also the name of the popular approach to yoga taught by Pattabhi Jois of Mysore, India, and practiced worldwide. The complete name, Ashtanga Vinyasa yoga, identifies Jois's method of yoga practice, which for Jois is firmly grounded in the Yoga Sutras. The origin of this method has been somewhat mystified. We are told it is an ancient system of practice written down by the sage Vamana Rishi in the Yoga Korunta, one of several texts said to have been transmitted orally to Tirumalai Krishnamacharya in the early twentieth century by his teacher, Rama Mohan Brahmachari. The Yoga Korunta is said to have contained lists of asanas grouped into what are now the six "series" of Ashtanga Vinyasa, each a set sequence of poses, along with original teachings on vinyasa, *dristi,* bandha, mudra, and philosophy. Told by Brahmachari that the original text could be found in the Calcutta Central Library, Krishnamacharya is said to have spent a year there in the mid-1920s researching the Korunta and transcribing what he could from the badly damaged original text.

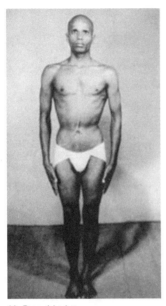

K. Pattabhi Jois

Jois says this was the source of the system he learned from Krishnamacharya. Jois's version of the practice was first published in 1962 as *Yoga Mala* (Jois 2002).[5]

Ashtanga Vinyasa yoga is traditionally taught in "Mysore style," in which each student in a class moves through a sequence of asanas on their own while the teacher gives individualized guidance. The practice is done every day except Saturdays, new moons, and full moons. Sunday mornings, the teacher usually guides the class through the Primary Series. Although this is the beginning level, most students new to Hatha yoga still find it difficult. Indeed, there are many asanas in that series that are considered advanced in other approaches. Conversely, some poses in the intermediate and advanced Ashtanga Vinyasa series are considered relatively simple.

Through the regular practice of the Primary Series, an intense series of postures also called *yoga chikitsa,* meaning "yoga therapy," the body's energy pathways (nadis) are opened and prana flows throughout the body, ridding it of toxins and relaxing the nervous system. The second or Intermediate Series, called *nadi shodhana,* meaning "nerve cleansing," focuses intensively on the spine and pelvis, further opening and balancing energy channels in and around the spine. In the Advanced Series, called *sthira bhaga* and which encompasses four sequences, students integrate the strength and balance of the practice (Flynn 2003). When the teacher senses a student's ease and steadiness in a pose, he or she gives the student the next pose, and when the student performs the entire series with steadiness and ease, the first pose of the next series is introduced. Advanced students continue to do the Primary and Intermediate series.

Ashtanga Vinyasa is a highly focused practice.[6] The practice of dristana, in which one gazes steadily upon a specified point in and between each asana, lends to pratyahara, a more internal awareness. Ujjayi pranayama is maintained throughout, creating a steady rhythm in the breath that is sustained evenly from pose to pose, its sound and sensation creating a mantra that fosters greater mental focus and acuity. Bandhas are employed in most of the practice, assisting in the regulation of pranic energy flowing through the body. The practice is tied together through vinyasa, the conscious connection of breath to movement that helps generate a "balance of strength and flexibility, lightness and heaviness, movement, and stillness" (Swenson 1999, 11).

To teach Ashtanga Vinyasa with authorization, one is required to study for several years directly with Jois's grandson Sharath Rangaswamy in Mysore, India, and with one of his small cadre of authorized teachers. As a general principle, you must be two series ahead of the series you teach. Thus, to teach Primary Series you are expected to be in Third Series. Following the traditional model as taught by Jois, those interested in teaching typically apprentice for a year or more with an experienced Ashtanga Vinyasa teacher after completing the Intermediate Series, learning adjustments and other intricacies of the practice. Many devoted *ashtangis* in the Primary or Second series begin teaching when they feel the inner inspiration, often taking teacher-training courses outside the Ashtanga Vinyasa system to learn more about alignment, modifications, use of props, and other essential teaching skills that are not routinely taught in the Ashtanga Vinyasa practice.

Bikram Yoga

Very few approaches to yoga in the West are named for their leading teacher. B. K. S. Iyengar, Ana Forrest, and Bikram Choudhury are the only ones to name a system after themselves. Perhaps more than any other yoga teacher, Choudhury is unabashedly boastful in describing his personal accomplishments both on the mat ("I am beyond Superman") and off the mat, frequently reminding others of his financial success. Whether from authentic megalomania or a brilliant public relations ploy (or both), Choudhury and his approach receive extensive coverage in the media. With hundreds of Bikram's Yoga College of India and Hot Yoga studios dotting the planet, many thousands of students religiously follow the Bikram method of Hatha yoga.

In his now-classic *Bikram's Beginning Yoga Class* (2000), Choudhury tells the reader that he or she "will learn the Hatha yoga asanas (postures) as set down by Patanjali over four thousand years ago." Putting aside for a moment that Patanjali wrote approxi-

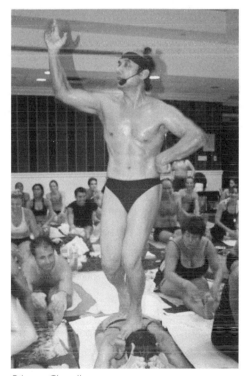

Bikram Choudhury

mately two thousand years ago and never described a single specific asana, we can allow that Choudhury developed his twenty-six pose and two breathing exercise routines during what he describes as "years of research" following his initial training with Bishnu Ghosh, Paramahansa Yogananda's younger brother. Sent to Bombay by Ghosh to teach Hatha yoga to sick people, Choudhury (2000, xii) tells of researching all the diseases and postures, drawing on the methods taught to him by his guru as well as "modern medical measurement techniques," and designing his sequence to heal "no matter what condition you are in, what chronic diseases you may have, or how old you are."

The basic Bikram yoga class is specific. The room temperature is set to at least 105 degrees Fahrenheit. Each of the twenty-six poses is performed twice, most for either thirty seconds or a minute, in a set sequence. There are no inversions and no arm balances. Although each posture is said to have "a particular way that constitutes correct breathing for that posture," neither Choudhury's book nor many classes in his studios explain the breath specifically for each pose. The basic Bikram breathing technique is called "normal breathing," in which you take a full breath, go into the pose, let out twenty percent of the breath through your nose, then complete the exhale. If the 20:80 technique proves too difficult, students are encouraged to breathe as needed.

Railing against other forms of Hatha yoga in the West as ill-informed, inventive, and dangerous, Choudhury asserts that his method is "the right way" to do yoga. Asserting that "using props to help you do the postures only makes matters worse and not better," he warns that American students are "getting ripped off, even getting hurt" in practices that deviate from the true system of yoga he claims was given in the Yoga Sutras. Concerned that Americans are "making up posture after posture, making up names for them," Choudhury says he wants students to learn "true Hatha yoga," which apparently he alone offers. Ironically, the one and only prop allowed by Choudhury—an extremely heated room—is itself a source of injury. Stretching in an environment heated to such an extreme as in Bikram yoga allows a person to stretch much further than would otherwise be possible for his or her body. The problem is that this extended stretching ability is often beyond what the body is ready for, often resulting injuries (A. Stephens 2005).[7]

Bikram yoga responds well to the powerful impulse in Western culture to feel quick results from any effort. In taking a Bikram yoga teacher-training course, you learn the twenty-six pose routine, the two breathing techniques, the claimed medical benefits of each pose, and the prescribed narrative overlay to each class given by Choudhury. You will gain certification to teach one of the most popular styles of Hatha yoga that thousands of Westerners rave about as the most powerful workout around.

Integral Yoga

The basic aim of integral yoga is the integration of many different yoga paths (hatha, raja, bhakti, karma, jnana, and japa) into one with overall integrity, yet ironically there are two separate integral yoga movements, one founded by Aurobindo Akroyd Ghosh (1872–1950), the other by Ramaswamy Satchidananda (1914–2002). Known respectively as Sri Aurobindo and Swami Satchidananda, both established large followings through their writings and networks of teaching centers and ashrams.

Educated at Cambridge University, in the early 1900s, Aurobindo was a leader in the Indian nationalist group known as the Extremists for its advocacy of independence from Britain and its willingness to use violence as a means to gaining that independence. Imprisoned for his political activities, his spiritual journey began, he says, while meditating on the Bhagavad Gita and being visited during his meditations by Swami Vivekenanda. Once free, he studied deeply and started publishing his extensive writings (Van Vrekhem 1999). *The Synthesis of Yoga* was published in serial form between 1914 and 1921, outlining the practice of integral yoga. The central purpose of yoga, he wrote, is "Transformation of our superficial, narrow, and fragmentary human way of thinking, seeing, feeling, and being into a deep and wide spiritual consciousness and an integrated inner and outer existence and of our ordinary human living into the divine way of life" (Satprem 1968). The practice itself draws broadly from India's spiritual traditions and synthesizes them with its own methods. Since the goals of this yoga are attained only through divine guidance, each individual's specific path differs. The basic approaches are karma yoga, jnana yoga, bhakti yoga, and what Aurobindo called "the yoga of self-perfection," where cultivation of the mind into an "overmind" of higher consciousness allows the practitioner to perfect all aspects of his or her life.

Looking on this practice as "the art of harmonious and creative living on the basis of the integral experience of Being," integral yoga aims at "opening the springs of creative inspiration hidden in the human psyche" and the "active participation in the being of the world with a view to the outflowering of the Divine in the march of civilization" (Chaudburi 1965, 15–16). This concept of integral practice not only has led to yoga classes and all the integrally related practices in some centers, but also has inspired the creation of institutions like the California Institute of Integral Studies, a private graduate school founded in 1968. All of this pales by comparison with Auroville in the southwest of India, a city-ashram with more than two thousand residents from around the world giving full material and cultural expression to integral yoga.

Winning the trademark to "Integral Yoga" in 1985, the Satchidananda group has strongly established itself in the North American yoga community and worldwide, even creating "Yogaville" in Virginia. Rooted in the teachings of Ramaswamy Satchidananda, this integral philosophy of yoga arises from the *sannyasa* order, which, in studied contrast to Aurobindo's tantric-oriented philosophy, renounces all worldly thoughts and desires. (Ironically, Satchidananda was the welcoming speaker at Woodstock in 1969.) As a young adult the wealthy Brahman-born Satchidananda was not involved in spiritual matters until after his wife died a few years following the birth of their second son. This led Satchidananda to a spiritual quest, traveling across India to meditate and study with spiritual teachers, including Aurobindo, Ramakrishna, and Ramana Maharishi. Traveling north to Rishikesh in the Himalayas, Satchidananda met and became a disciple of Swami Vishwananda Sivananda (1887–1963) and was initiated into the Holy Order of Sannyasans, a renunciate order. After teaching in India for many years, Satchidananda was invited by New York artist Peter Max to the United States, where he stayed, gaining citizenship, and established the Integral Yoga Institute at Yogaville.

Critiquing pure Hatha yoga for its "overemphasis on the physical side of existence" in which "the body is sometimes almost deified," the integral yoga of Satchidananda, like that of Aurobindo, goes far beyond the physical practice of yoga postures to include meditation, mantra, service, devotion, and deep study, integrating the major branches of yoga. As a pure Sannyasan renouncing all worldly thoughts and desires, Satchidananda's interpretation of the Yoga Sutras is clearly distinguished from the tantric influences found in Aurobindo. For example, in his translation of saucha, one of the niyama practices, Satchidananda gives us this: "By purification arises disgust for one's own body and for contact with other bodies" (Satchidananda 1978, 142).[8] In Satchidananda's approach to Hatha yoga, postures, breath control, relaxation, and cleansing practices are used to purify and strengthen the body and mind. The approach to asanas is very gentle, with most classes offering pranayama, chanting, *kriyas,* and meditation. In inspiring students to go beyond the physical practice of yoga asana, this integral yoga method encourages students to integrate the mind, body, and spirit so they can live happier and more peaceful lives with others.

Iyengar Yoga

Belur Krishnamachar Sundararaja (B. K. S.) Iyengar was born in 1918 into a difficult situation. His family was poor at a time when escape from the influenza pandemic then sweeping across India was an option only for the wealthy. Throughout his childhood he suffered from general malnutrition as well as tuberculosis, malaria, and typhoid fever. His father died when he was nine years old, leading him to live with his brother in Bangalore. In 1932 he was invited by his sister to live with her and her husband, Tirumalai Krishnamacharya, in Mysore, where Krishnamacharya taught yoga at the local palace. Iyengar never describes the specific content of that practice in writing. However, a newsreel published on the YouTube Web site in 2006 showed Iyengar and Krishnamacharya in 1938 doing what appears to be part of the Ashtanga Vinyasa yoga Advanced (Third) Series.[9] After five years of studying yoga with Krishnamacharya and showing improvement in his health, Krishna-macharya asked Iyengar to go to Pune to teach.

In the early years of his teaching, Iyengar was often less proficient in asana than his students. In a practice he describes as having incorrect technique, he was often in pain. He began experimenting with the various props and modifications for which his method is well known. With the publication of *Light on Yoga* in 1966 (with a foreword written by Yehudi Menuhin), Iyengar's precise instruction of asanas, including very specific alignment in each pose, began to change the practice of Hatha yoga worldwide. While rooted in Patanjali's Yoga Sutras, Iyengar innovated in his practice and teaching of asana. His approach to the practice is given more refined explication in his later writings.[10]

In explaining his focus on physical practices, Iyengar makes reference to the Kathopanishad, one of the Upanishads written around 300 BCE that compares the body to a chariot, the senses to the horses pulling it, the mind to the reins, the intellect to the charioteer, and the soul to the master of the chariot itself. All must be functioning well for the chariot to move forward. With many approaches to yoga slighting the body, Iyengar (2001, 16) affirms his commitment to all eight limbs of Patanjali's ashtanga yoga, including asana. Rather than a "one size fits all approach," he emphasizes, "asanas cater to the needs of each individual according to his or her specific constitution and physical condition." Going beyond the concept of a "pose," Iyengar (2001, 17) stresses "an asana is achieved when all the parts of the body are positioned correctly, with full awareness and intelligence," with the benefits of the asana coming when "you are absolutely comfortable in that final posture." The idea of the "perfect pose" runs throughout Iyengar's writings and teachings. In his

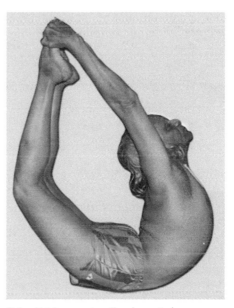

Belur Krishnamachar Sundararaja Iyengar

translation of the Yoga Sutras II.27 (1993), he writes: "Perfection in an asana is achieved when the effort to achieve it becomes effortless, and the infinite being within is reached." It should be noted that no other published translations of this

Sutra—including from others in the Krishnamacharya lineage such as his nephew Desikachar—use the term *perfection*.

In contrast to the Ashtanga Vinyasa path taught by Krishnamacharya to Pattabhi Jois (and to Iyengar as well), in Iyengar yoga poses are typically held for a much longer duration. It is in holding asanas that alignment is perfected along with energetic actions that refine the asana. In the beginning stages of practice, Iyengar stresses grasping the whole asana, striving for stability rather than getting lost in the finer details. From this strong foundation, with the body under control, the practice should become more reflective and meditative. "You must become aware of your tissues, organs, skin, and even individual cells. . . . Your mind must flow along with all these parts" (B. K. S. Iyengar 2001, 43). Finally, one reaches a stage of intimate knowledge when "the mind ceases to be a separate entity, and the intelligence and the body become one." With a balance between movement and resistance, one's intelligence engaged at every level, a sense of spaciousness and subtlety of perception, the body symmetrical, here one is in asana.

This approach is one of disciplined practice for cultivating ease and health in a stressful world where ailments and physical limitations are very common. The use of props—anything that helps stretch, strengthen, relax, or improve the alignment of the body—is one of the most distinctive elements of Iyengar yoga, enabling students to attain the perfection that Iyengar sets as a goal in the asanas. Experimenting with walls, chairs, stools, blocks, bolsters, blankets, and straps, Iyengar discovered that the props helped retain key movement and adjustments of the body. "Ultimately," he says, "yoga with props creates a feeling of peace and tranquility, and culminates in a fresh perspective and renewed strength" (B. K. S. Iyengar 2001, 165).

Many students and leading teachers, even those whose approach is different from Iyengar's, pay homage to Iyengar as a yoga master. "His legacy has not only made yoga accessible to all regardless of needs and limitation," writes Vinyasa Flow teacher Shiva Rea (2007, 250), "but has offered a path of conscious embodiment at the heart of yoga." Although he is criticized by some for compromising the spiritual spirit of practice amid technical detail, even those who departed his system defend him as a deeply spiritual and wise teacher. Describing his practice with Iyengar in 1976, Erich Schiffmann (2007, 84) emphasizes that "The whole point of all this hard physical work—and it was very physical and very demanding—was to get into a deep meditative state. And for me," Schiffmann continues, "*it* worked."

Teaching Hatha yoga with the Iyengar method begins with years of consistent practice under the close guidance of a certified Iyengar teacher. To gain certification as a teacher requires many more years of in-depth study through an authorized Iyengar institute or senior certified instructor. The Iyengar organization maintains a precisely defined hierarchy of certification levels that correspond to demonstrated skill and knowledge at increasingly complex levels of the practice. At the most senior levels of certification you must be repeatedly invited to study directly with Iyengar in Pune, India. At even the most junior level of Iyengar certification, there is assurance that the teacher has proven his or her competence in teaching yoga the Iyengar way.

Krishnamacharya Yoga

Tirumalai Krishnamacharya (1888–1989) may have influenced the practice of Hatha yoga more than any other teacher dating back to the Hatha Yoga Pradipika in the fifteenth century. A five-foot, two-inch Brahman born in a small south Indian village, when barely five years old he started learning about the history, philosophy, and practices of yoga from his father, who told him they had descended from a great ninth-century sage, Nathamuni. After the passing of his father while he was still a young boy, Krishnamacharya sought out yoga instruction at a nearby temple, learning basic asanas. At age sixteen, he says he ventured out to Nathamuni's shrine at Alvar Tirunagari, where he had what he describes as a mystical experience in which he was greeted by Nathamuni and received a transmission of the Yoga Rahasya, a long-lost ancient yogic text in which Nathamuni gave the essence of the practice. After his return home his family moved to Mysore, where he began formal studies, eventually going to the university at Benares. During breaks in his studies he would venture into the Himalayas seeking out teachers, eventually finding Ramamohan Brahmachari, whose yoga school was in a cave at the foot of Mount Kailash. Staying there for seven years, Krishnamacharya studied asanas and pranayama, memorized the Yoga Sutras, and began his deep study of the therapeutic aspects of yoga. After re-

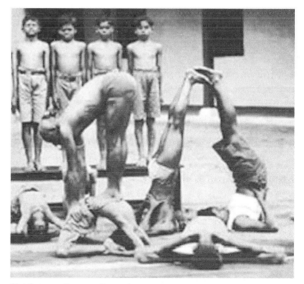

Krishnamacharya at work

turning from Tibet, Krishnamacharya began studying *ayurveda,* the traditional medical practice of India. These studies deepened his individualized yoga instruction as he recognized the unique conditions of his students. In 1924 the Maharaj of Mysore invited Krishnamacharya to teach at the Mysore Palace. Tailoring the practice to the condition of his young Brahman boy students, Krishnamacharya taught them Ashtanga Vinyasa yoga.[11] At the same time he taught more gentle and therapeutic practices to others at the Palace.

Some of Krishnamacharya's students would go on to become some of the world's most renowned teachers—Pattabhi Jois, B. K. S. Iyengar, Indra Devi, and his own son, T. V. K. Desikachar, who writes that the essence of his father's teaching is "not that the person needs to accommodate him- or herself to yoga, but rather the yoga practice must be tailored to fit each person" (Desikachar 1995). Desikachar and A. G. Mohan, also a student of Krishnamacharya, would go on to further develop yoga as a therapeutic practice. This approach has increasingly influenced teaching worldwide, primarily through the Desikachars' Krishnamacharya Yoga Mandirim and International Association of Yoga Therapists (IAYT).

Krishnamacharya Yoga is grounded in Patanjali's description of asana as sthira and sukham: steadiness and ease. While many approaches to asana encourage students to push hard, the *Krishnamacharya* approach says that without sthira and sukham, there is no asana. If, in going into a pose, you feel tension or pain, you are not ready for that pose. Accepting one's self as one is in the present moment and practicing poses patiently and progressively, a sequence of poses is created depending on one's immediate needs and goals. This allows a variation in practices for seasons, daily routines, energy levels, and whatever else is happening in the person's life right then. Guided by the breath and attuned to the balanced presence of sthira and sukham, a person can then bring varying degrees of dynamism into his or her practice, perhaps flowing with continual movement in and out of poses, or holding poses longer to explore them more deeply (Desikachar 1995, 25–31). Using a step-by-step process to move in the right way, asanas themselves are adapted to ensure the integrity of the spine, joints, organs, and breath. Using *pratikriyasana,* or counterposes, to help to integrate an overall practice, Desikachar (1995, 27) stresses that "It is not enough to climb the tree; we must be able to get back down." With balanced attention to asana modifications, a variety of pranayama techniques, the application of ayurvedic analysis in prescribing a practice, and attention to the unique conditions and intentions of each student, teaching this approach asks the instructor to possess both broad and deep knowledge of yoga and related practices in crafting classes for individual students. As IAYT and others work to establish yoga therapy as a legitimate healing modality, more and more teachers are finding this approach a viable profession.

Kundalini Yoga

Kundalini yoga might seem like a distant cousin of Hatha yoga because the emphasis is less on the asanas than on breath, chanting, and meditation. While some Hatha yoga practices make oblique reference to the connection between breath, physical movements, and the movement of energy through the chakras, these are the focus of kundalini. Considered supremely powerful and potentially dangerous, the kundalini techniques were historically practiced in secret. Brought to the West in 1969 by Harbhajan Singh Puri, known affectionately as Yogi Bhajan (1929–2004), this "yoga of awareness" is primarily shared through 3HO, the Healthy, Happy, Holy Organization established by Yogi Bhajan. The yogic lifestyle and practices taught by 3HO and embraced by most Kundalini yoga teachers are closely associated with the Sikh faith, an eclectic system of religious philosophy founded in northern India in the fifteenth century.

In kundalini practice, a variety of techniques are used to move energy up through the chakras using several different asanas, pranayamas, mantras, and mudras. Most practices begin sitting, where focus is brought to the first chakra and an awareness of acceptance. With the shifting of positions, focus is gradually brought into the second chakra, where an awareness of creativity and human relations is nurtured. In the third chakra, awareness is brought to commitment, where balance is found in the core of the body. As the "lower triangle," these first three chakras are seen as forming the foundation of our physical and energetic form. With the awakening of the fourth chakra in the spiritual heart center comes kindness and compassion, a sense, Yogi Bhajan says, of "the healing activity of God within the being flows" (Khalsa 2000, 94). With awareness moving from "me" to "we," a new sound is created in the mantra practice: "Hum," which means "we" or "that." In the fifth chakra comes an awareness of one's truth. Singing freely, positive words are created as one is filled with the healing light of truth. From here, as a sense of clear rises through the sixth chakra, confusion dissolves and clarity sets in, leading to a sense of boundlessness, the mandala of supreme consciousness flowing forth at the sahasrara chakra.

Kundalini is an intense practice. One is invited to move through what might feel like painful intensity, holding the arms aloft for long periods, stretching the breath seemingly beyond limits, sitting still for extended periods of meditation. In this way it is a tapas-oriented approach, stoking the inner fires of transformation through the intensity of practice. The promise in this practice is immediate experience of the fruits of yoga (Narayanananda 1979).[12] Yet Yogi Bhajan describes mastery of this practice as arising from teaching it: "If you want to learn something," he says, "read it. If you want to know something, write it. If you want to MASTER something, Teach it!" (Bhajan).

Power Yoga

Power yoga fully arrived on the yoga scene in 1995 with Beryl Bender Birch's release of *Power Yoga: The Total Strength and Flexibility Workout* (1995), Bryan Kest's series of *Power Yoga* videos through Warner Brothers, and Baron Baptiste's launch of Power yoga in New England. What most distinguishes Power yoga from other styles is its detachment from traditional yoga philosophy in exchange for an emphasis on yoga as a vigorous workout drawn primarily from the Ashtanga Vinyasa method. Recognizing that most students struggled to a point of frustration with beginning-level Ashtanga Vinyasa, Power yoga pioneers saw that this vigorous practice could appeal to fitness buffs if given a familiar language and presented in whatever form seemed doable. As with much of Power yoga, many asanas are taught in modified forms that make them more accessible to students interested in a physical workout.

Power yoga is very popular across the United States, especially in gyms and fitness centers, and is gaining a following in Europe and Asia. Sometimes it is given a slightly different name, such as power Vinyasa, power flow, hot Power yoga, etc. It typically attracts students looking for an intense workout free of strange Sanskrit words, chanting of *aum,* or sitting in meditation. Emphasizing a powerful workout, many Power yoga classes give little attention to alignment. Combined with a "go for it" attitude, this results in a high rate of injury that is similar to that sustained by students in the Bikram and Ashtanga Vinyasa systems. While some Power yoga teachers—including in recent years Birch, Kest, and Baptiste—encourage students to explore meditation and other contemplative practices, this is a small part of the Power yoga subculture.

In her book *Power Yoga,* Birch (1995, 274) sets forth the "Axioms of Power Yoga," the first of which she says comes from Ashtanga Vinyasa but is more akin to Bikram yoga: "You must be hot to stretch." She suggests that this is a five-thousand-year-old insight, but that as recently as 1980 she was "practically the only one" saying this (Birch 1995, 23). For emphasis, she stresses that to stretch you have to be "not only warm, but hot and sweating." Birch's second axiom, that "strength, not gravity, develops flexibility," is somewhat more curious because no one claims that gravity by itself is the source of flexibility. In Power yoga classes, many still go with Birch's replication of the Ashtanga Vinyasa Primary Series, while many others have introduced other poses and sequences. Because physical strength, power, and getting a physical workout are the primary aims of the practice, most classes include long sets of standing balancing poses sequenced for their intense workout effect rather than safe opening of the body.

After years of instructing, many Power yoga teachers are encouraging a more well-rounded practice. In an online interview with the Web site About.com, Baptiste emphasized the importance of "adaptation," saying that the practice is "to challenge you to experience a transformation, but starting from where *you* are presently, and steadily building to a place that allows you to authentically experience the yogic rewards of being stronger, more supple, relaxed, and stress-free" (Pizer 2007). In *Beyond Power Yoga,* Birch (2007) has refocused her emphasis away from "hot and sweating" and instead fixed her attention on spiritual philosophy, meditation, and bliss. And on his Web site, Kest (2007) says "Power Yoga is about working hard sensitively. It's about feeling good, not just looking good. The tone and shapeliness you attain from this work is a by-product. The focus here is balance and healing."

Sivananda Yoga

The author of nearly three hundred books on yoga, metaphysics, religion, philosophy, fine arts, ethics, health, and many other topics, the man who came to be known as Swami Sivananda (1887–1963) had an enormous influence on Hatha yoga practice. Born Kuppuswami in Tamil Nadu, he attended medical school, ran a medical journal called *Ambrosia,* and practiced medicine for many years in Malaya before setting out in 1923 on a spiritual quest that eventually brought him to Rishikesh in 1924. There he met his guru, Vishwananda Saraswati, and was initiated into the renunciate Sannyasan order. Settling in Rishikesh, Sivananda immersed himself in Sannyasan practice while continuing to offer medical services. He traveled extensively throughout India, visiting among other places the Aurobindo Ashram. In 1936 he started the Divine Life Foundation, offering free spiritual literature and more formal spiritual guidance to the many seekers coming to visit him in Rishikesh. Calling his approach "the yoga of synthesis," paying homage to Aurobindo's *The Synthesis of Yoga,* Sivananda stressed the practical application of yoga philosophy over abstract thinking. The synthesis represents a balanced integration of the four principal paths of yoga taught by Krishna to Arjuna in the Bhagavad Gita and embraced in Vedantic philosophy: jnana, bhakti, karma, and raja yoga. Whereas some interpretations of the Bhagavad Gita say that one might well choose one of the four paths, Sivananda taught that everyone should practice certain techniques from each path in accordance with individual temperament and taste.

One of Sivananda's many disciples, Swami Vishnudevananda (1927–1993) studied this approach to yoga with Sivananda for ten years before being asked to take the teachings to the West. Vishnudevananda then traveled and taught yoga throughout North America, first settling in Montreal to create the Sivananda Yoga Vedanta Centre in 1960 and then ultimately settling in Quebec. Numerous ashrams would follow, in the Bahamas, California's Sierra Nevada Mountains, the Catskills, the Indian paradise of Kerala, as well as many cities in the United States, South America, Europe, and the Middle East. Vishnudevananda's teachings followed closely those of Sivanada, adding the "Five Points of Yoga," interpreted elements that in combination give Sivananda yoga its full character: proper exercise, proper breathing, proper relaxation, proper diet, and positive thinking and meditation.

Sivananda's prescription for proper exercise is a basic asana practice that can be modified for age, special conditions, and ability. The traditional Sivananda yoga practice (which Sivananda yoga asserts is *the* traditional practice of asana) starts with relaxation in Savasana (Corpse Pose) before commencing with Surya Namaskara. This is followed by twelve asanas, each held for up to a few minutes before resting again in Savasana. Proper breathing, called "Full Yogic Breathing," is a slow, diaphragmatic technique in which the abdomen, then the rib cage, and finally the upper chest expand with the inhale, then reversing this with a slow exhale. Sivananda yoga also teaches kapalabhati pranayama and *anuloma viloma pranayama.* Vishnudevananda (1960, 203) describes three methods of relaxation. First, through a process of "autosuggestion" the entire physical body is brought into a state of deep relaxation in Savasana. Beginning in the toes and slowly progressing up through the entire body, this relaxation is finally extended to all the organs of the body. With slow rhythmic breathing, mental tension melts away, slowly giving way to a "floating sensation" and sense of inner calm. Still, tension remains until you go into spiritual relaxation, where from a state of deep physical and mental relaxation you withdraw yourself and come to identify with the "all-pervading, all-powerful, all-peaceful self, or pure consciousness within."

Vinyasa Flow Yoga

Vinyasa flow yoga is somewhat less definable than others approaches precisely because it embodies the continuous, dynamic, conscious evolution of the practice. It reflects the constant interplay of human beings in the flow of life, connecting our inner nature, life experience, and the received wisdom of tradition as we explore and discover new possibilities for creative expression and conscious living on this planet. The term *vinyasa* is derived from *nyasa,* meaning "to place," and *vi,* meaning "in a special way." The term *flow,* originally defined by Ganga White (2007, 114) in relationship to Hatha yoga, "implies a practice with a theme or purpose with poses linked or associated together." Taken together, Vinyasa Flow thus suggests a practice in which we consciously place the body-breath-mind in the constant flow of space and time. In *The Complete Book of Vinyasa Yoga*, Srivatsa Ramaswami (2005, xvii, 260), a longtime student of Krishnamacharya, defines *vinyasa* simply as "variation" or "variations and movements." Godfrey Devereux (1998, 253) offers two definitions: lowercase *vinyasa*, meaning "progression, continuity," and uppercase *Vinyasa*, meaning "a continuous sequence of breath-linked postures." At the heart of each of these definitions is a spirit and process that Vinyasa Flow teacher Shiva Rea describes as "one that awakens and sustains consciousness." She continues:

> In this way vinyasa connects with the meditative practice of "nyasa" within the Tantric yoga traditions. In nyasa practice, designed to awaken our inherent divine energy, practitioners bring awareness to different parts of the body and then, through mantra and visualization, awaken the inner pathways for *shakti* (divine force) to flow through the entire field of their being. As we bring the techniques of vinyasa to bear throughout our lives, we open similar pathways of transformation, inner and outer—step-by-step and breath-by-breath (Rea 2005, 6).

As in Ashtanga Vinyasa yoga, Vinyasa Flow moves steadily from pose to pose in sequences of movements synchronized with ujjayi pranayama, often pausing to hold poses for various lengths of time while maintaining the rhythmic flow of the breath. Unlike Ashtanga Vinyasa, each class usually offers a different sequence of poses, although most use some form of Surya Namaskara A and B from the Krishnamacharya lineage. Many classes also closely follow the basic standing poses and finishing sequence found in Ashtanga Vinyasa. Many Vinyasa Flow classes apply Iyengar alignment principles, energetic actions within poses, and use of props. The insights and methods of Krishnamacharya are seen in Vinyasa Flow's emphasis on vinyasa *krama*, *krama* referring to "stages" that create a deliberate sequencing of asanas. Vinyasa krama also refers to the staging of practice that accommodates differing intentions and abilities, so you start from where you are and move consciously—"in a special way"—as you progress from simpler to more complex asanas. Vinyasa Flow often applies the concept of pratikriyasana, meaning neutralizing or "counterposes." Working with the idea "to place in a special way," many Vinyasa Flow teachers highlight this concept in several relationships within the practice: being conscious of how the body is moved and placed within and between poses; conscious linking of breath and body-mind within and between poses; the way you approach your mat, set an intention, stay connected with that intention throughout a practice, get up from your mat, and move out into the larger world; paying attention to what you are doing while practicing—breathing, moving, feeling, watching, being in the flow; opening in a more intuitive way that expresses and embodies the feeling of pranic energy flowing in the universe.

Unlike most approaches to Hatha yoga, which have a fixed system, Vinyasa Flow is not a system. This allows creativity in sequencing asanas and offering a diverse array of themes in different classes. This freedom and dynamism help make

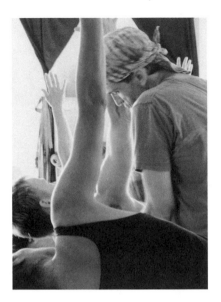

Vinyasa Flow one of the most attractive forms of yoga today, variously resonating with the spirit, intentions, and life experiences of different teachers and students. Like its cousin, Power yoga, there is no hierarchy, no leading guru as in Anusara, Ashtanga, Bikram, Iyengar, and many other approaches. Without gatekeepers as in the hierarchical systems, anyone can teach Vinyasa Flow yoga. Amid this freedom there can be misguided instruction, confused or ineffective sequences, even dangerous classes, but with a growing number of recognized teacher trainers who are respected for their depth of knowledge, wisdom, and skill, Vinyasa Flow teachers are increasingly finding rich sources of guidance along their own creative paths. In the ideal Vinyasa Flow class, the teacher will have substantial training and experience that combines skills and knowledge of yoga philosophy, subtle energetics, functional anatomy and physiology, the biomechanics of sequencing asanas, hands-on adjustments, and other areas of teaching, all the while opening to the spontaneity of life and immediate experience to share in the further evolution of yoga.

A TEACHER'S PALETTE OF STYLES

The various practices of yoga have continually evolved, creating many paths, with every Hatha yoga style or lineage today a fusion of approaches that came before. Most approaches have tapped into insights from outside the yoga world, drawing from various forms of dance found around the world as well as gymnastics, martial arts, physical therapy, and functional anatomy to further develop and refine their approach. Although some of the approaches we have reviewed here insist that their way is ancient, pure, and correct, all have changed within the past generation alone. With evolution and refinement have come attempts to differentiate and rate, with many leaders claiming their way to be the best way, to which one might reply, "For whom?" Each style and tradition has something to offer; how it is offered is often just as significant as the style itself. The best teachers are those attuned to their students' needs and capable of teaching in a way that addresses those needs while safely introducing them to new challenges and possibilities. If, as a teacher, you are committed to one approach, then acknowledge that to yourself while appreciating that you will have many students for whom another approach is probably better suited. Broadening your repertoire of skills and knowledge will enable you to more easily recognize these fits and help you prepare to respond in the most effective, appropriate, and honorable way. Sometimes that might involve offering variations and modifications, other times suggesting a completely different practice or teacher. If you are committed to a certain lineage, this will help define who you are as a teacher. If you are more independent in your approach, how you choose to relate in your teachings to the many lineages and styles of yoga will go far in defining your own teaching. But no matter your perspective in relation to gurus, systems, and approaches, what will always most define you as a teacher is how you choose to relate as a human being with your students. With compassion, knowledge, and skills, you will be the best teacher you can be.

CHAPTER THREE

SUBTLE
ENERGY

Let the beauty that you love
be what you do.
—*Rumi*

In Chapter One we saw how the rise and spread of tantra eventually gave rise to Hatha yoga as a practice of conscious embodiment. Rather than starting with meditation or other practices, the original Hatha yogis worked with the immediate experience of their physical bodies to move through the layers of being that seemed to separate their sense of individual being, including body and mind, from connection with all of nature or the divine. Drawing from the deep well of ancient wisdom found in the Upanishads and a wide variety of esoteric traditions handed down through ritual, songs, and stories, they undertook this exploration with an expanding map of consciousness and being that today still gives us the primary concepts of anatomy and physiology from a traditional yogic perspective. For many these concepts are treated literally, while others view and use them in practice and teaching as symbolic ideas that help chart the pathway of self-transformation through Hatha yoga practice.

The earliest motivation of yoga, expressed by Krishna in his conversation with Arjuna on the edge of the battlefield in ancient India, was to move beyond the illusion of the self and unite with the real Self, or atman. In the Yoga Sutras, Patanjali gives a more refined explanation of the nature of this self-illusion—*kleshas*—that traps us in a confused state of alienated being. This ignorance—or *avidya*—keeps us trapped in a sense of self that is identified with our mind and material existence. Across centuries of trial and error, yogis "discovered they could unwind the painful misidentification, retracing the steps of the human self back through the layers of reality, from the most gross, physical plane with which we now identify, to the most refined planes of pure consciousness" (Cope 1999, 67). In this process of discovery, the ancient yogis described in vast detail a system of energetic being that could be consciously cultivated, elaborating a complex system of scientific medicine with theories of anatomy and physiology that are at once mystical, symbolic, and practical. Here we will look at the major elements of this system and how they are interrelated. In this overview of koshas, prana, nadis, bandhas, chakras, *gunas,* and doshas, we will pause along the way to consider how to bring these concepts alive in our teaching.

THE FIVE SHEATHS

An overarching concept in subtle anatomy is that the energy of each embodied being is contained in a set of five interrelated sheaths, or koshas, that define the three "bodies." First mentioned in the Taittiriya Upanishad (Gambhirananda 1989), the kosha model helps to map the inner journey of yoga.

TABLE 3.1—**The Three Bodies and Five Sheaths**

THE THREE BODIES (SHARIRAS)	THE FIVE SHEATHS (KOSHAS)
Physical body (sthula)	Annamaya—food
Subtle body (sukshma)	Pranamaya—energy
	Manomaya—mind
	Vijnanamaya—intellect
Causal body (karana)	Anandamaya—bliss

Starting on the periphery of the physical body and moving toward the core of your being as an embodied soul, the koshas are not a literal anatomical model of the body but rather, as Shiva Rea (2002) puts it, "a metaphor that helps describe what it feels like to do yoga from the inside—the process of aligning what in contemporary language we often call the 'mind, body, and spirit' or 'mind-body connection.'" Using this typology to conceptualize the nature of being, yoga helps bring the body, breath, mind, wisdom, and spirit (bliss) into harmony. Existing as an energetic whole, all aspects of all five sheaths are simultaneously present, interwoven like a tapestry. Hatha yoga is a means for becoming consciously aware of this interwoven fabric of existence, connecting the physical and subtle bodies, bringing awareness more and more to a place of blissful being.

Physical Body

Annamaya kosha is the sheath of the physical self, named for the fact that it is nourished by food (*anna* means "food"; *maya* means "full of"). In Hatha yoga it is here that we start our practice, exploring the physical body. But this is just the beginning. This is a dimension of existence in which we experience matter that is a combination of energy and consciousness, even if we are not yet fully conscious of this interconnection. Yoga starts to happen as we begin to explore and experience the physical body in its manifold connections with the energetic, intellectual, and blissful bodies.

Subtle Body

The *pranamaya* kosha, or energy sheath, connects the physical body with the other koshas, vitalizing and holding together the body and mind. Composed of prana, the vital life force, it pervades the whole organism, physically manifesting in the constant flow and movement of breath. Part of the subtle body, prana cannot be seen or physically touched as it moves through thousands of nadis, or energy channels, sustaining the entire physical and energetic system. As long as this vital element exists in the organism, life continues. The pranamaya kosha is associated on a physiological level with the respiratory and circulatory systems but is neither reducible to, nor coterminous with, them. In teaching pranayama, we can guide students in expanding and directing this energy to cultivate a more fluid and harmonious interaction among their koshas, integrating body, mind, and spirit. Working with the breath in the physical body in exploration of asanas—playing with the asanas, holding them, refining them, letting them go—expands our awareness beyond the physical body. With prana as the source and guide, we begin to discover its more subtle expressions, called "prana vayus," each with a unique movement and effect.

The *manomaya* kosha is composed of *manos*, or "mind," and the five sensory faculties, conveying the powers of thought and judgment. Associated with the brain and nervous system, manomaya kosha distinguishes humans from other living organisms. Endowed with the ability to differentiate, it is the cause of distinctions such as "I" and "mine" from which it creates freedom or bondage. Breath mediates the interaction between this sheath and the physical body, which we sense when mental strain compromises breath and wellness, or when the breath leads to a sense of oneness between body-mind and a sense of inner peace.

Vijnanamaya means "composed of *vijnana,*" or "wisdom," referring to the reflective aspect of consciousness that discriminates, determines, or wills. Associated with the organs of perception, this sheath gives us our sense of individuality.[1] The reflective aspect of consciousness, vijnanamaya is present to our consciousness when we begin to experience deeper insight into ourselves and the world. Sometimes referred to as the "wisdom sheath," vijnanamaya is still identified with the body, subject to change, insentient, and thinking. As the physical and subtle bodies are felt as one, there is a deepening insight into the unity of self and nature, ego and the divine. When this experience is shrouded over by memories, manos, the identity is still with the ego, the vijnanamaya kosha, not the supreme Self. But when "the witness of the experience dissolves into the experience of the moment," as Shiva Rea says, *anandamaya* is shining through.

Causal Body

From *ananda,* meaning "bliss," in the Upanishads the anandamaya kosha is known as *karana sharira,* or the "causal body." It is the consciousness that is always there, that always has been and always will be there, even when the mind, senses, and body are sleeping. It manifests itself by catching a reflection of the divine, which is absolute bliss, felt in moments of calm inner peace and tranquility.

PRANA

Prana has many descriptions: the energy permeating the universe at all levels; physical, mental, intellectual, sexual, spiritual, and cosmic energy; all vibrating energies; all physical energies such as heat, light, gravity, magnetism, and electricity; the hidden or potential energy in all beings; the prime mover of all activity; the energy that creates, protects, and destroys; vigor, power, vitality, life, and spirit; the principle of life and consciousness; the breath of life of all beings in the universe; the hub of the Wheel of Life; being and nonbeing.

These are just a few definitions of *prana,* which collectively we can take as referring to the vital life-sustaining force permeating living beings and vital energy in all natural processes of the universe. If nothing else, we are reminded of its importance, as we can gather from an old Vedic story about prana in the Chandogya Upanishad (Nikhilananda 2008). The five main faculties of our nature—the mind, breath (prana), voice, ears, and eyes—were arguing over which was most important, reflecting the ordinary human condition in which our faculties are not integrated, instead competing for our attention. To resolve the dispute, they each agreed to leave the body and see whose absence was most missed. To make the story short, prana won the argument: no breath, no life. But while prana is associated with the breath, it is more than simply respiratory air. From the Vedas through the Sutras to the Pradipika, the breath is seen as a gateway to the world of vital energetic currents generated in the human body and controlling all the biological processes. Prana was first expounded in the Upanishads, where it is part of the worldly physical realm, sustaining the body and the mother of thought and thus also of the mind. Described in the Taittiriya Upanishad, prana has five energetic expressions, or functions, called vayus (Gambhirananda 1989, I.vii.1):

TABLE 3.2—**Prana-vayus**

VAYU Here the general term describes the particular	MANIFESTATION
Prana-vayu	Prana moves inward, entering the body through the breath, and is sent to every cell through the circulatory system. Responsible for the beating of the heart and breathing. This energy sets things in motion and guides them along the way.
Apana-vayu	Moving downward and outward, apana moves in the lower abdomen and controls the elimination of urine, semen, menses, and feces. This energy eliminates negative experiences.
Samana-vayu	Moving from the periphery to the center through a swirling and churning action, samana stokes the gastric fires, aides digestion, and creates a caldron integrating other energies. Responsible for the digestion of food and the repair and manufacture of new cells.
Udana-vayu	Moving upward, udana works through the larynx and pharynx to control the vocal cords, the exchange of air, and the intake of food. Responsible for producing sounds through the vocal apparatus, as in speaking, singing, laughing, and crying. It also represents the conscious energy required to produce the vocal sounds corresponding to the intent of the being. It is the main positive energy stimulating the evolution of consciousness.
Vyana-vayu	Moving outward while pervading the entire body, vyana distributes the energy derived from air and food throughout the body. Responsible for the expansion and contraction processes of the body, including circulation and voluntary movements, vyana assists all other pranas in the work.

There are several effective ways to bring greater awareness to the vayus in guided classes.

- *Prana-vayu,* centered in the spiritual heart center, is awakened with ujjayi pranayama that distributes it throughout the body. Governing the area from the throat to the heart center, prana-vayu is associated with *jalandhara bandha,* regulating the intake of breath and energy. Guiding students in the flow of conscious ujjayi pranayama is an effective way of helping them bring about more subtle awareness to jalandhara bandha, which in turn will help them to effect the balance of energy they are experiencing in their practice.

- *Apana-vayu* is the energetic force of exhalation that governs the elimination of waste, working in the kidneys, colon, rectum, bladder, and genitals to help maintain balance in the system. Its functioning is enhanced by the rooting actions of standing asanas and the cultivation of *pada bandha* and *mula bandha.* Guiding students to give more awareness to these energetic actions and to the full completion of each and every exhale leads to a stronger sense of grounding, and with it greater decisiveness and clarity of action.

- *Samana-vayu* governs the area from the heart to the navel. It is the energy that stokes our inner fire, associated with the *manipura* chakra and our willfulness in the world. In asana practice you can guide students' awakening and balance of samana-vayu through abdominal core work, in which students are encouraged to explore moving energy broadly and deeply in the center of their belly. Overstoking the fire with gripping in the belly will lead to a lack of discrimination and even a fiery anger in how one manifests his or her energy in the practice and in life. Kapalabhati pranayama is an effective tool for stoking the fire but should be done with a sense of lightness. Exploring a sense of steadiness and ease while working strongly in the core will create more balance in samana-vayu.

- *Udana-vayu* governs the area from the throat into the head. Associated with the *vishuddha* chakra, udana-vayu is the energetic force that expels the breath and allows us to express ourselves vocally. When out of balance, it leads to disjointed or incoherent speech. The purifying effects of asana and pranayama practice allow the more balanced flow of udana-vayu. Teaching students how to practice ujjayi pranayama that is both strong and soft is an effective way of helping them find the deeper energetic balance that allows clearer and easier self-expression. In leading guided visualization and meditation practices, you can offer students even more refined exploration of udana-vayu.

- *Vyana-vayu*, associated with the water element, runs through the entire body, serving as a unifying force with all the other prana-vayus. It is that quality of energy that gives one a feeling of being whole and integrated. While it functions at the surface of the body to give us a sense of boundaries in social interaction, it also governs our inner sense of balance and coordination. The balanced practice of asana, pranayama, and meditation leads to vyana-vayu being more in balance and the creative expression of life—seated in the *svadhisthana* chakra—flowing more naturally. Teaching energetically balanced classes that encourage creativity and playfulness, strength and flexibility in each student's exploration of yoga is an effective way to enhance the balanced flow of vyana-vayu.

NADIS

The life-force energy of prana flows throughout the pranamaya kosha via a network of fine, subtle channels called nadis, meaning "channel" or "vein," derived from the root *nad,* meaning "flow" or "motion." First mentioned in the Upanishads around the seventh century BCE as part of a mystical physiology, we cannot physically detect or show the precise number or location of the nadis. Still, traditional literature gives specific numbers and even maps of the channels in what appear as incredibly dense lines running throughout the body: 72,000 in the Hatha Yoga Pradipika, 200,000 in the Goraksa Paddhati, 350,000 in the Shiva Samhita; 72,000 is the commonly accepted number, probably from the influence of Arthur Avalon's *The Serpent Power* (Avalon 1974, 115). All are rooted in the *kanda* ("bulb") near the base of the spine. Ten are emphasized in the Sita Samhita and up to fourteen are said to be particularly important in the Goraksa Sataka and Hatha Yoga Pradipika. The original descriptions tend to be obscure, typically shrouded in language that attempts to express in words phenomena that resist verbal description except in the most flowery symbolic terms, as we can see in some of Avalon's book.

Among thousands of nadis, three are most important: sushumna, *ida*, and *pingala*. The Sat-Cakra-Narupana, one of the earliest

TABLE 3.3—**The Principal Nadis**

LEFT SIDE	CENTRAL	RIGHT SIDE
Ida	Alabusha	Pingala
Shankhini	Kuhu	Pusha
Gandhari	Vishvodhara	Payasvini
Hastijihva	Varuna	Yashasvati
	Sarasvati	
	Sushumna	

Source: Frawley 1999, 147.

texts on subtle energy, calls these nadis *sasi, mihira, susumna.* Sushumna nadi moves up from the base of the spine "beautiful like a chain of lightning and fine like a lotus fibre, and shines in the minds of the sages. She is extremely subtle; the awakener of pure knowledge; the embodiment of all Bliss, whose true nature is pure Consciousness" (Avalon 1974, 12). Prana-vayu moves through the sushumna nadi, energizing the spine, nerves, and brain, while collecting the pranic energy of all the other nadis in the third eye. Ida and pingala nadis crisscross back and forth as they rise from the kanda "like the double helix of our DNA" (Bailey 2003), branching out from the third eye to the left and right nostrils. Beginning and ending on the left side of the physical body, the cooling, vibrating quality of ida nadi nourishes the body with pranic energy. Commonly referred to as the "moon" channel for its gentle nature, the ida nadi is said to regulate the sympathetic nervous system, calm the mind, and nourish our softer aspects. Pingala nadi, beginning and ending on the right side, is referred to as the "sun" channel, conveying strong energy. It governs the parasympathetic nervous system.

When the nadis are blocked, prana is kept from flowing freely through the subtle body, causing imbalances in our physical and mental processes. Put in more purely yogic terms, when there is dysfunction in the pranamaya kosha, the annamaya and manomaya koshas are further disturbed and disconnected. Opening all the nadis, cultivating the balanced flow of energy through the ida and pingala nadis, and bringing awareness to the movement of prana—in the form of *kundalini-shakti* energy—up through the sushumna nadi leads to blissful ecstasy (Vasu 2004). Nadis are effectively purified and opened through asana, pranayama, and meditation practices.

BANDHAS

First described in tantric literature, bandhas (meaning "to bind") are muscular contractions in the physical body that retain the circulation of prana in the subtle body. Three primary bandhas—mula bandha, *uddiyana* bandha, and jalandhara bandha—are described in the Hatha Yoga Pradipika and the Gheranda Samhita. All are described as being done while sitting, primarily in conjunction with pranayama practices but never in conjunction with other asanas. The three major bandhas are classically instructed as follows:

- Mula Bandha—the Gheranda Samhita says that "the wise yogi should apply pressure to the perineum with the heel of the left foot and carefully push the navel plexus against the spine" and "tightly press the penis with the right heel.

> This mudra destroys decrepitude [!] and is called Mulabandha" (Mallinson 2004, 66). The Hatha Yoga Pradipika adds "forcefully contracting the anus so that apana vayu moves up . . ." (Muktibodhananda 1993, 340).

- Uddiyana Bandha—meaning "to draw upward," the Gheranda Samhita says to "draw the abdomen backwards above the navel so that the great bird [shakti] flies unceasingly upward. This is uddiyana-bandha, a lion against the elephant of death" (Mallinson 2004, 62). The Pradipika emphasizes "making the navel rise" (Muktibodhananda 1993, 334).

- Jalandhara Bandha—the Pradipika and the Gheranda Samhita instruct the yogi to "contract the throat and put the chin on the chest" (Muktibodhananda 1993, 352; Mallinson 2004, 62).

When practiced together, the three major bandhas create *mahabandha* (the "great bandha"): "By contracting the anus, performing uddiyana bandha, and locking the ida and pingala with jalandhara, sushumna becomes active. By this means prana and breath become still. Thus death, old age, and sickness are conquered" (Muktibodhananda 1993, 359). This is said to be the most assured way for establishing balance and union between mind and body. Many contemporary teachings emphasize use of the bandhas throughout asana practice, but there are varying (even conflicting) views about how, when, and to what degree. There are also widely varying views about the muscular actions and other physical body elements with each bandha, as well as their effects. In later chapters we will discuss how to teach the activation and application of bandhas in asana and pranayama practices.

CHARRAS

According to Hatha yogis, the junctions of the major nadis as they spiral and rise along the spine give rise to chakras ("wheels"), the major psycho-spiritual-energetic centers of the subtle body. As with everything in the world of yoga, with chakras there are numerous contrasting and even conflicting views about what they are, how they work, their number, location, and even whether location is a relevant concept. Different chakra models found in historical, philosophical, and literary works have as few as five chakras or infinite chakras throughout the subtle body. In the traditional yogic literature the number varies from chakras at the intersection of every nadi to the identification of the major chakras, usually said to number between five and eight. The tantric model, developed around the eleventh century and described in the Sat-Cakra-Nirupana, is the most widely accepted, giving seven chakras described as emanations of divine consciousness (Avalon 1974, 318).

Just as the movement of prana is felt in the physical body and in our mental awareness despite being invisible, the chakras are psychic centers of energetic and spiritual experience, not physical locations that can be palpated, x-rayed, or detected with magnetic resonance imaging technology. "Concentration on physical organs or spots in the body as prescribed by many spiritual masters," says Harish Johari, "is misleading, for the chakras are not material" (Johari 1987, 15). Yet the chakras may correlate with the major nerve plexuses of the physical body; some schools of thought associate chakras with particular sensations in the body.[2] More commonly they are correlated to psychological, emotional, and mental qualities. Lecturing in 1932, Carl Jung emphasized that "they symbolize highly complex psychic facts which at the present moment we could not possibly express except in images" (Shamdasani 1996, 61). Whether the relationships indicated by these symbols are useful is a question best answered in personal practice. Presently we will consider all of these elements, as they can be helpful in creatively mixing the teaching palette.

Chakras are part of a much higher energy system than the physical body. Traditionally it is said that awakening of the chakras depends on opening a higher source of energy than the physical body can provide, that it takes a concentrated quality level of awareness (Frawley 1999). Awakening of kundalini requires that prana enters the sushumna—the central energetic channel of the subtle body. So long as one's life energy and consciousness are identified with the physical body, prana can't come into the sushumna channel. Arousing kundalini involves a state of samadhi—a trancelike condition of awakened being that is the eighth limb of ashtanga yoga. At the root of yoga is the concept of kundalini-shakti, the latent life-force energy resting in the subtle body. During normal consciousness, this energy is dormant. When awakened through the conscious movement of prana through the ida and pingala nadis uniting the feminine and masculine elements of one's nature, this cosmic energy rises through the sushumna channel, creating ecstatic bliss. For this to happen there must be balance in each of the chakras where ida and pingala cross.

- *Muladhara chakra*—found around the base of the spine, between the anus and genitals, the muladhara chakra symbolizes our present psychic condition, bound as we are in normal consciousness to the physical body and caught in the web of earthly forces. It is related to the cohesive power of matter, inertia, instinct, security, survival, and basic human potential.

- *Svadhisthana chakra*—found around the base of the genitals, the svadhisthana chakra is related to base emotion, sexuality, and creativity. With the stirring of kundalini-shakti, our emotions are stirred in ways that have physical expression, opening us to sensations of physical control, pleasure, and expression. In sublimating sexual desire, here we can cultivate and enjoy the simple flow and flavor of this energy as the movement of delight.

- *Manipura chakra*—found in the lumbar region at the level of the navel (epigastric plexus). It is related to the transition from simple or base to complex emotion, energy, assimilation, and digestion, and is held to correspond to the roles played by the pancreas and the outer adrenal glands, the adrenal cortex.

- *Anahata chakra*—found in the area of the heart, the seat of prana. It is related to emotions, compassion, love, equilibrium, well-being, and going beyond personal emotions to understand the love in all emotional fluctuations, becoming love itself.

- *Vishuddha chakra*—found in the throat, it is related to communication and growth, growth being a form of expression, as well as being silent, losing one's personal voice in the divine word.

- *Ajna chakra*—situated between the eyebrows, ajna is held as the chakra of time, awareness, and light as well as learning to live as pure insight, not requiring a body.

- *Sahasrara chakra*—located at the top of the head. It is generally considered to be the chakra of consciousness, symbolized by a lotus with one thousand petals, and represents becoming one with the infinite.

See Table 3.4 The Chakras, page 58.

GUNAS

In Samkhya, one of six classical schools of Indian philosophy, the universe is divided into *purusha,* or consciousness, and *prakriti,* or nature/matter. Prakriti consists of three qualities known as gunas, which describe the natural tendencies of the mind and emotions that are the expression of the manomaya and vijnanamaya koshas. The unique expression of the gunas within each person gives that person his or her self-identity. It is also a way of describing the relative contentment we find in our emotional relationship to desire. This model is a useful tool in analyzing and understanding the patterns of our thoughts and emotions, with direct application in our practice and teaching of yoga. The three gunas are *sattva, rajas,* and *tamas:*

- Sattva describes a calm and clear state of mind, a sense of being complete and fulfilled. Filled with this sense of levity, clarity, and tranquility, you are more kind and thoughtful toward yourself and others. Yoga philosophy describes

TABLE 3.4—**The Chakras**

CHAKRA	COLOR	PRIMARY FUNCTIONS	ELEMENT	LOCATION
Crown Sahasrara	Violet	Union, bliss, sense of empathy	Space/thought	Top of the head
Third eye Ajna	Indigo	Direct perception, intuition, imagination, visualization, concentration, self-mastery, extra sensory perception	Time/light	Between the eyebrows
Throat Vishuddha	Azure	Creativity, communication, expression, eloquence, intuition, synthesis, hearing	Life/sound	Base of the throat
Heart/Lung Anahata	Green	Love, wisdom, stability, perseverance, mental patience and equilibrium, pleasure, compassion, touch	Air	Center of the chest
Solar plexus Manipura	Yellow	Will, determination, assertion, personal power, laughter, joy, anger, sight	Fire	At the mouth of the stomach
Sacrum Svadhisthana	Orange	Creativity, sexual energy (for women), desire, pleasure, stability, self confidence, well-being, taste	Water	The lower belly
Root Muladhara	Red	Survival, grounding, sexuality (for men), stability, smell	Earth	The base of the spine

this as our natural state of mind. We can act in the world with ease because our mental balance is not dependent on something external. This allows us to move about in our lives in harmony with others.

- Driven by desire, rajas revolves around the feeling of needing or losing something, even to the point of becoming obsessed by it. If we do not act, we fear losing what we feel we need. If successful in attaining whatever is driving our desire, then the mind will return to a balanced sense of calm (or potentially flip into fear of loss). Rajas involves a sense of intense dynamism, stimulating you to act in the world with excitement and passion, the mind always imbued with anxiety or expectation about how things might turn out.

- Tamas reflects a confused mind that leads to indecision, lethargy, and inaction. This is the feeling of not knowing what you are feeling or what you want or need. Caught in this tendency, your behavior can become self-destructive or harmful to others. Yet tamas also allows us to calm down, relax, and restore our energy through rest and sleep.

Taken together, the three gunas are always present to some degree in everyone's life, forming your attitude, nature, and potential. Rather than judging these tendencies as good or bad, we can look upon them for insight into how we feel within ourselves and how we interact with others in our lives. In our normal life we tend to be attracted to things and people in the world. There is nothing wrong with this. More important is the *quality* of that attraction. Whatever we tend to be attracted to preoccupies our mind. If our intention is to move into a place of clarity, being aware of where our attention and energy are focused in the simplest of life activities gives insight into what stands in the way of that clarity. If you find yourself preoccupied with endless ruminations or fantasies, you might find your energy takes you further away from other values that you may hold, such as living simply or aligning with the divine.

David Frawley (1999) offers the metaphor of an oil lamp for grasping the essential interplay of the gunas. The heavy basin containing the oil rests stably on the ground, seemingly inert in its tamasic nature. The oil, with properties of movement or flow, symbolizes the rajasic tendency. The wick, made of clean white cotton, symbolizes sattva. The interplay of these elements produces the flame. A healthy balance in life involves all three, with each predominating at the appropriate time. Without tamas we would never sleep. Without rajas we would never move. Without sattva we would never calmly shine forth in the world.

We can become more conscious of the balance of our gunas by paying attention to the tendencies that arise while practicing yoga. Attuned to the sensations in the physical body (annamaya kosha), consciously moving prana with the breath, we can yoke the body-breath-mind in a way that directly affects manifestation of the gunas. In the same way we can encourage our students to be more self-reflective in their practice, offering them questions that help them to become more self-aware: Where are your senses directed? How are you breathing? Where are you gazing? What do you hear? Is there a pattern in your thoughts and feelings? What is associated with those patterns? Does the feeling tend to arise with some asanas more than others? Are the patterns affected by the time of day, time of the month, certain others or types of others in the room?

DOSHAS

As prana manifests in the physical body, it moves in different ways in different people depending on all of life's circumstances. In ayurveda the manifestation of prana in the body is described by the energetic interplay of the universal elements: air, fire, water, earth, and ether. The elements give us several qualities, from hot to cold, dry to wet, light to heavy, hard to soft, as well as functional tendencies such as grounded or floating, spacious or constrained. How these elements interact creates patterns in three expressions of prana in the physical body called doshas (literally "deviations"). The three main doshas are vata, pitta, and kapha, which together comprise the *tridoshas* ("three doshas"). All processes in the physical body are governed by the balance of doshas. One dosha tends to be dominant in any individual, giving him or her a specific doshic constitution. Sometimes two are equally present, or when all three are in balance one's constitution is described as "tridoshic." Ayurveda provides a science of the body that is largely predicated on looking at individuals through the prism of their doshic constitution. It is in the combination of the basic elements that the doshas are determined:

- Vata, similar to vayu, arises from the combination of air and ether, creating the subtle energy of movement in the mind and body. It governs breathing, the flow of blood, muscle and tissue movement, even the movement of thoughts in the mind. In activating the nervous system, when vata is in good balance it is a source of creativity, enthusiasm, and flexibility. With excessive vata one becomes fearful, worrisome, and prone to insomnia.

- Pitta arises from fire (and some air, as fire requires air), creating the heat that governs digestion, absorption, metabolism, and transformation in the body and mind. Put differently, heat in the body is the product of metabolic activity, thus placing this process under pitta. In balance, pitta is a source of intelligence and understanding, helping us discriminate between right and wrong. Excessive pitta lends to anger and hatred.

- Kapha, formed from earth and water, creates the body's physical structure—bones, muscles, tendons—and cements the body together. Kapha supplies the body with water, lubricating the joints, moisturizing the skin, reinforcing the body's resistances, helping to heal wounds and give biological strength. Associated with emotions, Kapha is expressed as love, compassion, and calmness. Out of balance, it creates lethargy, attachment, and envy.

The relative constitution of the balance of doshas is affected by diet and lifestyle. Ayurvedic doctors give advice and treatments to help cultivate doshic balance. Yoga is one important part of balancing the doshas. There is an expanding literature on how to adapt one's yoga practice for doshas, which is tricky given the diversity of doshic types in most classes.

Vata types—filled with air, tending toward being dry and cold, flexible when young but typically stiff and prone to arthritis later in life—benefit from exploring poses more gradually and steadily, moving very slowly through their Sun Salutations, focusing more on grounding in standing and balancing poses, and lingering longer than most in deep asanas. Nadi shodhana (alternate nostril breathing) emphasizing the right nostril in the morning for energy and warmth and the left at night to promote calm and sleep should be done in a gentle and grounding way.

Pittas tend to push hard and gravitate toward hot, vigorous practices. In cultivating balance, pittas benefit from letting go of their competitive tendencies, tapping into asana as a cooling, nurturing, and relaxing practice. Rather than moving quickly into the next pose, the pitta student benefits from a longer pause, especially after strong sequences, being mindful of relaxing and letting go of tension. Rather than going for the hot and sweaty practice, pittas are better advised to go slow and learn to relax deeply by moving more slowly and consciously in their practice. Cooling pranayamas such as *sitali* can help with further balancing, allowing them to come away from the practice with a calmer, clearer mind and a lighter, more relaxed body.

Kaphas, inclined as they are to lethargy and heaviness of movement, benefit most from a warming and flowing practice to stimulate their metabolism and circulation. Starting practice with a warming pranayama such as kapalabhati helps kaphas get their energy up for the asanas. Starting with simple flowing sequences to further warm the body and keep energy flowing, kaphas benefit from moving into sustained asana sequences requiring (and thereby cultivating) strength and stamina. Standing pose sequences that involve heart-opening variations benefit kaphas by further stimulating circulation and the movement of mucus. Sustained backbending sequences further stimulate circulation and the movement of energy in the chest and head, lending to more balanced energy and a clearer, more active mind.

HIGHLIGHTING SUBTLE ENERGY IN CLASSES

The entire yogic process awakens, moves, balances, and integrates subtle energy. The integration arises from a sense of apparent disintegration, or separation of body, mind, and breath. While a few students have the blessing or luxury of pacing their day around yoga—or *as* yoga—this is the rare exception. Most students arrive to class after dropping their kids off at school in the morning, during a break in the day, or after hurrying from work to make it to class on time. Even weekend classes tend to be squeezed in around errands, family activities, and other commitments. This presents teachers with a special opportunity for guiding students in how to move subtle energy easily and gracefully to experience wholeness, inner peace, and bliss.

The essential source of wholeness is prana, which we tap into and move with the breath. Using the breath as the starting point and focus of yoga practice, it is important to create space at the beginning of each class for students to check in with how they are breathing and feeling—which is connected. When students first arrive to class and sit on their mats, they are most likely "in their heads," whether scattered, focused, overloaded, depressed, agitated, or in some other mental or emotional condition. Asking them to tune in inside to the natural rhythm of their breath initiates the invitation to more conscious awareness of the connection between the breath and their overall energetic sensation. This is the starting point for consciously cultivating subtle energetic awakening and balance in the practice, as explored in Chapters Five, Six, Seven, and Eight.

CHAPTER FOUR

BODY STRUCTURE AND MOVEMENT

Once you have flown,
you will walk the earth
with your eyes turned skyward,
for there you have been,
and there you long to return.
—*Leonardo da Vinci*

Teaching Hatha yoga effectively involves guiding students in, through, and out of asanas in a safe, clear, and efficient way. Describing yoga asana requires describing the anatomy of stable and easy movement in the human body. As with any specialized description, there is a specialized language—the language of anatomy. Presently we will look more closely at the major joints in the body, including their structure and movements. These insights will be expanded and related to the real-practice complexities of individual asanas in Chapter Seven. They also inform asana sequencing, part of the vinyasa krama that makes up an entire class or set of classes as discussed in Chapter Ten.

THE FEET

With twenty-six bones that form twenty-five joints, twenty muscles, and a variety of tendons and ligaments, the feet are certainly complex (Netter 1997, plates 488–499). This complexity is related to their role, which is to support the entire body with a dynamic foundation that allows us to stand, walk, run, and have stability and mobility in life. In yoga they are the principal foundation for all the standing poses and active in all inversions and arm balances, most backbends and forward bends, and many twists and hip openers. Meanwhile they are also subjected to almost constant stress, ironically one of the greatest stresses today coming from a simple tool originally designed to protect them: shoes. Giving close attention to our feet—getting them strong, flexible, balanced, aligned, rooted, and resilient—

is a basic starting point for building or guiding practically any yoga practice, including seated meditation.

In order to support the weight of the body, the tarsal and metatarsal bones are constructed into a series of arches. The familiar medial arch is one of two longitudinal arches (the other is called the lateral arch). Due to its height and the large number of small joints between its component parts, the medial arch is relatively more elastic than the other arches, gaining additional support from the tibialis posterior and peroneus longus muscles from above. The lateral arch possesses a special locking mechanism, allowing much more limited movement. In addition to the longitudinal arches, there are a series of transverse arches. At the posterior part of the metatarsals and the anterior part of the tarsus these arches are complete, but in the middle of the tarsus they present more the characters of half-domes, the concavities of which are directed inferiorly and medially, so that when the inner edges of the feet are placed together and the feet firmly rooted down, a complete tarsal dome is formed. When this action is combined with the awakening of the longitudinal arches, we create pada bandha, which is a key to stability in all standing poses (and a key source of mula bandha).

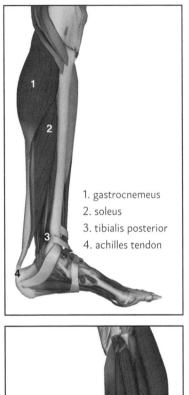

1. gastrocnemeus
2. soleus
3. tibialis posterior
4. achilles tendon

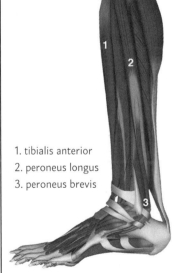

1. tibialis anterior
2. peroneus longus
3. peroneus brevis

Primary lower leg muscles (lateral views)

However, the feet do not stand alone, even in Tadasana, nor do they independently support movement. Activation of the feet begins in the legs as we run lines of energy from the top of our femur bones down through our feet. This creates a "rebounding effect." Imagine the feeling of being heavier when riding up in an elevator, or lighter when riding down. The pressure of the elevator floor up against your feet not only makes you feel heavier, it has the effect of causing the muscles in your legs to engage more strongly. Similarly, when you intentionally root down from the tops of your thighbones down into your feet, the muscles in your calves and thighs engage. This not only creates the upward pull on the arches of pada bandha (primarily from the stirrup-like effect of activating the tibialis posterior and peroneus longus muscles) but creates expansion through the joints and a sense of being more firmly grounded yet resilient in your feet while longer and lighter up through your body.

TEACHING PADA BANDHA

- Bring the class to standing with their feet together at the front of their mat.
- Ask them to look down at their feet and lift and spread their toes wide apart.
- Keeping the toes lifted, guide your students to feel the inner edges of the balls of their feet (about an inch in from the space between the big toe and the fourth toe) and to press that point more firmly down into the floor.
- Now ask students to repeatedly release the toes down and lift them up while keeping the inner edges of the balls of their feet rooting down, noticing how, with the toes lifted, the inner ankles and ankles automatically lift.
- Encourage the class to try to keep their inner arches and ankles lifted and to feel how this creates a sense of lifting the center of each foot like a pyramid, awakening pada bandha. The challenge arises in trying to maintain this awakening of the feet while allowing the toes to release softly down and spread into the floor.
- With pada bandha active, draw their attention to the rebounding effect, feeling the stronger activation of their leg muscles, awakening of their inner thighs, and lengthening up through their entire body.

It is helpful to divide the feet into the "heel foot" and the "ankle foot." The "heel foot" derives from the lateral arch, which is connected to the fibula bone in the lower leg, a non-weight-bearing force distributor. Positioned in relation to the calcaneus and cuboid bones, and from there to the fourth and fifth metatarsals and phalanges, it creates more direct grounding and stability. The "ankle foot," relating the tibia to the talus, navicular, cuneiforms, and first three metatarsals and phalanges, is more resilient and a source of refined movement. Thus, in standing balance asanas such as Vrksasana or Virabhadrasana III, you can guide more stable balance by asking students to bring more awareness to grounding down through the inner heel of their standing leg. At the same time, rooting through all four corners of each foot while cultivating pada bandha gives greater overall balance and stability amid a feeling of more resiliency.

To point or flex? In many asanas we either "point" or "flex" the foot, movements that in anatomy are described respectively as "plantar flexion" and "dorsiflexion." Dorsiflexion creates greater stability in the ankle joint as the wider (anterior) part of the wedge-shaped talus is lodged in the space between the fibula and tibia.

In plantar flexion the narrower part of the talus moves into this space, creating less stability but an easier sense of radiating energy out through the feet.

THE KNEES

Connecting the femur to the tibia, the knees receive considerable stress from above and below, making their stabilizing muscles and especially ligaments among the most frequently strained in physical yoga practices. Athletes, runners, even committed sitting meditators discover that the stress created in the knees from their athletic or spiritual avocation can lead to debilitating injury, especially when lacking the beneficial effects of a balanced, appropriate practice of physical asanas. Even in a balanced yoga practice, the knee still has to handle considerable forces, primarily from bearing weight but also due to twisting forces exerted from above and below (Cole). In more strenuous yoga practices, the knee has to handle very powerful physical forces. Primarily a hinge joint capable of extension and flexion, with minor capacity to rotate when flexed to about ninety degrees, sudden or excessive movement in any of these motions can tear one of the supporting ligaments or cartilage. Understanding and honoring the knees is one of the keys to guiding a sustainable yoga practice. Let's take a closer look at the knee, which is actually two joints:

- the femorotibial joint, which links the femur and tibia;
- the femoropatellar joint, where the patella is situated within the anterior thigh muscle and a groove it slides through on the front of the femur.

The distal femur and proximal tibia are expanded into condyles that increase their weight-bearing capacity and offer larger points of attachment for supporting ligaments. The convex shape of the femoral condyles articulates with the concave tibial condyles. The joint is cushioned by articular cartilage that covers the ends of the tibia and femur as well as the underside of the patella. The medial meniscus and lateral meniscus are C-shaped intra-articular pads made of fibrocartilage that further cushion the joint, functioning as shock absorbers between the bones and preventing the bones from rubbing each other. Tears in the medial meniscus are common in yoga, whether originally injured during an asana or exacerbated in an asana such as Padmasana or others where forced rotation at the hip joint can transfer stress into the knee when the foot is held in place by the floor or another part of the body. With little or no blood supply, they heal slowly—if at all. A set of ligaments, all of which are in the fully stretched position when the knee is extended (leg straight), help to stabilize the knee. When the knee is flexed, the ligaments are softened (shortened), allowing rotation in poses such as Padmasana.

The medial and lateral collateral ligaments (MCL and LCL) run along the sides of the knee and limit sideways motion. The MCL, extending vertically from the femur to the tibia, protects the medial side of the knee from being bent open by force applied to the outside of the knee, such as when a student presses down on the outside of the knee of the back leg in Parsva Dhanurasana. The LCL protects the lateral side from an inside bending force, such as when a student inappropriately places the heel of the right foot against the inside of the left knee in Vrksasana. Both of these ligaments are supported by muscles that run outside them.

1. vastis lateralis
2. vastis intermedius
3. vastis medius
4. patela tendon
5. fibula
6. condyles of the tibia
7. LCL
8. MCL
9. lateral meniscus
10. medial meniscus

The knee joint (anterior view)

Inside the knee joint are two cruciate ligaments. The anterior cruciate ligament, or ACL, connects the tibia to the femur at the center of the knee. Its function is to limit rotation and forward motion of the tibia away from the femur; without it the femur would slide forward off the knee. We will revisit this when looking at a variety of poses, especially lunges such as Warrior I or II, where the ACL is both a crucial source of stability and at considerable risk if the knee is not properly aligned. The posterior cruciate ligament, or PCL, located just behind the ACL, limits excessive hyperextension (backward motion) of the knee joint. Injury to the PCL is rare, especially in yoga, where there are no asanas that place great force on this ligament. The patella ligament is sometimes called the patellar tendon because there is no definite separation between the quadriceps tendon, which surrounds the patella, and the area connecting the patella to the tibia. This very strong ligament helps give the patella its mechanical leverage and functions as a cap for the condyles of the femurs.

The muscles acting on the knee from above—the abductors (primarily the glutei and tensor fascia latae, acting through their attachment to the iliotibial band), adductors (primarily the gracilis), the quadriceps (for extension), the hamstrings (for flexion), and the sartorius (a synergist in flexion and lateral rotation)—help the ligaments to stabilize the knee when contracting from their various origins on the front, back, and bottom of the pelvis. The gluteus and tensor fascia latae attach to the iliotibial band, which in turn attaches to the lateral tibial condyle below the knee, contributing to lateral stability. The medial side of the knee is given more balanced stability through the actions of the gracilis, sartorius, and the semitendinosus (one of the hamstrings) as they pull up and in from their attachments on the medial tibia just below the knee: the gracilis from the pubic ramus at the bottom of the pelvis, the sartorius (the longest muscle in the body) from its origin at the anterior superior iliac spine (ASIS), and the semitendinosus as it runs up the back of the leg to its origins in the ischial tuberosity (most commonly known as the sitting bones). These medial and lateral stabilizers also play a small part in the rotation

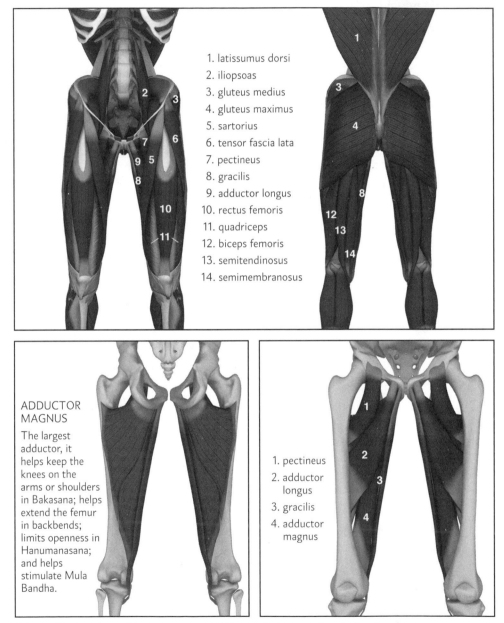

1. latissumus dorsi
2. iliopsoas
3. gluteus medius
4. gluteus maximus
5. sartorius
6. tensor fascia lata
7. pectineus
8. gracilis
9. adductor longus
10. rectus femoris
11. quadriceps
12. biceps femoris
13. semitendinosus
14. semimembranosus

ADDUCTOR MAGNUS

The largest adductor, it helps keep the knees on the arms or shoulders in Bakasana; helps extend the femur in backbends; limits openness in Hanumanasana; and helps stimulate Mula Bandha.

1. pectineus
2. adductor longus
3. gracilis
4. adductor magnus

Primary hip muscles and knee extensors and flexors (anterior and posterior views)

of the tibia on the femur when the knee is flexed and the foot drawn toward the hip in poses such as Vrksasana or Padmasana.

While lending stability to the knee, the quadriceps and hamstrings are the most powerful muscles involved in knee extension and flexion. The most powerful muscle in the body, the quadriceps (so named in Latin for its "four-headed" origins) has just one foot as the four parts combine to form the quadriceps tendon, which extends across the front of the knee to become the patellar tendon and inserts on the proximal edge of the patella, which then transfers their action via the patellar tendon to the tibia. Three of the four—vastus medialis, vastus lateralis, and vastus intermedius—originate from the femoral shaft, while the rectus femoris arises from the top front of the pelvis, giving the rectus femoris a strong role in hip flexion as well as knee extension. This combined action is involved in Utthita Hasta Padangusthasana. Their collective power in knee extension is increased through the fulcrum-like structure of the patella. Their concentric or isometric contraction extends or holds the knee in extension to stretch the hamstrings in a variety of standing and seated poses and contributes to lifting the body through eccentric contraction in backbends such as Setu Bandha Sarvangasana and Urdhva Dhanurasana.

STRETCH REFLEX

Some movements involving voluntary muscle contraction happen automatically as a reflexive response to intended movements or external stimulation. Here the body is acting before you can think about it. When a muscle contracts in response to stretching within the muscle, this is called a stretch reflex. For example, the hamstrings stretch while eccentrically contracting in trying to hold the body against the force of gravity when folding into Uttanasana. In folding forward we ideally relax the hamstrings, allowing them to stretch more easily. But before we know it, the hamstrings are actively engaging to control the weight of the upper body moving forward and down. It is as if the hamstrings want to pull the body back up into its natural anatomical position, fully upright and stable. Stretch reflexes limit the development of flexibility and must be circumvented through countervailing muscular actions in order to cultivate full flexibility. When students move very quickly in and out of asanas, they are likely to trigger stretch reflexes that not only limit flexibility but also increase the risk of straining muscles or tearing ligaments. As we will explore in some detail when discussing how to "play the edge," listening to the body's natural feedback through the breath, heartbeat, and nervous-system messages is the key to moving with ease and stability.

The three-and-a-half hamstrings are the principle flexors of the knee. The semimembranosus and the semitendinosus originate from the ischial tuberosity and run down to the medial side of the knee, giving medial support to the knee as well as assisting in medial rotation. The biceps femoris originates on the back of the ischial tuberosity and the back of the femoral shaft, merging along the way before crossing the lateral side of the knee—contributing to lateral stability—and inserting via a common tendon on the head of the fibula. The partial origin of the biceps femoris (its "short head") on the back of the femoral shaft also leads up to the attachment of the adductor magnus, giving the adductor magnus a "half hamstring" function that, when tight, adds further limitation to wide-angled forward bends such as Upavista Konasana.

THE PELVIS

Mediating between the upper body and the legs, the pelvis is the hub of the body. Cradled within we find our deep abdominal organs and the resting place of the kundalini-shakti energy long ago revered by the ancient yogis. As a principal center of stability and ease, we both originate key movements and cushion the impact of those movements through the bones, muscles, ligaments, and energetic actions emanating from within and around this vital structure. As a strong stabilizing structure, pelvic postural imbalances, traumas, and injuries tend to manifest below in the knees or above in the spine and upper body, although wear and tear in the hip itself can cause debilitating pain that in some cases finds relief only through replacement of the joint. When strong, balanced, and flexible, it lends these same qualities above and below. With around thirty muscles giving support to hip movement and stability, there is much here to work with in nearly every family of asanas.

At the lower front side of the pelvis is the acetabulum, the hip socket that receives the ball of the femoral head in creating the hip joint, joining the thighbones to the pelvis and supporting the weight of the body while allowing mobility through its ball-and-socket structure. It is formed at the intersection of three bones that are fused into one in infancy: the ilium, ischium, and pubis. The articular portions of the acetabulum and the femoral head are covered with cartilage, allowing smooth movement of the femoral head. The outer rim of the acetabulum has a strong fibrocartilaginous ring, the labrum, which increases the depth of the socket and lends to greater stability in the joint. This capsule is reinforced by four ligaments that wind around the head of the femur, twisting and untwisting as we move the femur bone to create stability that also limits the range of motion. In Virabhadrasana 1 and Ashta Chandrasana the tension created by these ligaments, especially the iliofemoral ligament, limits the depth of the lunge and/or causes the pelvis to pitch forward, creating lordosis as well as possibly excessively pressuring the intervertebral disks of the lumbar spine. These same ligaments are also what keep the thigh-

bone from popping out of the hip socket in Virabhadrasana II when the back leg is fully extended and externally rotated. The length and girth of the femoral head and neck vary by individual, giving further limitations to the allowable movement of the femur that shows up in a variety of poses, especially when the femur is fully abducted in poses such as Upavista Kona-

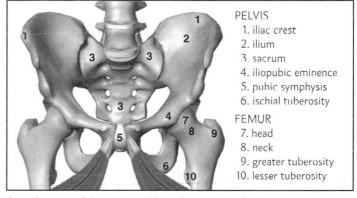

PELVIS
1. iliac crest
2. ilium
3. sacrum
4. iliopubic eminence
5. pubic symphysis
6. ischial tuberosity

FEMUR
7. head
8. neck
9. greater tuberosity
10. lesser tuberosity

Bony features of the pelvis and hips (anterior view)

sana. Women's acetabula are generally wider apart than in men, another factor affecting range of motion and stability. The left and right hips are joined at the pubic symphysis by a fibrocartilage disk and to the sacrum by the sacroiliac joint.

The hips gain further stability in supporting the weight of the body plus precision mobility through a complex set of muscles running in every direction. Six deep lateral rotators with various origins inside the pelvis insert on different parts of the greater trochanter of the femoral head, creating several refined movements of the femur: piriformis and quadratus femoris create lateral rotation when the sacrum is fixed and the thigh is extended, or cause adduction when the thigh is

flexed (as in Vrksasana); obturator internus and externus along with gemellus superior and inferior give more refined lateral rotation movements depending on the position of the femur. The muscles you feel being stretched in Upavista Konasana and Baddha Konasana are primarily the five hip adductors: adductor magnus, the largest and strongest of the adductor group; adductor longus and adductor brevis, which extend from the medial pubis to the linea aspera; pectineus, running from the lateral pubis to a line connecting the lesser trochanter to the linea aspera; and gracilis, a long, thin muscle running from the medial pubis to the tibia just below the medial condyle. The strength of the adductors is crucial in

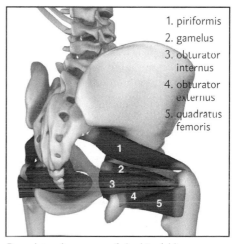

1. piriformis
2. gamelus
3. obturator internus
4. obturator externus
5. quadratus femoris

Deep lateral rotators of the hip (oblique anterior view)

a variety of poses, from arm balances such as Bakasana to Salamba Sirsasana, where their ability to draw energy to the medial line of the body is essential.

The psoas, as Mabel Todd expresses in *The Thinking Body* (1937), is the most important muscle in determining upright posture. Arising from the vertebral bodies of T12 through L5, its fibers run downward through the anterior pelvis, where they join in a common tendon with the iliacus muscle, which arises from inside the ilium. The iliopsoas then reaches down to the lesser trochanter of the femoral head, creating the prime flexor of the hip joint—you feel it in Navasana—and one of the prime limiters in hip extension asanas such as backbends and lunges like Anjaneyasana. When the femur is fixed, as when sitting in Dandasana, the psoas and iliacus create different movements (lumbar flexion and hip adduction plus anterior pelvic rotation, respectively). In creating lumbar flexion, the psoas acts on the SI joint relatively independently of the position of the hips (Myers 1998, 82). When short and tight, it causes potentially severe lumbar lordosis and compression of the intervertebral disks in the lower back. When weak it can contribute to a flat back. As we will see later, the iliopsoas also plays an important role in deep core stability as well as the integrity of breath and movement in the upper body, in part due to its shared connection at T12 with the crura of the diaphragm and the lower fibers of the trapezius.

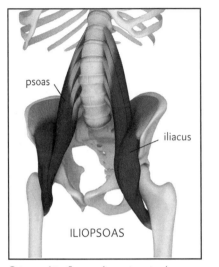

Primary hip flexors (anterior view)

The pyramid-shaped piriformis muscle originates on the anterior sacrum, passes under the sciatic notch (inflammation can cause painful pressure on the sciatic nerve) and inserts on the top of the greater trochanter. With the sacrum fixed, the piriformis laterally rotates the extended leg or abducts the flexed thigh, helping open the hips in poses such as Padmasana. If the femur is fixed, its contraction tilts the pelvis back, opposing the action of the psoas and creating more balanced stability and movement in the sacroiliac joint.

Earlier we looked at the role of the hamstrings and gluteus muscles in relationship to the knee; they also bear significantly on the pelvis, primarily as extensors. Contraction of the hamstrings brings the pelvis into a posterior tilt when the femurs are fixed, or bring the legs into extension when the pelvis is fixed. Tight hamstrings limit forward bending by bringing the sitting bones (the ischial tuberosities, where the hamstrings originate) closer to the back of the knees in poses such as Uttanasana or Paschimottanasana. Weak hamstrings contribute to lumbar lordosis when the hip flexors are tight.

The largest muscle in the body, gluteus maximus is both a hip extensor and a lateral rotator, creating different movements depending on which of its fibers are activated. Its upper fibers are lateral rotators, helping open the hips out in poses such as Virabhadrasana II. Its lower fibers act as prime movers in hip extension, along with the hamstrings, assisting the movement into backbends such as Salabhasana or Urdhva Dhanurasana, where we want to rotate the femurs internally as a means of softening pressure on the SI joint. Typically students will squeeze the entire gluteus maximus in backbends as they create hip extension, thereby creating the unintended effect of internally rotating the thighs—which, as a teacher, you will see plainly as the student's feet turn out in poses such as Setu Bandha Sarvangasana. With insertions on the iliotibial tract, gluteus maximus is an important stabilizer of the hip in standing poses. The lesser-known gluteus medius is one of the primary stabilizing muscles in one-legged standing poses such as Vrksasana and Ardha Chandrasana. As an abductor it is also the prime mover in abduction of the hip into Ardha Chandrasana. Even lesser-known gluteus minimus, a small muscle laying superficial to gluteus medius, assists gluteus medius in abduction of the hip and also assists in hip flexion and medial rotation.

THE ABDOMINAL CORE

We can usefully begin our exploration of the abdominal core by considering the belly button. The umbilicus is an important landmark on the abdomen in part because its position is relatively uniform among people, the motionless center of human gravity as represented in Leonardo da Vinci's *Vitruvian Man*. Perhaps even more important is the psychophysiology of this center of the belly, the portal of nutrition and development in the nine months of our embryonic life. Throughout life it is a potent well of emotion and for many a focus of obsessive attention and sculpting connected to feelings or projections of sexuality and power. It is also the home of the manipura chakra, the subtle energetic source of willfulness in the world.

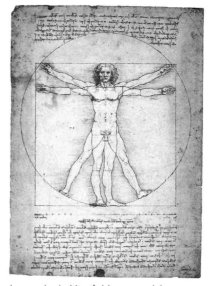

Leonardo da Vinci's Vitruvian Man

Looking more deeply, we find the vital abdominal organs: liver, spleen, pancreas, stomach, large and small intestines, gallbladder, and appendix. Four abdominal muscle groups combine to completely cover these organs: rectus abdominus, transverse abdominus, internal oblique, and external oblique. Looking inferiorly into the bowl of the pelvis, we find the reproductive organs and a supporting structure of muscles and ligaments that are the physical source of mula bandha and uddiyana bandha, two of the essential energy locks first described hundreds of years ago in the earliest writings on Hatha yoga. Superiorly we have the diaphragm, the principal respiratory muscle. Long erector spinae muscles at the back of the torso lie parallel to the vertebral column, and deep to these muscles the multifidi lie in the gutter next to the spinous processes. Psoas, iliacus, piriformis, and quadratus lumborum also play vital roles in the body's core. When in balance this group of muscles supports standing with stability and ease, allows full and safe range of motion in the lumbar spine, supports the internal organs without compressing them, and allows the breath to flow strongly and freely.

Transverse abdominus (TA) is the deepest of the four main abdominal muscles. Its fascia wrap all the way around the waist to attach to the transverse processes of the lumbar vertebrae, while in front it is joined by a fascial sheet at the linea alba, thus giving its horizontal fibers a girdling effect as if a single muscle. It attaches below to the inguinal ligament, running from the iliac crest to the pubic tubercle. When you laugh until your belly aches, you are feeling your TA. It is also the muscular focus of kapalabhati pranayama, discussed in Chapter Eight. When properly toned, this muscle keeps your organs in place while giving support to the lumbar spine. When habitually gripped, it compresses the organs and lends to abdominal hernias, urinary incontinence, and digestive problems.

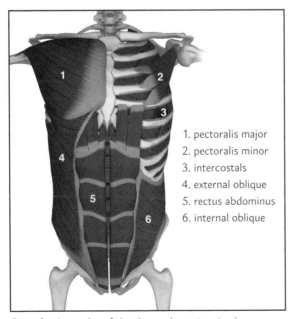

1. pectoralis major
2. pectoralis minor
3. intercostals
4. external oblique
5. rectus abdominus
6. internal oblique

Superficial muscles of the thorax (anterior view)

The internal and external oblique muscles (IO and EO, respectively) rotate the ribcage on the pelvis or the pelvis under the ribcage. The IOs are just outside the TA, with most fibers running anteriorly and superiorly from the lower ribs to the hips. When contracted together (right and left sides) the IOs flex the spine and compress the belly. Contracting one side causes side-bending such as Parivrtta Janu Sirsasana and assists the opposite-side EO in rotation of the lower trunk to the same side as the contracted IO. The EOs run anteriorly and inferiorly from the outer surfaces of ribs 5–12, superficial and roughly perpendicular to the IOs, with fibers heading to the linea alba, inguinal ligament, or the pubic bone. Contracting both sides compresses the abdomen and flexes the trunk, while contracting one side causes either lateral flexion or twisting.

The most superficial abdominal muscle is the rectus abdominus (RA). Attached to the pubic symphysis and xiphoid process and located inside a sheath formed by the TA, IO, and EO, RA contracts to shorten the distance between these attachment points, pulling equally on both ends to flex the spine. When highly toned, its transverse grooves at three tendinous intersections create what is popularly called "six-pack abs" (actually a four-pack). Overemphasis on strengthening this muscle makes it hypertonic, overwhelming other muscles as it pulls the ribs closer to the pubic bone, pulling the ribs out of shape, restricting the breath, and lending to kyphosis and neck problems. As RA travels down to the public bone, it becomes less superficial—anatomically as well as functionally for the bandhas. A few inches below the belly button, the obliques and TA all pass in front of the RA, with the RA suddenly becoming the deepest abdominal muscle and one that plays an important role in uddiyana bandha. In looking at the

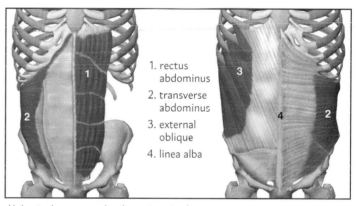

1. rectus abdominus
2. transverse abdominus
3. external oblique
4. linea alba

Abdominal core muscles (anterior view)

anatomy and actions of uddiyana bandha, we must first return to the feet and the deep pelvis to explore the relationship between actions lower in the body and in the abdominal core.

THE SPINE

The spine is at the center of yoga. In the traditional yogic literature we find it as the sushumna channel, carrying life-force pranic energy up through the subtle body. Its relative stability, mobility, and overall functioning are among the primary sources motivating people to try yoga initially. More than any other part of the skeleton, the spine is directly involved in every asana. Weakness in support for the spinal column is a leading source of distraction in sitting meditation. With greater and more stable range of motion in the spine we experience more ease and sensory awakening throughout the entire body. "At its essence the spine is really a system of skeletal, neurological, electrical, vascular, and chemical input that when balanced and

MULA BANDHA AND UDDIYANA BANDHA

Earlier we looked at the cultivation of pada bandha, the energetic awakening of the feet through the stirrup-like effect of contracting the tibialis posterior and peroneus longus muscles on the lower leg. The fascial attachments of these two muscles interweave with those of the hip adductors, which have origins in and around the ischial tuberosities (the sitting bones). The sitting bones are the lateral aspects of the perineum, with the pubic symphysis at the front and the coccyx at the back. The front half of this diamond is the urogenital triangle, a landmark for the urogenital diaphragm, a hammock-like layer that is created by three sets of muscles: transverse perineal (connecting the two sitting bones), bulbospongiosus (surrounding the vagina or bulb of the penis), and ischiocavernosus (connecting the ischium to the clitoris or covering the penile crura) (Aldous 2004, 41). Contracting this set of muscles awakens the levator ani muscle, another hammock-like layer composed of the coccygeus, iliococcygeus, and the pubococcygeus muscles. When these muscles contract, they pull the entire pelvic floor up and naturally stimulate the awakening of core abdominal muscles with attachments at the pubis (including the TA and RA). This is the muscular action of mula bandha, which creates a feeling of grounded levity in the asana practice, supports the pelvis organs, creates an upward movement of energy, and stimulates uddiyana bandha. With practice, mula bandha can be accessed directly (i.e., independently of pada bandha) and steadily maintained throughout asana practice.

Uddiyana bandha is among the most misunderstood aspects of practice, owing in part to very different definitions and instructions from different traditions and teachers. In its basic form, uddiyana bandha involves pulling the entire abdominal region strongly back toward the spine and then up toward the breastbone when completely empty of breath. Its engagement is part of specific pranayama and kriya practices, not asana practice, yet many teachers instruct students to engage it while doing asanas. In asana practice we want the breath to flow smoothly, continuously, and fully, which requires the full, natural functioning of the diaphragm. However, uddiyana bandha prevents the diaphragm from expanding naturally, thus severely restricting the inhalation of breath.

The confusion about uddiyana bandha arises from a very different breath-related muscular action in the lower abdomen that we do want to cultivate in asana practice. With each and every complete exhale the major abdominal muscles naturally contract (primarily the TAs but also the obliques and the RA). When this occurs along with mula bandha,

the very light, subtle engagement of these abdominal muscles can accentuate, deepen, and give more stability and ease to the body in many
(but not all) asanas and asana transitions. Indeed, in some asanas we
want the belly to be quite relaxed in order for the spine, pelvis, and
breath to move appropriately for those asanas. We can refer to this as
"uddiyana bandha light" to distinguish it from the full form of uddiyana
bandha done in pranayama.

Mula bandha and uddiyana bandha are tools that can be variously
engaged to support different energetic actions in the practice. In no situation do we want to grip the belly as in full uddiyana bandha, which
restricts the breath in asana practice. Nor do we want to create tightness in the pelvic floor. Rather, mula bandha and uddiyana bandha are
best cultivated as light and steady energetic lifting actions that draw energy up and into the core of the body while allowing that energy to radiate out and fuel the practice. The balance of these qualities comes with
practice, and with time is increasingly subtle yet pervasive in its effects.

connected," Susi Hately Aldous (2004, 30) enthuses, "creates magically fluid movement, much the same way a well-balanced and connected orchestra creates awe-
inspiring music." When unbalanced due to overdeveloped or weak muscles,
repetitive stress, organic tension, or emotional gripping, we begin to see a variety
of problems: lordosis, kyphosis, bulging or herniated disks, and other painful conditions that compromise the delicate balance, stability, and mobility of the spine.

A column of thirty-three vertebrae, the spine curves up from the coccyx to
the base of the skull. Viewed laterally, the vertebral column presents four curves
corresponding to different regions of the spine: sacral/coccygeal, lumbar, thoracic,
and cervical. The sacral/coccygeal curve consists of four separate coccygeal vertebrae and five fused sacral vertebrae, the latter forming the sacrum. Twenty-three
intervertebral articulations allow it to bend and rotate in a variety of directions
while its central column protects the delicate spinal cord that branches off into
nerves sending and receiving information to and from most of the body. Viewed
from the back, the spine looks like two pyramids, one short and inverted at the bottom (the coccyx and sacrum), the other tall and increasingly slender with each successively higher vertebra in the lumbar, thoracic, and cervical segments. This
pyramid-like structure gives the spine its inherent structural stability.

The vertebrae in each segment are numbered from top to bottom: C1–C7 (cervical spine), T1–T12 (thoracic spine), L1–L5 (lumbar spine), and S1–S5 (sacral spine).
The vertebrae in each segment of the spine have certain unique distinguishing features, starting at the bottom with the sacrococcygeal segment. Four vertebral

remnants at the tail of the spine make up the coccyx, commonly referred to as the tailbone. Although most anatomy texts describe the bony segments as fused (and indeed sometimes they are ossified), a number of studies show that a normal coccyx has two or three movable parts that gently curve forward and slightly flex if we slump back in poses such as Dandasana or Navasana. It provides an attachment for nine muscles, including the gluteus maximus and the levator ani. The top of the coccyx articulates with the sacrum (from the Latin *sacer,* meaning "sacred"), a large inverted triangular set of five usually fused vertebrae wedged between the hip bones (the ilia) to complete the pelvic ring. The bodies of the first and second sacral ver-

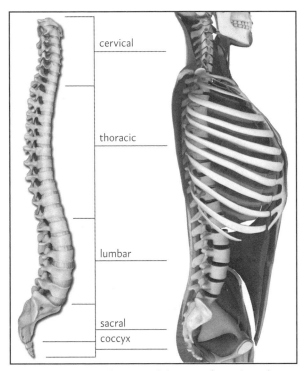

Segments and natural curves of the spine (lateral view)

tebrae may not be fused. In most people the sacroiliac points are tightly bound and immobile, although some have the ability to rotate the sacrum a few degrees forward or back (nutation and counternutation, respectively). In women the sacrum is shorter, wider, and presents a slightly different curvature and tilt than in men.

The fifth lumbar vertebra rests on the slanted top of the sacrum, creating natural shear forces in the lower lumbar spine that are ideally balanced by muscles and ligaments in the lower back and abdominal areas. The lumbar vertebrae are the largest and strongest of the movable vertebrae, bearing more body weight than their vertebral siblings above as well as having the most flexibility, a dual role that makes this segment the most susceptible to injury and strain. The spinal cord comes to an end between L1–L2, splitting off into nerve roots that exit between each of the lumbar vertebrae and gather together lower down to form the sciatic nerve. Compressed or herniated intervertebral disks in the lumbar spine, often caused by an excessive lordotic curve (remember that tight psoas muscle?), can affect these nerve roots and contribute to sciatica, which is experienced as pain radiating down the back of each leg into the feet.

The twelve thoracic vertebrae are unique in articulating with the twelve pairs of ribs. Increasing in width from T12 up to T1, they are distinguished by facets on the sides of their bodies for articulation with the heads of the ribs and by facets on the transverse processes of all but T11 and T12 for articulation with the tubercles of the ribs. T1 closely resembles the wide cervical vertebrae resting above while T11 and T12 approximate the size and shape of the lumbar vertebrae.

The cervical vertebrae are the smallest true vertebrae and can be most readily distinguished from thoracic and lumbar vertebrae by a hole in each transverse process through which the vertebral artery passes. C1, called the atlas, rotates left and right on top of C2, called the axis, giving the cervical spine most of its rotational capacity. C3–C6 are similar to one another, all small and broader from side to side than front to back. C7, called vertebra prominens, is unique in its longer and more prominent spinous process.

Intervertebral disks cushion each vertebra, forming a joint that allows slight movement of the vertebrae while keeping them separated. The disk is formed by a ring called the annulus fibrosus, formed by layer upon layer of fibrocartilage, each layer running in a different direction. This ring surrounds the inner nucleus pulposus, a gel-like substance that absorbs impact in the spine. The intervertebral disks allow the spinal column to be flexible while absorbing shock from walking, running, and other physical activities. In deep forward bending (flexion) of the spine, the front of the disk compresses and pushes the nucleus back as the posterior side of the disk expands; just the opposite happens in extension (backbending), while in side-bending poses such as Parighasana (Gate Pose) the nucleus moves to the opposite side. Injury and aging can cause the expanding side of the disk to bulge and possibly herniate. This most commonly occurs in the posterior part of the disk, precisely where major spinal nerves extend out to different tissues and extremities. While the herniation tends to happen more commonly in forward-bending asanas, the associated pain is more likely felt when standing or in backbending.

Along with the malleable intervertebral disks, a complex and finely integrated system of ligaments and muscles bring further stability and mobility to the spine. Three ligaments extend the entire length of the vertebral column: the anterior and posterior longitudinal ligaments and the supraspinous ligament. In spinal flexion (think of folding forward) the posterior longitudinal ligaments absorb some of the pressure from the disk nucleus pressing back, although with excessive pressure, bulging occurs just to the outsides of the ligament (laterally). The anterior and posterior longitudinal ligaments limit extension and flexion, respectively. Other vertebral ligaments connect adjacent vertebrae. All create stability while limiting the degree of rotation, flexion, extension, and lateral flexion.

The two psoas and two posterior transversospinal muscles form four muscular bundles arranged around the lumbar spine that can contract together to create balanced lengthening in the lower back. Some have suggested that the upper and lower segments of the psoas lend to this balance because the lower fibers pull L5 and L4 anteriorly into lumbar hyperextension while the upper psoas fibers pull T12 and L1 toward the groin in lumbar flexion.[1] But the psoas as a whole pulls the lower lumbar vertebrae forward, bringing the sacrum along in tilting the pelvis forward. Recalling that the psoas is a powerful hip flexor (bringing the knee toward the chest), we can appreciate how hypertension in this powerful muscle not only potentially compresses the lumbar disks but creates a major limitation in all backbending asanas. Also note that when the psoas on one side contracts alone, this creates side-bending or rotation of the spine. If it is relatively more tense on one side, then a variety of asymmetries arise that cause imbalance or strain in the SI joint and up through the spine, many of which we can easily observe when a student is standing in Tadasana or inverted in Salamba Sirsasana I. A strong yet supple and balanced psoas is thus one of the most important sources of overall stability and mobility in the spine and the body as a whole. Asanas such as Anjaneyasana, Virabhadrasana I, and Supta Virasana stretch the psoas, while Navasana and Utthita Hasta Padangusthasana strengthen it. A close neighbor of the psoas, quadratus lumborum originates from the posterior iliac crest and inserts on the transverse processes of L1–L5 and rib 12. With ipsilateral contraction (or hypertonicity on one side) it draws the pelvis and ribs on one side closer together; with bilateral contraction it creates spinal extension that is opposed by the psoas and abdominal muscles.

Several layers of deep muscles run up along the posterior spine, some connecting one transverse process to the next (intertransverse muscles), some connecting spinous processes (interspinales), some connecting transverse processes to spinous processes (transversospinales). At the neck a set of muscles very similar to the transversospinales, the rectus capitis and oblique capitis, connect the spine to the lower rear part of the skull at the occiput. Depending on how these muscles are contracted, they can assist in extension, side-bending, and rotation of the spine. Superficial to the deep muscles of the spine are a set of erector spinae muscles and associated tendons that lie in the groove along the sides of the spinal column. In the lumbar region they arise from the thick, fleshy, tendinous mass of the lumbar aponeurosis, then split into three parallel columns of muscle rising along the spine. The primary action of these muscles is extension of the spine in poses such as Salabhasana and Pursvottanasana. In flexion these muscles control rather than produce movements, then they fall silent while being stretched in full forward-bending poses such as Paschimottanasana or Uttanasana. In twists and side bends, they are active on both sides in both producing and controlling movement. With each muscle crossing several segments of the spine, their contraction or relaxation has an effect in multiple vertebrae. They are most fully contracted and strengthened in prone backbends such as Salabhasana.

At the neck the erector spinae muscles are complemented by several other muscles that stabilize and mobilize the head on top of the spine like guy-wires, including the splenius capitis, levator scapulae, longus colli, rectus capitis, scalenes,

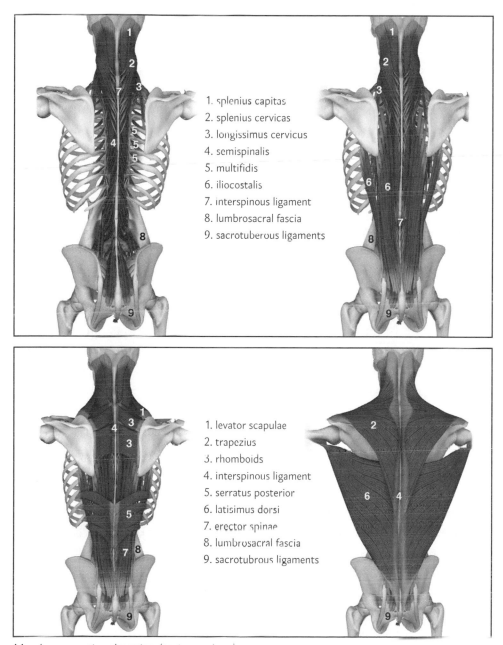

1. splenius capitas
2. splenius cervicas
3. longissimus cervicus
4. semispinalis
5. multifidis
6. iliocostalis
7. interspinous ligament
8. lumbrosacral fascia
9. sacrotuberous ligaments

1. levator scapulae
2. trapezius
3. rhomboids
4. interspinous ligament
5. serratus posterior
6. latisimus dorsi
7. erector spinae
8. lumbrosacral fascia
9. sacrotubrous ligaments

Muscles supporting the spine (posterior views)

sternocleidomastoids (SCMs), and the upper fibers of the trapezius. Here we find a fascinating world of nerves, muscles, and movements that for many yoga students is a common area of tension and strain. Typically overworked due to postural imbalances elsewhere in the body (and often excessively recruited in breathing), "pain in the neck" is very easily caused in some of the simplest asanas.

Three other muscles of the back—the latissimi dorsi, rhomboids, and trapezius—are discussed in detail in below. For now we will summarize how they act on the back. The latissimi dorsi are the most expansive muscles in the body, covering almost the entire back and giving greater structural integrity to the trunk as a whole. The rhomboids draw the vertebrae toward the scapulae or release to allow easier movement into shoulder flexion backbends such as Urdhva Dhanurasana. The trapezius, with fibers running in three directions, can produce spinal extension as well as side bending.

THE SHOULDERS, ARMS, AND HANDS

Much of human life and consciousness is predicated on our ability not just to erect elaborate structures or actions in our complex mind, but also on our ability to fashion those ideas into material reality in the world. In this creative expression we largely depend on the manipulative abilities of our arms and hands, the relatively free movement of which rests on the mobility of our shoulders. While it is the most mobile joint in the human body, it must also be strong enough to allow us to lift, push, pull, twist, and move with or against force in multiple directions. Indeed, human consciousness itself and the very fabric of human thought is inextricably intertwined with this uniquely human ability to engage creatively with the physical world in often fine and elaborate ways allowed by the shoulder, arms, and hands. The humble shoulders, where we carry much of our responsibility, or sometimes a chip (and where the Hindu god Shiva carries a resting cobra), determine much about our posture and movement in the world, on and off the mat.

Anatomically, the shoulder is not a joint but a complex structure comprising three bones—the humerus (upper arm bone), clavicle (collarbone), and scapula (shoulder blade)—tied together by muscles, tendons, and ligaments. The articulations among the three bones give us the three joints of the shoulder: glenohumeral, acromioclavicular, and sternoclavicular. Working together they give the arms tremendous range of motion and stability, a balancing act that when off-kilter creates a variety of problems largely unique to this part of the body.

The glenohumeral joint is the primary joint of the shoulder, where the head of the humerus rests in the glenoid fossa of the scapula, much like a golf ball on a tee. A ball-and-socket joint that allows the arm to rotate circularly or hinge out away from the body, four muscles form a "rotator cuff" around the humeral head to keep it secured to the glenoid fossa: supraspinatus, infraspinatus, subscapularis, and teres minor, often referred to as SITS. The tendons of these muscles connect to the capsule of the glenohumeral joint, lending it further stability. Still, the shallowness of the glenoid fossa makes this one of the most commonly dislocated joints in the body, and inappropriate hands-on adjustments in poses such as Urdhva Dhanurasana have been known to cause this joint to dislocate. The smooth movement of the upper arm bone in the glenoid fossa depends on the balanced strength, flexibility, and neurological functioning of the rotator cuff muscles along with the soft tissue capsule that encircles the joint and attaches to the scapula, humerus, and the head of the biceps. Lined by a thin synovial membrane, the capsule is strengthened by the coracoclavicular ligament.

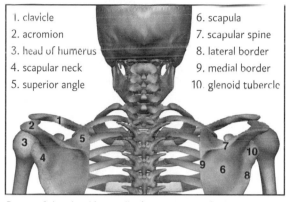

1. clavicle	6. scapula
2. acromion	7. scapular spine
3. head of humerus	8. lateral border
4. scapular neck	9. medial border
5. superior angle	10. glenoid tubercle

Bones of the shoulder girdle (posterior view)

The acromioclavicular joint is at the top of the shoulder, located between the acromion process of the scapula and the distal end of the clavicle, and is stabilized by three ligaments: the acromioclavicular ligament attaches the clavicle to the

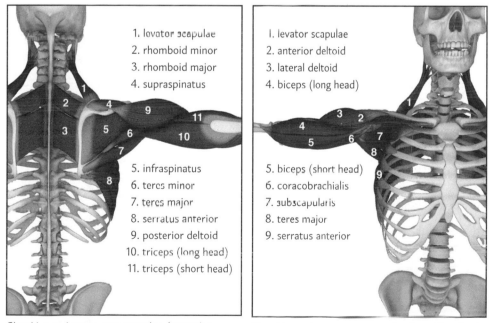

1. levator scapulae
2. rhomboid minor
3. rhomboid major
4. supraspinatus

5. infraspinatus
6. teres minor
7. teres major
8. serratus anterior
9. posterior deltoid
10. triceps (long head)
11. triceps (short head)

1. levator scapulae
2. anterior deltoid
3. lateral deltoid
4. biceps (long head)

5. biceps (short head)
6. coracobrachialis
7. subscapularis
8. teres major
9. serratus anterior

Shoulder and upper arm muscles (posterior view)

Shoulder and upper arm muscles (anterior view)

acromion of the scapula; the coracoacromial ligament runs from the coracoid process to the acromion; and the coracoclavicular ligament runs from the scapula to the clavicle. The movement of this gliding synovial joint allows the arm to rise above the head, helping the movement of the scapula and giving the arm greater rotation for asanas such as Urdhva Hastasana and Adho Mukha Svanasana. At the medial end of the clavicle is the sternoclavicular joint, where the convex shape of the manubrium interfaces with the rounded end of the clavicle. The scapula is a flat and roughly triangular-shaped bone placed on the back of the rib cage, forming the posterior part of the shoulder girdle. The relatively thicker lateral border of the scapula contains the glenoid fossa, home to the upper arm bone's proximal end. The various physical features of the scapula allow the attachment of seventeen muscles that give this bone its stability and six basic movements that allow greater range of motion of the arm:

TABLE 4.1—**Movements of the Scapula**

MOVEMENTS	MUSCLES	EXAMPLES OF ASANAS
Elevation	Upper trapezius	Adho Mukha Vrksasana
	Rhomboids	Adho Mukha Svanasana
	Levator scapulae	Adho Mukha Svanasana
Depression	Lower trapezius	Virabhadrasana II
	Serratus anterior	Anjali mudra
Adduction	Rhomboids	Gomukhasana
	Mid-trapezius	Phalakasana
Abduction	Serratus anterior	Adho Mukha Svanasana
		Chaturanga Dandasana
Upward rotation	Upper trapezius	Urdhva Hastasana
	Serratus anterior	Adho Mukha Svanasana
Downward rotation	Rhomboids	Tolasana
	Levator scapulae	Bakasana

Muscles that attach the humerus to other parts of the shoulder create movement of the upper arm bone. The infraspinatus muscle, assisted by the teres minor, externally rotates the arm, as when standing in Tadasana and turning the palms out or when wrapping the triceps side of the arm toward the ear in Utthita Parsvakonasana. The subscapularis adducts and rotates the arm medially, a rare movement in Hatha yoga (there is some internal rotation in Parsvottanasana). The supraspinatus abducts the arm, as when bringing the arms out and up into Virabhadrasana II. Again, these four muscles work collectively as the rotator cuff to stabilize the glenohumeral joint, keeping the humeral head in the glenoid cavity.

EXTERNAL AND INTERNAL ROTATION

Imagine standing in Tadasana and rotating your arm bones to turn your thumbs in and back. This is internal rotation. Now try to maintain strong internal rotation, keep your shoulder blades depressed, and try to extend your arms out and up (in abduction) all the way overhead into Urdhva Hastasana. Unless you are extremely hypermobile in your shoulders, you are unable to lift your arms higher than your shoulders. Now externally rotate your arms and repeat the movement, noticing that your arms now easily move overhead into full flexion relatively free of constraint. Yet with your arms overhead the external rotation action appears to be just the opposite. This is a common source of confusion in asanas such as Utthita Parsvakonasana. Once in the asana, the verbal cue to "externally rotate the upper arm" often results in students doing just the opposite, consequently jamming their humerus into their acromion process, which is not funny. That is why it is helpful to instruct students to extend their upper arm down toward their hip, externally rotate the arm while positioned there, and then maintain that rotation while bringing their arm overhead. Now Utthita Parsvakonasana makes more sense.

Two bones form the elbow joint: the distal humerus of the upper arm and the proximal ulna of the forearm. A second forearm bone, the radius, articulates proximally with the radial notch of the ulna and distally with the carpal bones of the wrist. The forearm can move in (1) flexion and extension (through hinge-like movement at the articulation between the humerus and ulna), and (2) pronation or supination, as when turning the palm alternately face up or face down while the humerus is fixed. The simple hinge joint of the elbow is made more complex by the articulation of the ulna and radius and the way these three bones share synovial cavities and ligaments. Like the knee joint (also a hinge joint), the elbow is very prone to hyperextension, a cause of misalignment and injury especially in weight bearing arm support asanas.[2]

Flexion and extension of the elbow joint arises from contraction of muscles from above: biceps, brachialis, and brachioradialis create flexion, while the triceps is the primary extensor. In pronation and supination movements, the ulna and radius cross over each other to rotate the palm up and down. The pronator teres and pronator quadratus muscles are the primary pronators (assisted by brachioradialis from a supinated position) while the biceps and supinators create supination. The difficulty of pronation is evident when attempting to keep the palms fully rooted down in Pincha Mayurasana, which is more challenging when the biceps muscles are tight.

Human evolution is largely due to our ability to hold and manipulate objects, an ability crucially afforded by our opposable thumb. Along with qualities of spirit, verbal cues, and demonstration of asanas, the hand is perhaps our most important teaching tool, enabling us to communicate with tactile precision, subtlety, and sensitivity. In asana practice, it provides one of the most important foundational anchors, included in all the arm balances, many backbends, even leveraged hip openers, twists, and forward bends. Given considerable mobility by the wrist joint, this precious tool is also one of the most vulnerable parts of the human body, and the wrist one of the most commonly injured in asana practice.

The hand consists of five metacarpal and fourteen phalange bones linked by ligaments and surrounded by muscles, nerves, vessels, fascia, and skin. The wrist consists of eight small carpal bones, two of which articulate with the distal radius bone and four with the metatarsal, all essentially wrapped by transverse ligaments. The arch-like structure of the wrist bones creates a central compartment containing flexor tendons, their sheaths, and fascia that support the positioning of the tendons. Movements of the wrist joint are seen in the hand: flexion draws the hand toward the inner forearm (which tends to elongate the fingers), extension draws the hand toward the top of the wrist (causing the fingers to tend to tighten, as in the tendency for the fingers

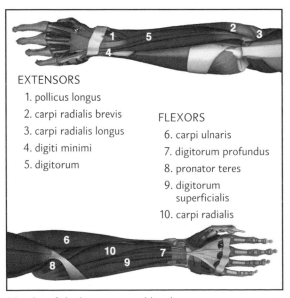

EXTENSORS
1. pollicus longus
2. carpi radialis brevis
3. carpi radialis longus
4. digiti minimi
5. digitorum

FLEXORS
6. carpi ulnaris
7. digitorum profundus
8. pronator teres
9. digitorum superficialis
10. carpi radialis

Muscles of the lower arm and hand

and knuckles to rise from the floor in Adho Mukha Svanasana), abduction turns the thumb out when the palm is turned up, and adduction the opposite. The thumb has considerable mobility in extension, flexion, abduction, and adduction.

The primary muscles acting on the wrist and hand originate along the forearm bones (radius and ulna), with long tendons inserting on the more distal bones of the wrist, metatarsals, and phalanges. Several small muscles intrinsic to the hand (four dorsal, three palmar) originate on the metatarsals or flexor tendons and insert on the phalanges, allowing flexion and extension of the palm and fingers. Several other small muscles cross over from the base of one finger to the first joint of the neighboring finger, allowing the fingers to abduct and adduct. Especially notable among these for our purposes are the thenar muscles, which move the thumb and its metacarpal; while we want to spread the fingers wide in cultivating *hasta bandha* in asanas such as Adho Mukha Svanasana and Adho Mukha Vrksasana, abducting the thumb out as wide as possible easily strains the thenar muscles and possibly the palmar branch of the median nerve.

ANATOMY IN TEACHING

Most anatomy books describe the structure of the body observed in most people. Teachers are often frustrated because students in their classes do not neatly conform to the illustrations or texts they have studied. Skeletal structure will differ due to the varying shape, length, and thickness of bones. There is variation in the size, shape, and attachment of muscles and tendons. There are differences between men and women, different age groups, as well as differences arising from congenital anomalies. Rather than ignoring variations and trying to produce conformity to a standardized structure, it is important to maintain a sense of open-minded curiosity and a spirit of exploration and learning when you encounter students whose anatomy differs from textbook depictions.

Furthermore, the body never functions as the set of isolated parts depicted in most anatomical discussions. It is always a whole, even if it might not feel that way. What is happening in our feet affects what is happening in our spine no less than what is happening in between our ears affects sensation in our bodies. As we continue to weave together the fabric of the human physical body using technical concepts and terms, bear in mind that if that is all you do as a teacher, your classes will tend toward technical tedium that misses the deeper spirit of the practice. Still, detailed technical instruction is important. Giving it with softness and clarity depends on learning how the body works, including the functional anatomy, biomechanics, and kinesiology of any asana or sequence of asanas. Using your broader palette of knowledge and insights in yoga, you can convey this information to your students as part of a narrative overlay to your classes that weaves other elements into the fabric of your teaching.

CHAPTER FIVE

CREATING SPACE FOR SELF-TRANSFORMATION

What if our religion was each other,
if our practice was our life, if prayer our words?
What if the temple was the earth, if forests were our
church, if holy waters—the rivers, lakes, and oceans.
What if meditation was our relationships,
if the teacher was life, if wisdom was self-knowledge,
if love was the center of our being?
—*Ganga White*

The early Hatha yogis discovered that awakening and moving energy in the body gave them a feeling of radiant well-being and wholeness while opening wide the portals of conscious being. But the pathway of yoga—to yoke, to make whole—may not reveal itself automatically. Indeed, our tendency as human beings is to separate the body, breath, and mind, a disconnection that creates suffering as we become alienated from our essential nature as whole beings.[1] This alienation is expressed in everything from stress and confusion to disease and despair. Hatha yoga offers an array of tools for unraveling the knots that bind us to this limited sense of self. "The transformation that yoga brings makes you more yourself," Joel Kramer (1980) intones, "and opens you up to loving with greater depth. It involves a honing and refining which releases your true essence, as a sculptor brings out the beauty of form in the stone by slowly and carefully chipping away the rest."

The primary roles of a yoga teacher are showing students a yogic pathway and offering them guidance along that path. Doing this with inspiration, knowledge, skill, patience, compassion, and creativity defines a good teacher. The many elements of teaching—creating a safe space for self-exploration, crafting sequences of asanas and pranayama practices that take students on physical and energetic journeys, cueing students in their process of refinement, offering practical guid-

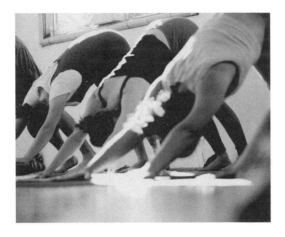

ance in meditation, offering examples for extending the practice off the mat—collectively lead to the same thing: yoga as a process for awakening to the truth of one's being, to an abiding sense of equanimity amid the shifting tides of daily experience and the seasons of one's life. If yoga were a practice of attainment in which we were all aiming for a certain goal, the role of the teacher would be much simpler. We would tell students what to do and how to do it. We would draw from our knowledge of yoga philosophy, energetics, anatomy, and psychol-

ogy to craft classes and instructions that correctly orient students in moving toward the goal. In the physical practice, instruction would focus on the perfection poses; in pranayama we would teach the perfection of breath and energetic balance; in meditation we would teach students to still the mind. But yoga is not a practice of attainment; it is an unending *process of self-discovery and self-transformation.* In this process, teachers are facilitators and guides who offer insightful encouragement along each student's unique path as it evolves, breath by breath.

All one really needs to practice yoga is intention. This is the most basic quality of the practice and the starting point of teaching. When a teacher has clarity of purpose, all the other qualities of teaching become clearer and more aligned. So the first question to ask one's self is, Why do I want to teach? For many teachers, the core intention is simple: to create a space where students feel safe and supported in their practice. Below are the tools for creating that space.

THE PHYSICAL SETTING

It is possible to practice yoga anywhere. On one level the idea is to be doing yoga all the time—being conscious of breath, body, and mind as a seamless happening that brings about an abiding sense of inner peace and joy. You could be doing yoga while waiting in line at the market, driving, walking, or sharing conversation. I have taught yoga in federal prisons amid loud banging and chaotic yelling, on the desert floor under the blazing sun, at high altitude in the Andes in freezing cold wind, in urban yoga studios where jackhammers and sirens punctuated the quiet rhythm of the breath, in tropical yoga *shalas* surrounded by the melodies of jungle life. All these settings presented a different opportunity for the practice of pratyahara. They also presented different opportunities for appreciating the richness of life and cultivating clarity amid whatever is happening. Still, we can identify certain environmental conditions that are favorable to the practice. Consider the following:

Dedicated space: Creating a place exclusively devoted to yoga lends to the overall ambiance of the practice and helps to ensure the ideal environmental elements suggested below.

The floor: The optimal yoga floor is made of smooth wood, preferably hardwood or a wood-like laminate. Ideally it is "sprung" like a dance floor, providing a stable yet slightly flexible and warm foundation. A mushy carpeted floor does not provide a stable foundation for standing and balancing asanas and is a source of wrist strain in asanas that place substantial weight on the hands. Carpeted floors are perfectly suitable for "easy does it" classes in which students rarely stand, balance, or place much weight on their hands.

Walls: Many asanas are best introduced or refined with practice at a simple wall free of obstructions (such as artwork, vents, windows, switches, and lights). Elaborate yoga walls can be designed with built-in straps that, ideally, are removable so that the space can also be used without them.

Air: Some students want a constant flow of fresh air in order to breathe fully, while others think the slightest breeze tightens their muscles and inhibits safe opening. This is a common tension in most classes. While some classes are designed to be extremely hot, most classes and students will benefit from a moderately warm room with good circulation of fresh air.[2]

Light: The use of skylights and horizontal windows high up on the walls allows natural light without reducing precious wall space. Use dimmer switches and candles to add a warm and soulful quality.

Music: Some styles and traditions strongly discourage music in classes, while in others music is an essential part of the overall experience. If you choose to use music, still give primary consideration to the audibility of your verbal cues and, more importantly, your ability to hear your students as they breathe and speak. Craft a variety of playlists to harmonize with the arc and moods of your classes, and try them before using them in class.

Aroma: In the 1960s, yoga and incense were often found in the same sentence and room, largely giving way to yoga and aromatherapy in the 1980s and beyond. Many students enjoy the way certain scents transport their awareness to a yogic mood or feeling, while others find these scents distracting or even nauseating. Just as we encourage students to attend class free of fragrance, it is best to offer a room that is filled with fresh and natural air that's free of artificial smells.

Props: The practical application of props is addressed in Chapter Seven, "Teaching Asanas." Here are the basic props:

- *Mats* are the only prop deemed acceptable in some styles of yoga; all students should own one. There are several factors for students to consider in choosing a mat: its ecological construction and recyclability, firmness or softness, stability, weight, durability, and stickiness. In sweaty practices it is helpful to place an absorbent fabric over the mat to create a more stable surface and allow easier washing away of toxins.

- *Blankets* are a versatile prop that can be folded for varying heights of bolstering, rolled for various placements, opened for covering, and used in other creative ways. Firm wool blankets fold and roll most uniformly.

- *Bolsters* can provide stable and uniform support in a variety of asanas. Most bolstering can be done with alternately stacked blankets.

- *Blocks* are a multifunction prop: They can serve as a bolster in seated asanas, allow easier grounding of the hands in standing asanas, and help awaken and support energetic actions. Wood blocks are stable but heavy; foam blocks are light but can be flimsy.

- *Straps* are a versatile prop that extends reach without compromising the integrity of posture and maintains or stabilizes positioning in a variety of asanas. The "quick release" design offers greater versatility, allowing the strap to be more easily secured or released.

- *Chairs* are essential props with many students. It is possible to teach an entire class with students seated in chairs, with which you may find yourself teaching prenatal or postnatal classes or working with elderly practitioners or others who have limited mobility or stability. There are also a variety of benches and stools that can be utilized in various asanas.[3]

- *Sandbags* add weighted traction to limbs in asanas such as Supta Baddha Konasana. They also serve as a versatile elevating or grounding prop for the heel in asanas such as Virabhadrasana I, which is especially helpful to students with recent ankle sprains.

CLASSROOM SETUP AND ORIENTATION

The physical shape and layout of the room will determine the ideal way to orient yourself and your students. Along with the safety concerns discussed below, your primary consideration should be your ability to easily see students—and their ability to see you. If you are in a rectangular room, positioning yourself in the middle of a long wall will maximize visibility. Orienting the other way will create too much of a front-back orientation to the room, with newer or less secure students tending to take a spot toward the back and farthest from an open visual line to your demonstrations. While some teachers prefer to have more experienced or proficient students in front as models, this can create a problem because some experienced students tend to show off in their practice, often in ill-informed and potentially dangerous ways, which many beginning students will interpret as the model of what to do. Meanwhile, the newer or relatively less proficient students will have greater difficulty observing your demonstrations. This is also why it is preferable to have taller students further to the sides or back of the room. For a variety of reasons, many students like to be in a particular place in the room. Students with special needs, including newer students, those with certain injuries, pregnancy, physical limitations, or greater balance challenges, are best set up next to a wall where they can more easily access the wall as a prop and should be given priority for those spaces. This might involve asking a regular or random student to give up his or her preferred space to accommodate the student with special needs. A few simple words of explanation usually make this an easy shift.

Positioning your own mat away from the room's main entrance enables students to see you more easily when entering, thus allowing you to see and greet them more easily. This orientation also usually results in less distraction when students enter or leave the room during practice. Bear in mind that once the class starts you will be moving around the room observing, cueing, and interacting with students. Anticipate that with some asanas or asana sequences you might ask students to turn sideways on their mat, thus facing in a different direction. As we will explore in the next chapter, the "front" of the room—the place where you generally first demonstrate an asana—will shift accordingly, with all the same considerations shifting along with you.

In crowded classes, it is helpful to alternately stagger mats, creating more lateral space for students when they extend their arms out and less entanglement with their immediate neighbors when turned to the side and folding forward with arms overhead. Staggering works well whether the entire class is oriented toward the front of the room or toward each other in two long, opposing rows. The latter orientation works best in classes in which there is a set sequence that students repeat in each practice on their own, thus minimizing the extent of class-wide demonstrations of asanas. Some teachers prefer perfect lines of mats, military style, which creates order and clear, uniform angles; this setup allows them to more easily perceive alignment. Others prefer a more community-oriented energetic vibe by arranging students in a circle or semicircle without losing their ability to easily observe alignment.

CLASS LEVELS AND PREREQUISITES

Should anyone be able to attend any class? What if a beginning student drops in for an advanced class? Or a self-identified advanced student, enthusiastic ego intact, drops in on a beginning class? What about "all levels" classes? And to what degree should Hatha yoga be presented through a sequential curriculum in which some observed or measured degree of proficiency is a prerequisite for advancing to the next level? There are very strong and divergent opinions about these issues. Some teachers are adamant in limiting classes to only certain students and accomplish this in part by requiring preregistration and prior teacher approval.[4] Offering classes for preset periods of time, much as a school divides classes into terms or semesters, adds further structure. This requires students to make a commitment, gives greater cohesion to the class, and allows the teacher to deliver a preplanned curriculum designed to take students progressively from one place to another in their practice, fostering students' self-discipline in the process.

But there are just as many good reasons to offer open classes. First, while discipline is an important value, a relatively open class structure—one that allows students to drop in—makes it easier for most students to attend class. Many people want to explore the river by wading or diving in at various points rather than starting at the top in slow, shallow waters and going only as far as allowed by a predetermined time frame or set program. Students come to yoga with widely varied backgrounds and might be well suited in an intermediate class even if they are entirely new to yoga. Many have life situations that prevent them from committing to a specific schedule for weeks or months at a time. Many experienced students find benefit in taking different kinds of classes from day to day. If a studio offers a variety of class levels throughout the week, as well as different teachers and styles, these students can explore more freely. Drop-in students, especially brand-new students or those with exceptional challenges, require more of the teacher. But even in the most highly structured classes, regular students show up with new needs that require just as much special attention. A strict policy prohibiting students from dropping in to classes can be just as discouraging as being indiscriminate about who is in your class. When you first meet a new student, part of your initial conversation should include asking about his or her prior experience with yoga, injuries and other physical conditions that might limit that person's practice. If you perceive the student as unfit for the class, first explain the nature of the class and describe more appropriate alternatives on the schedule or elsewhere in your local yoga community. If the student still wants to take the class, show him or her Balasana and emphasize the importance of taking it easy. Offering an open schedule of classes with different levels and styles can be complemented by "intensives" that offer more structured teaching. The intensives can be structured for introduction to yoga, specific levels, or specific audiences. Teachers can then refer drop-in students to the intensives as appropriate while generally allowing students the freedom to participate in whatever classes they want to take.

CLASS ETIQUETTE

Your effectiveness as a teacher and the ability of your students to refine and deepen their practice in your classes depends in part on the conduct of everyone else in the room. By and large, most students will never have an issue in honoring the basic etiquette that allows you to teach and every student to practice. Issues usually arise from not knowing that certain conduct disrupts or distracts the class. It is therefore important to clearly state basic standards of conduct, including:

- *Cleanliness:* Students should be encouraged to wash their body before practicing. If this is impractical, they should be encouraged to "freshen up" before coming into class, as strong body odor can make it difficult for other students (and you!) to breathe comfortably. Discuss this issue privately and supportively.

- *Scents:* Whether perfume, cologne, deodorant, or an essential oil, what smells good to one person might cause nausea to another. The simple solution is to ask all students to refrain from wearing any scented products on their skin or clothes while in class.

- *Attire:* Yoga is best practiced in comfortable clothing. When practiced in a group setting, clothing should be simple and not a source of distraction. From a teaching standpoint, it is helpful to be able to see the contours of students' bodies.

- *Bare Feet:* Ask students to remove their shoes before entering the yoga room, honoring the cleanliness and (for many) the sacred quality of the *shala.*

- *Talking:* Encourage students to stay focused on the sound of the breath and your verbal cues. If a student frequently talks during class, discuss this with him or her privately after class. If two or more students are having a conversation during class, simply saying to the entire class, "Try to stay in your practice," will usually quiet the talkers. Remember, however, that all students should be encouraged to ask questions about the practice you are doing at any time. While you might simply want to acknowledge the question at that moment and say when you will address it, it is important to be open in your teaching by addressing questions and using them as an opportunity to provide more thorough explanations and instructions. Teachers who refuse to take questions not only come across as arrogant and authoritarian; their refusal to engage openly with students can also make students feel less safe and trusting in their relationship with the teacher.

- *Arriving/Departing:* Invariably, some students will arrive late or leave early, possibly distracting students and disrupting the flow of your teaching. Some studios and teachers insist on strict policies, turning students away if they arrive more than a certain number of minutes late. Many teachers who begin the practice with a period of silent or guided meditation ask late-arriving students to wait until the meditation has ended before entering the room. Others encourage students already in the room to use such potential distractions as an opportunity to stay present amid whatever might occur, further encouraging them to practice "karma yoga" by kindly opening up space in a crowded room

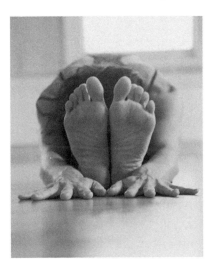

for others. While students should be encouraged to arrive at least five minutes early and stay to the end of class, in an often hectic and unpredictable world, even the most disciplined student will occasionally arrive late or need to leave early. Opening your space and heart to accommodating them can go far in conveying to all of your students that your intention is to be supportive, demonstrating flexibility and ease. When an existing student arrives late, encourage that person to do whatever he or she needs to get into his or her body rather than insisting that the student begin doing what the rest of the class is doing. If a new student arrives late, guide that person into Balasana until you feel it is appropriate for him or her to join in.

WAKING UP THE SPIRITUAL ENVIRONMENT

Creating a safe, nurturing space for students is among the most important roles of a yoga teacher. There are innumerable sources in the literature of yoga and spirituality offering guidance in the practice of knowing one's self. Because most traditional yoga spiritual teachings arose in a Hindu religious culture, they typically articulate Hindu-oriented assumptions about the spiritual path, usually described as being at one with brahman or the divine. We find many contemporary writings on yoga that embrace these traditional teachings as the sacred word of the divine, offering a form of fundamentalist yoga that takes on the air of religion. When we casually draw from these sources with only scant understanding of their religious underpinnings, it is easy as teachers to find ourselves expressing beliefs that, on closer examination, we might find far from how we really think or feel about matters of life and spirit. But we can also look to these and other sources as tremendous wellsprings of insight about life and yoga that are rich with metaphor, myth, and archetypes that as teachers we can make concrete and relevant to our students without a religious tone.

Many yoga teachers—indeed, much of the worldwide yoga community—take the Yoga Sutras of Patanjali as articles of religious faith and the foundational beliefs of their practice, teaching, and lives. Taking exception with the Sutras or other traditional texts or concepts, or applying them selectively or with liberal interpretation, is seen by some purist yogis as sacriligious. However, "the spiritual is not religion," says Rachel Naomi Remen (1993, 40):

> A religion is a dogma, a set of beliefs about the spiritual and a set of practices, which arise out of those beliefs. There are many religions and they tend to be mutually exclusive. That is, every religion tends to think it has "dibs" on the spiritual—that it's "The Way." Yet the spiritual is inclusive. It is the deepest sense of belonging and participation. We all participate in the spiritual at all times, whether we know it or not.[5]

In many traditional and contemporary yoga teachings there is a religious belief in "oneness" and a prescribed practice that requires renouncing desire, attachment, and individuality as "The Path" to spiritual being. Ganga White (2007, 200) reminds us that the "core belief in this perspective is that the underlying truth and reality in life is the One, and that the everyday world of diversity and individuality in which we live is actually an illusion, called *maya*." But is it really an illusion? White goes on to suggest that "it may be wiser to learn to live intelligently with these inherent dimensions of ourselves rather than try to annihilate them." When we let go of yoga fundamentalism we can creatively tap into gems like the Sutras and the Bhagavad Gita in offering spiritual insights and space that acknowledges the equally valid reality of life as it is experienced right here and now. In teaching yoga, this approach opens up the spiritual dimension to be more inclusive of whoever is in your class, regardless of his or her beliefs, faith, or views of spirituality and religion. "To the soul," Thomas Moore (1994, 203–205) notes, "the ordinary is sacred and the everyday is the primary source of religion." He continues, offering that "just as the mind digests ideas and produces intelligence, the soul feeds on life and digests it, creating wisdom and character out of the fodder of experience."

Most people are first drawn into the practice to reduce stress, develop flexibility, heal a physical or emotional injury, explore new social connections, or pursue physical fitness. But once in the practice, connecting body-breath-mind, something starts to happen. Students begin to experience a clearer self-awareness, a sense of being more fully alive; they feel better, more in balance, more conscious, clearer. The yearning that we have as human beings for a happy, wakeful, meaningful life and a sense of connection with something greater than our individual selves starts to become a powerful motivation for practicing over the long run of one's life.

When used as a tool for self-transformation and a path of spiritual being, yoga starts the moment a student first pays attention to what he or she is doing in the practice. If a student is unsteady, falling, in pain, or distracted by discomfort, the tendency will be to go back into his or her analytical or agitated mind. Sthira and sukham—steadiness and ease—give the asanas their transformative foundation. Being steady does not mean being perfectly still in a pose that you hold for a very long time. Indeed, a "pose" is static, something a model does for a camera. Asanas, by contrast, are alive, in each moment a unique expression of the human being doing them.[6] Opening one's self to a feeling of inner peace amid the relative intensity of the asana practice—being calm and soft while strong and stable—takes the practice to a deeper level.

Even when staying with an asana for a long time and cultivating steadiness and ease, there is always movement: the heart is beating, breath and prana are flowing. An expanded view of asana practice thus takes in a practice of movement within and between what are often described as separate asanas, movement in which one is just as present, just as steady in body-breath-mind, just as at ease. The breath itself starts to become as though a mantra in the movement meditation that is asana practice. In this way the practice is that of mindful meditation, in which one is fully present in the moment.[7] This experiential process—not the religious worship of a deity or insistence on precise form in held poses—is what makes asana practice itself a spiritual practice. And it is precisely here, in creating a space that encourages mindfulness, that the yoga teacher becomes a spiritual facilitator. In guiding yoga classes that encourage self-reflective awareness, each asana, each moment within and between the asanas, every breath, every sensation, and every thought and feeling become windows into the nature of the mind, consciousness, and spirit. The practice becomes a process offering insight into the "stickiness and delusions of the mind," which, Stephen Levine (1979, 69) writes, "are seen more clearly when viewed from the heart." This is where doing yoga asanas becomes a practice of self-transformation and healing, and a profound sense of conscious awakening and connection begins to emerge.

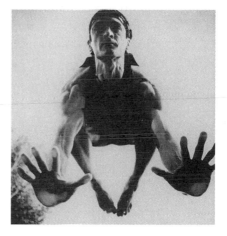

There are many ways to encourage this more conscious approach to yoga practice. Recognizing that some students are uncomfortable chanting "aum" while others are deeply into a bhakti practice, use your judgment in deciding how to create a safe space for everyone while remaining true to your own sensibilities. How you approach this will surely change as you evolve in your teaching. Try to keep yourself open to playing with how you hold a spiritual space, watching and listening for how your various approaches create different reactions in your students. Here are several ways to create a more spiritually awakening class:

Greeting your class: Try to greet each student as he or she enters the room. (See Chapter Six for detailed guidance on querying new students.) Make eye contact and be present with that one student, even if only for a brief time. When ready to start, greet the entire class by saying "Welcome" or "Namaste."

Getting situated: Starting your classes with at least a few minutes of sitting still helps students to fully "arrive" and tune in to what they are feeling in their body, breath, mind, and spirit. Invite everyone in the class to come into a comfortable cross-legged or another sitting position. Encourage and demonstrate the use of a bolster to elevate the sitting bones as high as it takes to bring the pelvis into a neutral position. Ask students to begin tuning in inside, to feel the simple, natural flow of their breath. Ask them to feel their sitting bones, encouraging them to more firmly nestle their sitting bones down as if into the earth, giving a greater feeling of being grounded. Then ask them to bring their attention back to their breath, feeling the natural movements in their body from the movement of their breath. Encourage them to relax their face, their eyes, between their temples. From a place of ease and stability, ask them to begin very gradually to breathe more deeply, feeling the natural effects of the breath in their body, expanding and growing taller and more spacious with each inhale, relaxing and quieting more deeply inside with each exhale. Encourage them to pay attention to the spaces between their breaths, without holding the breath in or out, and to allow the quality of sensation they feel in the pauses to come with them as the breath flows along. With the calm, steady cultivation of the breath, ask your students to listen to the breath as it flows through their throat, a sound like wind breezing through the trees or like the ocean at the seashore. Encourage them to stay attuned to the sound, sensation, and balanced flow of the breath throughout their practice.

Setting intention: From the soft and receptive inner space created from sitting, breathing, watching, and feeling, invite your students to draw their palms together at their heart in *anjali mudra* (prayer position of the palms). Encouraging your students to stay connected with the breath, ask them to bring their fingertips to their forehead, symbolically connecting their head with their heart. From this place of connection, ask them to take a moment to reflect inside, to remind themselves why they are there and to give themselves a clearer sense of intention, inner purpose, in their practice. Considering your own intention and the class setting, you may want to:

- Offer a few minutes of sitting in silence or with guided meditation.
- Read a poem or other writing that sets the mood or suggests a theme.
- Lead a chant, which might differ from class to class or season to season.
- Awaken with pranayama—ujjayi is a must; nadi shodhana and kapalabhati are good options for the beginning of some classes (see Chapter Eight).

Here you can also create the space for students (and yourself) to dedicate their practice to someone or something that is important to them. Allowing this to be personal and private, rather than suggesting that the dedication be to some particular concept of the spiritual, students will feel more free and comfortable in this part of the practice. At natural intervals later in the class, such as pausing after an intense sequence of asanas, ask the students once again to bring their palms together at their heart, fingertips to their forehead, and to come back into their intention.

Chanting the sound of aum: Most students in yoga studio classes enjoy the shared chanting of the sound of "aum." *Aum* is a mystical or sacred syllable mentioned in the Vedas, Upanishads, and Bhagavad Gita, variously described as "the essential sound of the universe," the "voice of God," and "the originating sound of creation." In some forms of Hinduism, the letter *a* represents creation (issuing from

Brahma's essence), *u* the preservation of balance in the world (as the god Vishnu balances Brahma overhead on a lotus flower), and *m* the completion of the cycle of existence (when Vishnu falls asleep and all existing things dissolve into their essence).[8] It signifies the beginning of the yoga practice, setting the tone and helping bring awareness more inside. In more simple form, you may make the sound as "om." You might find some students expressing resistance to this through their body language; let it be and continue with your class, or take the time to explain the meaning of *aum* and the reason for chanting it.

Guiding asana practice as movement meditation: We often hear of asana, pranayama, and meditation as if they were separate practices. The full practice of pranayama, as discussed in Chapter Eight, is done while sitting, and some of the deepest meditation practices are done while sitting still (see Chapter Nine). But as discussed earlier, to truly do asana practice involves being present, which is the heart of meditation, while breathing consciously with ujjayi pranayama. Connecting the rhythmic flow of the breath with the rhythmic expansion and contraction of the body within and between asanas allows students to experience their asana practice as a moving meditation. Beginning with simple, slow, rhythmic movements helps students to feel and stay with the connection of body-breath-mind. Starting the moving asana practice with a flowing sequence such as Surya Namaskara is an excellent way for the class as a whole to feel the syncopated flow of breath, energy, and spirit. Frequently remind students to feel the rhythmic flow of sensation in their body with the breath, whether in the relative stillness of a held asana or when transitioning from one place to another.

Guiding dristana: The mind tends to go wherever the eyes lead. The practice of dristana, in which we focus our gaze softly and steadily on a single dristi point, helps to keep the mind focused during asana practice, lending to a deeper quality of pratyahara, in which we relieve our senses of their external distractions, and dharana, the sixth limb, in which the mind is completely focused. In some teachings the student is told to gaze at a specific point during and between every asana. The strength of this approach to dristana practice is that it soon comes to feel effortless; there is no question in the student's mind about where to gaze, just as there is no question about what the next asana is, thus drawing the student deeper into his or her practice. Rather than prescribing a specific dristi point for students, a softer yet no less effective cue encourages students to gaze

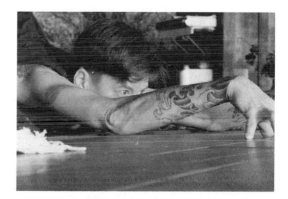

steadily at something nearby that is not moving, offering a general direction for the gaze without specifying the precise point.

Rhythms of nature: For tens of thousands of years the rhythms of human life were consciously connected to and even determined by the rhythms of the cosmos, especially the appearance and disappearance of light (sun and moon).[9] Since at least the early Greeks, scholars have been intrigued by seasonal influences on human experiences. Yet with the advent of modern civilization we have become increasingly alienated from the natural rhythms of the universe. Reconnecting our lives with the seasons and with the powerful influences of solar and lunar energy can help us feel the natural rhythms of our lives, and in this connection feel a deeper, steadier awakening of spirit. Creating class themes, sequences, and intentions that embody and honor how we feel at a particular time of the day, the seasons, and other cosmological rhythms helps to ground the practice in a natural form of spirituality, where body, breath, mind, and spirit are in syncopation with the flow of the cosmos. Exploring our feelings, sensations, and awareness in relationship to powerful natural energetic forces helps us tune in to the deeper rhythms of life. Creating the space for students to more consciously open the doors of their perception to human life and experience as a natural expression of the universe can then bring more light and clarity to the evolution of one's own spirit. With growing awareness in the practice, the rhythms and patterns of daily life can come to be felt more and more as the expression of spirit in the energetic pulsation of life itself.

Ambiance: Many yoga studios go to great lengths and expense in creating a spiritual ambiance. Walking into such a space can create an immediate sense of openness to the possibility of something happening in the heart or spirit. It can also turn away many students for whom these qualities feel out of sync with their conventional Western cultural sensibilities. Developing a sense of your clientele while honoring your own sensibilities will bring you to a balance of design elements that work in your space. Lighting even a single candle can help transform an otherwise cold industrial space into a temple of yogic awakening.

ARCHETYPES AND MYTHOLOGY

The verbal root *as* in *asana* includes the idea of ritual, a set of actions with symbolic significance that we can tie into practice to highlight certain areas of personal, emotional, spiritual, social, and ecological experience. When teaching yoga, you can accentuate these ties by emphasizing the symbolism expressed in different parts of the practice. One source of symbolism is the vast realm of mythological figures found across the world's diverse cultural landscapes. Whether we interpret myth as allegory and a "medium for or a flawed version of an immutable, eternal reality created by or for unsophisticated minds" or as "an essential function of the mind (conscious or unconscious) to express repressed needs and desires or to make sense out of life and resolve all conflicts therein," as Devdutt Pattanaik (2003, 161–162) contrasts, we can find within them profound wisdom about the conditions and circumstances of life and consciousness. (We will explore this in the following section.) Indian mythology is especially rich in tales, symbols, and rituals that are a reaction to and a communication of humans' understanding of nature and being. Part of the beauty of Indian mythology is that is it alive and evolving with new interpretations that relate to the quests of whoever delves into its seemingly endless stories. Many asanas are named for figures in these stories, offering a variety of metaphors that relate to daily life and yoga. The aim of Indian spiritual philosophy and mythology is to learn the secret of entanglement and dissolve the mental and emotional cobwebs that envelop our conscious being. Indian mythology offers abundant symbols found in the natural world that represent aspects of human life and experience: light and dark, mountains and rivers, trees and animals, wind and stars. Here are some of the ways that, as a teacher, you can tap into this mythological tradition, much of it found in the Ramayana and Mahabharata, making the practice more one of conscious awareness and self-transformation (Menon 2003; Dharma 1999).

Hatha as balanced integration: Reminding students of the essence of Hatha yoga as a practice of balanced integration of effort and ease is a powerful starting point for making yoga more transformational, especially as students begin to explore and discover how the practice can play with the apparent polarities of life. Although typically reduced to "physical yoga," the term *hatha* is made from the syllables *ha* and *tha,* which respectively signify the solar and lunar energies pulsating throughout the world.[10] Both sun and moon have rich symbolic significance in Indian mythology. The solar energies are expansive and invigorating, while lunar energies are more integrative and calming.[11] The term *hatha yoga* thus conveys the integration of opposites, the balance of effort and ease, a practice that is at once awakening and calming. Brought into asana and pranayama classes, these balanced qualities make yoga more sustainable and transforming.

Surya Namaskara—bowing to the inner sun: The Sun Salutations that initiate many yoga classes are rich in symbolism. Surya is the chief solar deity who drives his chariot across the sky each day as the most visible form of God that one can see. It is also the ancient Sanskrit term for "sun," which in most ancient mythology is revered, as Richard Rosen (2003) says, "as both the physical and spiritual heart of the world." *Namaskara* is from the root *namas,* "to bow" (as in "namaste"). In the myths of the Vedas, the gods use the sun's heat for many purposes, especially creation. Our "inner sun," the spiritual heart center, is seen as the source of light and truth along one's life path. In Surya Namaskara, we are bowing to the truth of who we are in our essence, releasing the head lower than the heart, connecting with our inner wisdom.

Nataraja—the dancing warrior: Shiva is usually represented in Indian iconography as immersed in deep meditation or dancing the Tandava upon the demon of ignorance in his manifestation as Nataraja, the lord of the dance (Zimmer 1972, 151–157). As an ancient form of magic, dancing induces trance, ecstasy, and self-realization. Shiva manifests in the form of Nataraja to gather and project his fran-

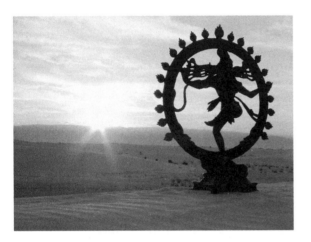

tic, endless gyrations in order to arouse dormant energies that are the creative forces shaping the world. Leading a class through a linked dance-like series of warrior asanas and vinyasas awakens students' creative energy as body and breath are synchronized in flowing movement. But Nataraja is also the god of destruction, manifesting the element of fire that symbolizes the destruction of illusions we hold about life and the world. In the balance of the dancing Shiva, we thus find a counterpoise of destruction and creation in the play of the cosmic dance, offering a pathway to enlightenment and equanimity.

Virabhadra—the fierce spiritual warrior: When Shiva's consort Shakti was killed by the chief of the gods, Daksha, Shiva tore out his hair in grief and anger, creating the fierce warrior Virabhadra from his locks. With a thousand arms, three burning eyes, and fiery hair, Virabhadra wore a garland of skulls and carried many terrifying weapons. Bowing at Shiva's feet and asking his will, Virabhadra was directed by Shiva to lead his army against Daksha to avenge Shakti's death, which he did with immediate success. Like Shiva, Virabhadra's aim in destruction is not revenge but to destroy the real enemy, which is the ego standing in the way of humility. Approaching the asanas named for Virabhadra—Virabhadrasana I, II, and III—we can encourage students to cultivate the mind of the spiritual warrior, aware of all sides, unattached to attainment, centered in one's being. Staying focused in the practice, holding on in the midst of fear and intensity, the spirit of Virabhadra helps students discover the strength and humility to explore challenges in their practice and life with greater courage and determination.

Shakti—the divine feminine: This is where we can infuse our classes with creativity and playfulness. Shakti is the creative power of existence, the cosmic energy that animates the universe, the source of energy, the mother goddess, representing the active, dynamic principles of feminine power. In some Indian traditions, every god in the panoply of Indian deities has his Shakti, the divine feminine energy without which the god would have no power. Shakti is the world-protecting, feminine, maternal side of god, symbolizing the spontaneous and loving acceptance of life's tangible reality. She is the creative joy of life, the beauty, enticement, and seduction of the living world, instilling in us surrender to the changing qualities of existence. She is the preeminent enigma to the masculine principle of spirit, symbolizing the way that the flow of experience in daily life casts mists around the clarity of being. As we constantly project and externalize our Shakti energy, we create the universe of our life, the small sphere of our immediate concerns. Like a painter covering a canvas, we populate and color the canvas of our lives, creating dramas and delights that are the illusions of our own Shakti energy. When we are entangled and captivated by what we feel are the vital, passionate issues in our lives, we are dealing with the projection of who we are, the spell of our creative being. Becoming aware of these creative projections, observing them just as we revel in them, brings dynamism to a life that might otherwise be quite boring. Rather than always guiding students into holding poses in a static mold, Shakti insists on liberating that dynamism in asanas, playing with the asanas, dancing with them, feeling them as fully alive, vibrant, and sensuous.

Astavakra—transcending misunderstanding: Kagola, a poor student of the Vedas, sat at night reciting aloud the sacred verses of the Vedas, his pregnant wife by his side in the dim light of candles. One late night he heard a voice laughing and correcting him for mispronouncing a verse. The tired and short-tempered father was enraged, cursing the unborn child, causing him to be born with eight crooks in his body, naming him Astavakra for the deformity (*asta* meaning "eight," *vakra* "crooked"). The crippled and humbled child sought to redeem himself to his father, studying deeply in the sacred philosophy of India and, in time, becoming a great Vedic scholar. But his deformities caused others to judge him for what they saw, not for his knowledge, wisdom, and simple articulation of the essence of mystical experience. While still a boy, King Janaka heard of Astavakra's wisdom and sought him out as a sage and teacher. When the boy's father learned of Astavakra's great scholarly accomplishments and the honor bestowed upon him by King Janaka of being the king's teacher, Kagola blessed him, his deformity vanished, and Astavakra stood straight. The story portrays the human tendency to dwell on appearances rather than on inner truths that are often concealed by what we see. In approaching

Astavakrasana, the asana named for Astavakra, students are usually intimidated by what appears to be a very complex and difficult pose. In reality, it is one of the eas-

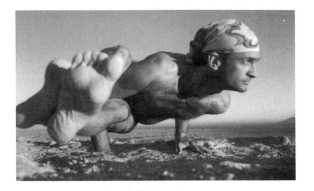

iest arm balances, requiring basic technique and knowledge of what to do. When we guide students to pause, breathe, watch, feel, and patiently explore with the knowledge of what we are sharing, they find a sense of liberation in Astavakrasana and other apparently challenging asanas. This extends into life off the mat, where we might shrink from certain actions in life out of misunderstanding the true nature of what is before us. With patience and learning, we can usually move forward with a renewed sense of freedom born of knowledge.

Ganesha—removing obstacles: Ganesha is the most popular member of the Indian pantheon of mythological deities. Represented as a short, potbellied man with yellow skin, four arms, and an elephant's head with one tusk, Ganesha is the second son of Shiva and Parvati (a form of Shakti). As with all the Indian gods, there are innumerable myths surrounding his creation and his role in the universe. He is the Lord of Obstacles, popularly worshipped as a remover of obstacles, although many stories have him both placing and removing obstacles.[12] Ganesha's elephant head symbolizes his unstoppable power and auspiciousness, his rotund body and potbelly symbolize abundance, and the subservient rat he rides symbolizes the wisdom that arises in the sublimation of selfish desires. While these qualities might seem to be in contradiction to one another, Ganesha represents balance in spiritual and material life. Loving, forgiving, and moved by affection, he can be ruthless when combating evil. If loved and respected, Ganesha is said to grant all wishes and ensure a steady path to success.

Vasistha and Vishvamitra—effortless grace and determined practice: The tale of Vasistha and Vishvamitra in the Ramayana tells of the dynamic tension in spiritual life between the ease that arises from contentment and the spiritual depth that can result from struggle and effort. Vasistha was an enlightened spiritual sage who established a peaceful, self-governing, cooperative society where all were happy. He had a "cow of plenty" named Nandini with the power to grant him whatever he wanted. The powerful ruler of a neighboring kingdom, Vishvamitra, was curious about Vasistha's society and went to visit with his army. Vishvamitra was impressed with Vashistha's cow and tried to take her away by force, but Vasistha's spiritual power—his tolerance and mastery of emotion—was too great for the many weapons that Vishvamitra used against him. In an epic battle between Vishvamitra and Vasistha, a hundred of Vishvamitra's sons were incinerated by Vasistha's breath. Vishvamitra eventually abdicated and committed himself to a simple ascetic life in pursuit of spiritual strength. Showing little hope for spiritual achievement, the very difficulty of his spiritual path led him to become a great sage himself, and Vasistha was among those who would come to pay homage to Vishvamitra. While the asanas named for these two sages are both difficult, Vishvamitrasana is considerably more challenging, requiring a deeper level of commitment, strength, and surrender.

Hanuman—leaping with devotion: Like Ganesha, Hanuman commands respect and veneration across Indian culture for his strength, humility, selflessness, devotion, determination, fearlessness, and commitment to spiritual discipline. The son of Vayu, the god of wind, and Anjana, a celestial being with the tail of a monkey (a *vanara*), Hanuman was the friend, confidant, and servant of King Rama. (Hanuman is also called Anjaneya, meaning "arising from Anjana," for whom the Anjaneyasana, Low-Lunge Pose, is named.) He accomplishes many feats in the Ramayana War. When Rama's wife, Sita, is kidnapped, Hanuman searches the world for her, eventually encountering the vast ocean. Everyone in the search party laments Hanuman's inability to jump across the water, and he too is saddened at the likely failure of his mission. But his commitment to his master is so great that Hanuman feels his powers, enlarges his body, and leaps across the ocean to find her. The story is one of purity of motive in uniting what has been separated, and the commitment to make whatever effort is needed to rise to the challenges we face in life. Hanuman reminds us that we can take larger steps in our lives if we open our awareness beyond the limitations of our immediate circumstances. The challenging asana named for Hanuman, Hanumanasana, allows us to embody these traits as we confront the apparent limitations we find in the flexibility of our hamstrings, quadriceps, and hip flexors. With patient devotion and openness to the possibility of going beyond what they think are their limits, students can invoke the spirit of Hanuman in exploring not just this difficult asana but other challenges in their lives as well.

CREATING A HAPPY SPACE

In describing the essential quality of yoga practice, Gérard Blitz, founder and president of the European Union of Yoga from 1974 to 1990, remarked that it is "to be firmly established in a happy space"[13] (Bouanchaud 1999, 131). This is echoed by Steve Ross (2003, 13), a Los Angeles–based yoga teacher whose highly popular and spirited classes have for nearly three decades embraced the idea that "happiness is found right where you are." But most traditional approaches to yoga are predicated on a rather different idea about happiness, one that assumes there is a certain pathway one must abide depending on the conditions in his or her life. As T. K. V. Desikachar (1998, 197–198) notes, "The path to happiness is a revelation of God as granted to a few of humanity's most inspired seekers," and to obtain it one must follow a set of prescriptions given in scriptural form in texts such as the Yoga Sutras of Patanjali that "take a very sophisticated approach to the search for happiness."[14] Here we will attempt to take a decidedly simpler approach that nonetheless draws from the received wisdom of ancient yogis, offering ways to create space in which students can experience the happiness in their essential nature here and now.

The ancient yogis were in many ways no different from people in the modern world. As part of ordinary life, they had moments of clarity and confusion, happiness and sadness, contentment and stress. Reflecting on the nature of their lives, they became more aware of their condition, recognizing that the incessant chatter in their mind was the source of their confusion—what Patanjali calls kleshas—and thus of many personal problems that flow from them.[15] As the kleshas manifest, the ancient yogis observed the tendency toward more rajasic or tamasic qualities of life: rajasic as we get really "high" with excitement, passion, agitation, and hyperintensity in our actions, tamasic when we feel "low" and get heavy, dull, depressed, and lazy, and act without considered reflection. Intrigued, they reflected even more deeply on the nature of the mind, seeking to unravel the mystery of existence. Like most students walking into yoga classes, they wanted to become clearer, happier, and more content. Deepening their self-study, they made some profound yet simple discoveries. One discovery is that a quieter mind—recall chitta vritti nirodaha, the first Yoga Sutra—brings about santosa, or contentment. Santosa was found to be associated with the third guna, sattva, or a more sattvic quality of life: lighter, clearer, more tranquil, a sense of moving into inner stillness, feeling more pure and

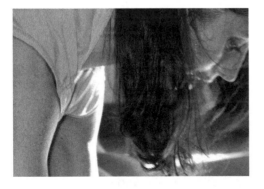

pleasant. Here one experiences a sense of personal integration and intrinsic authenticity, a sense of being at peace in life, aligned with the divine, at one with the universe—in a word, happy.[16]

Although motivated by wanting santosa and sattva, most students also embody strong rajasic and tamasic qualities. What you can offer them as a teacher is a *process* for refinement, what the ancient yogis called tapas, from *tap,* meaning "to burn or cook," in an environment of loving kindness, informed guidance, and freedom from judgment. Tapas arises when we make a commitment to being calmly present and reflective in the moment, when all the natural tendencies such as fear, boredom, excitement, anger, and distraction arise. An essential part of the self-transformative potential of conscious asana, pranayama, and meditation practices, this process has a seemingly magical way of making us happier.

A SPACE FOR HEALING AND AWAKENING

The emphasis on happiness might be construed as a glib take on the reality of human experience, especially given that many students come to yoga in crisis, as survivors of trauma, experiencing depression, or struggling in other ways. It is important to be attentive to this reality, providing gentle affirmation of each student's condition while offering guidance toward a yoga path that might help him or her to heal and reawaken to a new sense of santosa. While your role as a teacher is not that of a psychotherapist or doctor, you will have an effect on your students by virtue of how you create space and what you say and do in that space. The practice of yoga, as Carl Jung (1953, 529–530) wrote, "amounts to . . . a method of psychic hygiene." This psychic cleansing dissolves what the traditional yogic view calls our *samskaras:* essentially, emotional knots formed in the subtle energetic body from one's past and manifested in the physical body and the mind. The fabric of these knots is interlaced with the kleshas, mental-emotional fibers that cause pain and suffering. While the practice of yoga as a whole takes aim at samskaras and kleshas, we can highlight several techniques for getting at them as we hold a space for healing and awakening to a more holistic and integrated body, breath, mind, sense of self, and heart.

Practice of embodiment: Asana practice is inherently nourishing to the soul. As stated earlier, to truly "do asana" involves steadiness, ease, and being present in connecting body, breath, and mind in the moment. When we ask students to be present in their practice—to pay attention to what they are feeling in their body, to the movement of their mind, the flow of their breath, to "breathe into" areas of holding or tension— we are encouraging a practice of embodiment (Bailey 2003). Feeding the physical body—the annamaya kosha—with the *rasa* (juice) of conscious asana allows the release of the physical, mental, and emotional tensions that build up in the body during the normal course of life. In the mystical physiology of traditional yogic science, through asanas the nadis are opening, allowing the freer and more balanced flow of prana. This begins with the simplest experiences of bodily awareness: asking your students to lie on their backs and gradually bring awareness in through their toes, feet, ankles, lower legs, knees, thighs, pelvis, spine, heart, arms, fingers, neck, face, and head. In every asana, there is an opportunity to expand this simple awareness, going with the sensations that each asana naturally stimulates. Depending on a student's condition, the practice of embodiment through asana can be further varied by emphasizing different areas of asana. Most public classes should offer a well-rounded asana practice, helping students to cultivate overall balance and integration. Still, you might decide to give some classes a thematic focus that addresses particular aspects of healing or embodiment, such as a heart-opening through backbends. You can also design classes around the energetics and symbolism of chakras, intersperse sequences such as Dancing Warrior to accentuate emotional release and opening, or blend in pranayama techniques to bring more awareness to how energy is moving through the body. Creating a safe space for students to explore their body awareness, encouraging them to explore with self-disciplined intensity that brings their experience to a significant "edge"—where physical and emotional sensations are heightened—will allow them to move into deeper self-understanding, inner peace, and clarity.

Breath awareness: The breath is the vital link between body and mind, the essential source of feeling and thinking. When students learn to breathe consciously, they will use their breath to increase the awareness of sensation in their bodies. When attentive to breathing in the body, the body-breath-mind link is made complete as students concentrate their mind on the movement of their breath-body. With your students more subtly attuned to their breath, you can guide them in refining their breath awareness as they begin to move in the asana practice, connecting the pranamaya and annamaya koshas. As the breath becomes a source of guidance in asana, encourage students to continuously watch and feel it, thereby creating a sense of enveloping the mind in the breath while moving in the body.

Developing self-awareness: The manomaya kosha—sheath of the mind—is where we create differentiation in the world, distinguishing "I" and "mine," including a sense of "my breath" and "my body." It is from this place that we mentally perceive the world. Much of the struggle in life—*dukha*—comes from a lack of clear perception that arises from fear, anger, self-doubt, hatred, prejudice, and unconscious reactions to experiences that are colored by things that happened in the past. This creates a confused sense of self, leading to deeper manifestation of dukha as disturbance of body, breath, and mind. The practice of yoga offers a path of healing integration as we begin to rediscover the natural beauty of the body, the vital flow of the breath, and the clear processes of the mind. Guiding students along this path with an emphasis on mental clarity, you can encourage them in a process of self-study to help them develop a feeling of wholeness and healthiness. Some tools you can share include:

- Reflecting on how thoughts and actions are connected in daily life, giving more emphasis to daily affirmations that lead to acting more from a place of clarity;

- Tuning in to the natural mental reactions that happen during the asana practice, noticing how different asanas stimulate different kinds of emotional and mental reactions;

- Reading and reflecting upon spiritual, philosophical, or self-help writings as a means of gaining a clearer perspective on one's life;

- Learning to listen with refinement, opening to what is being expressed rather than always filtering everything through the prism of one's preconceptions.

Refining the personality: Even more refined than the manomaya kosha, the vijnanamaya kosha is where we find discriminating thought and qualities of judgment that, when acted upon, create a sense of personhood, or personality. *Vijnana* means "knowing." This sheath of being represents the wisdom that underlies the analytical, thinking, processing qualities of the mind. As we move along the path of yoga—embodied, energized, mentally connected—the full potential of our human character becomes more manifest. Gazing through the prism of a healthier body, awakened breath, and clearer mind, we find deeper integrity in our sense of self,

on the mat or off, walking alone or in relationship. Now we find ease in discovering clear insights about the nature of our true self.[17] Knowing who we are, we can move about in the world with an abiding sense of freedom. Meditation is a powerful tool for cultivating this awareness.

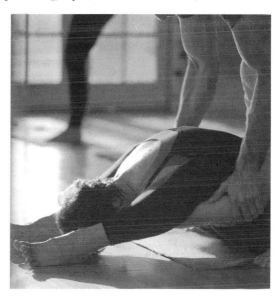

Opening to love: The most subtle of the five levels of the embodied self is the anandamaya kosha, the "sheath of bliss." The dimension of the spiritual heart center, it is here that our passions and potential for infinite joy come most alive. It is here that we discover bliss in the experience of love. How do we find it? Some say we don't, that instead love finds us in the mystery of life. "Because joy and love are intrinsic to the Self," Sally Kempton (2002, 40) shares, "the sages tell us that we can enter the experience of its expansive happiness through the doorway of our ordinary feelings of happiness and affection."

Indeed, where it most often and most fully blossoms for many people is in happy intimate relationships, in which we can cultivate the fertile soil of love in a variety of ways. As a teacher you can guide students in opening to their bliss by:

- Taking time at the beginning of class to draw the palms together at the spiritual heart center, setting clear and conscious intention in the practice that is sealed into the heart;
- Frequently reminding students to "breathe through the heart," expanding on this by emphasizing a feeling of the breath as if flowing in and out of the spiritual heart center;
- Asking students to think of those people in their lives who most inspire them;
- Leading guided meditations that focus on opening to the immediate experience of happiness, to the feeling of love, allowing that feeling to expand while letting go of whatever thought gave rise to the feeling, dwelling in the pure feeling itself;
- Creating living rituals in classes that instill a sense of communal experience, expanding everyone's capacity for bliss through shared experiences of asana, pranayama, meditation, chanting, and other group activities;
- Maintaining a warm human touch, greeting each student as he or she arrives to class, making eye contact, speaking with a soft yet clear and soothing voice.

HOLDING INTEGRATED SPACE

Skilled yoga teachers are talented multitaskers. They are attentive to the physical setting and the sense of energy in the room, creating and maintaining a space that is conducive to student comfort, focus, and ease. They are also aware of each student in the room, moving and adjusting their own positioning to help ensure that every student can easily observe demonstrations. Rather than working from a preconceived class plan that might or might not make sense for the students who are actually there, they strive to teach whoever is in the room with them. They create a safe and nurturing space for self-exploration that begins with greeting each student and encouraging conscious intention in the practice. They recognize and give support to students practicing with a wide range of intentions, encouraging deeper self-exploration and awareness of the emotional, mental, physical, and spiritual currents of the yoga experience. They support students in developing a more subtle awareness of the body-breath-mind connection, offering a variety of ways to explore this interconnection as a tool for deeper spiritual awakening, healing, and joyful life. Taken together, this set of qualities offers students an integrated space where they can most favorably take their personal practice wherever their intention and disciplined action leads. Doing this well requires practice. Holding this integrated space, you can then apply the fullest range of your skills and knowledge in guiding students in their practice, using the tools and techniques described in the following chapter.

CHAPTER SIX

TECHNIQUES
AND TOOLS
IN TEACHING
YOGA

*A good traveler has no fixed plans
and is not intent on arriving.*
—*Lao Tzu*

Teaching yoga is at once profoundly personal, predicated on sharing, and shaped by context. It is also inevitably surprising. We have no choice but to start from where we are and who we are, with whatever knowledge, skills, and experience we have in the moment. We also have little choice but to work with whomever shows up for class, teaching students whose conditions, intentions, learning styles, and needs are widely varied. On any given day, unanticipated events can make a class much different than what you might have envisioned. The changes that happen from class to class also have everything to do with whoever is in the class, the time of day, our own mood, and myriad other factors that invariably come into play in teaching. Indeed, if your classes are always perfectly predictable—if you feel the same, the students seem the same, the environment manifests as exactly the same—you might benefit from reflecting on the bubble you are in and how it is probably suffocating some aspect of the practice. It is precisely in the variability of every class and the unique experience of each new breath—even in fixed-sequence classes—that we find renewed stimulation of self-exploration and self-transformation, yet also the challenges that naturally arise in teaching. Going with the flow of change, you can draw from the richness of your teaching palette to inspire and guide your students along their yoga path.

This chapter presents a set of specific teaching techniques and tools that are applicable to every style of Hatha yoga, even while different styles often give more or less emphasis to certain other principles and techniques. This is not a blueprint for teaching; it is a flexible resource that you can draw from in your development as an excellent teacher, which starts with opening your awareness to the most authentic way you can teach yoga to others.

TEACHING WHO IS IN FRONT OF YOU

However much you prepare for a class, be just as prepared to improvise on the spot in order to teach a class that is appropriate for the students who are there. This requires assessing your students as thoroughly as you can within whatever time you have before the class starts and continuing that assessment throughout the class. Here are several ways to do the assessment:

Querying New Students

As part of introducing yourself to each new student, try to ask the following questions to inform your assessment of the student and how best to guide him or her in the practice.

1. *How you ever practiced yoga? If so, what style of yoga? For what period of time? How frequently?* This will give you an initial sense of the student's prior experience.

2. *Do you have any injuries or anything else going on with your body that I should be aware of? How are your ankles, knees, hips, back, shoulders, neck, wrists?* Always try to ask the follow-up question.

3. If a student reports having an injury or issue, follow up with more specific questions: *What is it about your knee? Have you had surgery? When? How does it feel now?* Based on the answers to these questions, give the student some initial guidance on how he or she might modify his or her practice. Use your knowledge but also be prepared to acknowledge that you do not know about the injury or issue, and encourage the student to take care of him- or herself.

4. *Are you pregnant, or have you recently had a baby?* Ask this of any woman you think is pregnant or who recently gave birth; share with her the basic trimester cautions described in Chapter Eleven.

5. *What is your work or daily life like?* This question can provide insight into chronic stress, pain, tightness, and weakness as well as larger lifestyle conditions that affect the body, breath, and mind.

6. *What do you do for exercise?* If the student runs, cycles, surfs, rock climbs, or engages in some other vigorous sports activities, this can tell you a lot about

chronic tightness or pain in the hips, legs, shoulders, back, wrists, and other places. If the student answers that he or she does not exercise, this is also important information for you to know.

Learning to Look and See

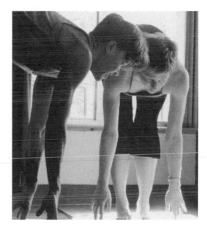

Self-reporting is not a guarantee that you will get accurate or complete information on a student's condition; many people are reluctant to share personal information with relative strangers, are unaware of a condition, or are in denial about its significance. Your ability to accurately see students in asana starts with learning to see bodies more generally, training the eye to see different bodies from various perspectives. This essential skill is best developed through anatomical and asana observation clinics in teacher-training workshops. Here we will look at three methods for developing these skills: (1) partner standing observation, (2) asana laboratory observation, and (3) practice teaching observation.

Partner Standing Observation

Partner up with another teacher or trainee, one in the role as the "looker" and the other as the "lookee." The looker uses a worksheet with three illustrations of the body in anatomical position (front, back, and side) to record their observations. There is no judgment about any of the findings. The lookees take a few marching steps forward and then stop and stand in a normal position as if waiting in line for a movie. They will be in this position for a few minutes. Ask them not to try to change or correct their posture as the "lookers" observe and record. Ideally the lookee's clothes allow his or her posture to be easily observed from foot to head. With "lookers" squatting behind their partners, the observation begins at the feet:

- *Feet:* Are the feet straight? One foot out, one foot in? Flat-footed or high-arched?
- *Achilles:* Do they align straight, veer toward the midline or toward the lateral?
- *Calves:* Look and feel. Is there more tension in one calf than the other? Is there more tension on the outside or the inside of the calf?
- *Knees:* Is the back of the knee hard or soft, flexed, extended, or hyperextended?
- *Hips:* Place the palms flat on the hips facing downward with thumbs straight across the sacrum. Are the hips level?

- *Arms:* Do they hang evenly at the side, or is one hand more in front than the other? Where are the palms facing? Is there a carrying angle at the elbow?
- *Shoulders:* Are they even or level? Does one shoulder ride higher than the other?
- *Head:* Is it centered between the shoulders? Does the head tilt or rotate to the side?

Now the lookers stand to the side of their partners (perpendicularly) and observe the following:

- Does the ear hole (external auditory meatus) line up over the shoulder? Does the head move forward or behind the shoulder? Are the shoulders either slumping forward or pulled back?
- Does the shoulder line up over the hip?
- Is the upper back hunched (kyphosis)? Is the chest collapsed?
- Does the hip line up over the knee? Is the pelvis pitched either forward or back?
- Does the knee line up over the ankle? Is it hyperextended?
- Does the ear hole line up over the ankle?

Now the lookers stand in front of their partners and observe the following:

- What do you notice about that person's feet? Are they noticeably different from this view?
- Do the kneecaps point forward? Do the knees collapse to the midline, are they straight, or do they bow to the side?
- Do the hips show rotation? How about the torso—any rotation there?
- Is one arm more anterior than the other? Where do the hands fall by the side?
- Are the shoulders still the same level?
- How about the person's head? What do you notice from this position?

Now take about five minutes to share the findings with the lookee, without judgment, then switch roles. If done as part of a group process, come together and ask, "Who had perfect posture?" You will find that almost everyone has some postural anomaly.

Asana Laboratory Observation

The yoga teacher-training asana laboratory is one of the most effective methods for learning to look at, see, and relate to students in the asana practice. Preparation for this exercise includes prior reading about the focus asana, study of its basic functional anatomy, alignment principles and subtle energetics, plus repeated practice in the asana. The basic method is to look separately at each of three or four "model" students—usually coparticipants in your teacher-training workshop—whose expressions of the selected asana display the different challenges typically found in a class of students: tightness, weakness, hypermobility, instability, misalignment, etc. Proceed as follows (here we use the example of Utthita Trikonasana):

- Honor your own needs for safety, comfort, and respect, and honor and support everyone else in feeling good about this exercise, commenting in a sensitive yet honest manner.

- Ask the model participant to come into the asana, reminding her that she can modify or come out of it at any time to take care of herself. Do not give any initial verbal cues, allowing her to guide herself into the asana. Encourage her to switch sides whenever she feels the need while trying to stay in it on each side as long as she comfortably can. If she modifies the positioning that you are expecting her to display (e.g., a hyperextended knee), cue her to move into that tendency to the extent that she feels comfortable.

- Take about a minute to observe the student, walking 360 degrees around her. Remember that asanas are an expression of unique human beings, not an ideal or static form or "pose."

- Bring your observation first to whatever is most at risk in the asana. While asking yourself what is happening there, ask the model participant how she feels in that part of her body.

Now look more comprehensively at the model student's entire expression of the asana:

- *Breath and general vibe:* How is she breathing? Does she look comfortable? Anxious? Balanced? Steady? At ease?

- *Feet and ankles:* How are they aligned? Is the front foot turned out ninety degrees? Does it appear that the feet are being rooted down? Where does the weight appear to be—inner foot, outer foot, balanced? Are the toes softly rooting or clinching? What is happening with the arches? Does pada bandha appear to be activated?

- *Knees:* Is the front kneecap aligned toward the center of the front foot? Is the knee bent into flexion or hyperextension? Is the kneecap actively lifted by the quadriceps? Is the back knee bent or hyperextended?

- *Pelvis:* Is it pitched forward in anterior rotation, back in posterior rotation, or close to neutral? Does she appear to be drawing the sitting bone of the front leg back and down as if toward the heel of the back foot?
- *Spine:* What is its position in the lumbar area as it extends from the pelvis? Is there an extreme lateral bend? Does there appear to be any compression in the spine? What curves do you see going up into the thoracic and cervical sections of the spine?
- *Rib cage:* Are the lower front ribs protruding out or softening in? Are the back ribs rounded? Are the upper side ribs protruding? What do these observations tell you about the spine?
- *Chest and collarbones:* Is the torso aligned straight out over the front leg, or is it leaning forward? Is the torso revolving open, lateral to the floor, or turned toward the floor? Is the chest expansive? Are the collarbones spreading away from each other?
- *Shoulders, arms, hands, and fingers:* Are the shoulder blades drawing down against the back ribs or tending to draw up toward the ears? Is the lower shoulder rolled forward or drawn back and down? Are the arms reaching out away from each other perpendicular to the floor? Are they fully extended? Are the elbows straight, bent, or hyperextended? Are the palms fully open and fingers fully extended?
- *Where is the model's energy?* Where does it appear she is applying herself with effort? Rooting down strongly from the tops of her thighbones down through her feet? Extending long through the spine and out through the top of the head? Radiating out from her heart center through her fingertips?

If you are facilitating this process with other teachers or trainees, this is an opportune time to address specific verbal cues and hands-on adjustments that reflect the observations. This process should include the sequencing of cues, how to combine verbal and physical cues, and where and how to demonstrate what you are cueing. Across the course of a teacher-training program, this can be done in round-robin style, with each participant taking turns giving what he or she sees as the most important cue, until the group has collectively guided the model student into and out of the asana. In debriefing this exercise, start with the model telling about his or her experience before repeating this exercise with a different student in the same asana.

Practice Teaching Observation

Guided practice teaching is an integral component of all strong teacher-training programs and an essential part of learning to see and guide students in their asana practice. Over the course of your training, you will ordinarily teach an increasing number of similar asanas, then more complex sequences that involve different asanas, and eventually a complete mock class.

Start by teaching a single asana to one other participant. Simulating the reality of an actual class, one partner takes the teacher role, and the other partner takes the student role. Using what you know (staying away from instructions you do not understand), guide your student into the asana. Go through the same process described above for asana laboratory observation, except that you are now observing *and* cueing. Start with purely verbal cues. As you become more comfortable in simultaneously observing and giving verbal cues, start to practice demonstrating while guiding your partner (we will cover demonstration below). Take your time (while honoring your partner's needs), staying attentive to what your partner is doing and giving verbal cues based on what you see and understand as the principles of the asana. Begin to weave verbal and physical cues together, always speaking to what you are encouraging with your physical cues.

As you progress from teaching one asana to one student to a few or several asanas to a small group, notice what happens to your observational practice, cues, and demonstrations. You will now experience seeing each student doing something slightly or very different from others in your group. Use this opportunity to hone your visual observation skills. Continue to give initial attention to the areas most at risk. Try to address those risks while maintaining your awareness of what is happening with others in your group. Notice the tendency to become so absorbed in something with one student that you momentarily lose sight and connection with everyone else. Here 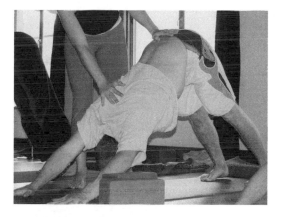 we come to a place where our personal practice of concentration and attention—being simultaneously focused and broadly aware—has tangible benefit in teaching.

Let your observational skills deepen as you progress into apprenticing and independent teaching. Apply them the moment you first meet and greet a new student. While not doing the comprehensive observation described above, notice the student's natural posture as you ask about his or her background. One benefit of bringing a class into Tadasana (Mountain Pose) at or toward the beginning of class is that it allows you to easily observe students' basic posture. Then expand your observation asana by asana. Notice how the tendencies evident in Tadasana likely manifest in more pronounced form as students move into more complex asanas. Use this observation to further refine your understanding of how different asanas increase the challenges seen in the more basic positions. Throughout this process of learning to see and relate to students, remember that you are teaching yoga, not trying to get people into poses. Keep coming back to the principle of yoga as a *practice of process,* not of attainment. Try to look at each student as the unique and beautiful person he or she is in the moment. Explore how you can share what you are seeing in a way that helps that student to see more easily and clearly and to feel his or her own body, breath, and practice. Remember the principle of sthira, sukham, asanam. Apply it to yourself while encouraging it in your students. Keep watching, keep breathing, feel your heart, and keep practicing your observational skills.

Learning Styles

The primary goal in teaching asanas is to enable students to perceive and understand more clearly what they are doing in developing a sustainable personal practice, whether in a class or independently. But there are many different ways of learning that require a varied approach to teaching. How people learn is closely tied to what educator Howard Gardner (1993) refers to as "qualities of multiple intelligence," which vary considerably in any given class of yoga students. In yoga classes, where the learning objectives include conceptual, emotional, physical, and metaphysical elements, the full range of multiple intelligences are in play. At the same time, a human being is more than his or her intellectual powers; motivation, personality, emotions, physical health, and personal will are more significant than a particular learning style in shaping how, where, and when one learns. This suggests that effective yoga instruction takes into account these variables in engaging with students while still appreciating the following learning styles:

- *Visual/spatial:* Tend to think in pictures and need vivid mental images to retain information, underlining the importance of demonstrating every asana.
- *Verbal/linguistic:* Tend to think in words rather than pictures and have highly developed auditory skills, thus needing clearly enunciated verbal descriptions of asanas.
- *Bodily/kinesthetic:* Process and remember information through interacting with the space around them and need to directly experience asanas.

- *Musically/rhythmically inclined:* Think in sounds, rhythms, and patterns and may be highly sensitive to environmental sounds. Can benefit from being encouraged to tune in more closely the sound and rhythm of their breath. They may also benefit from soft music that syncopates with the rhythm of a class.
- *Interpersonal:* Try to see things from other people's point of view; use both verbal and nonverbal cues to open up and maintain communication channels with others; need to feel a sense of genuine presence from their teacher in the learning process.
- *Intrapersonal:* Tend to be absorbed in trying to comprehend their feelings, dreams, relationships, strengths, and weaknesses; benefit from having more time and space to explore what an asana is about for them as they explore their practice.

VOICE AND LANGUAGE

Your voice and use of language are invaluable teaching tools. Considered from a chakra perspective, the voice manifests through the vishuddha chakra, which opens with ease and clarity when the body is grounded, the creative juices flowing, the willful center strong yet supple, the heart open, and the mind clear. How you speak as a teacher thus reflects where you are in your life, skills, and knowledge. Building from this natural foundation, there are several elements of voice to consider.

First and foremost, your voice should be sufficiently audible that everyone can hear you, yet not so loud that it interferes with students' attentiveness to the sound of their breath and sense of being in a tranquil space. If you choose to use music in your classes, control the volume of the music to be lower than you can comfortably project your own voice throughout the class. If you have a very soft voice or find yourself teaching very large classes, consider using amplification.

Explore how you can modulate your voice to match the mood or intensity of the asanas without resorting to a singsong quality of elocution. Your voice should flow along with the arc of the class, starting gently as students are warming into their bodies, reaching moderate crescendos accented by strength and dynamism as the practice moves through waves of intensity, softening and quieting as the class wanes toward Savasana. In a restorative class, try to maintain an even, relaxed tone that encourages letting go, allowing more space between statements so students can experience the freedom of silence.

Be aware of your tone of voice. Try recording and listening to one of your classes to become more aware of your tone. Many teachers are unaware that their voices sound a certain way. Speaking from your heart, let your technical instructions come across with the same even tonality as if you were speaking casually with a friend. At the same time, play with bringing enthusiasm and inspiration into your teaching through the current of your voice, balancing these qualities with assertiveness that tends more toward loving kindness than stern authority.

Language itself plays significantly in how students will hear and comprehend what you are saying. Try to use plain language that clearly describes what you intend to cue. It is usually much more effective to use direct, simple language than esoteric terms you learned studying anatomy, physiology, yoga philosophy, and psychology. Giving instructions in a concise manner is usually more effective in helping students to understand than flowery poetics or verbose statements. If you want your students to bring their feet together at the front of their mat, say, "Please bring your feet together at the front of your mat." That's all that's needed. Focus your initial cues on the basic foundational elements of the asana, saving more elaborate (yet still concise and specific) cues for the transition into the asana and refinements.

Different terms carry more or less weight. Verbs of action such as *press your fingers* or *breathe deeply* have more of a command quality than their noun forms, which tend to be more encouraging: *pressing your fingers* or *breathing deeply.* An even softer quality of instruction is expressed with terms like *feel, allow,* and *explore.* As a general approach, try offering the stronger verbs of action when cueing what you consider the most important foundational actions of an asana, then use softer language to cue refinements and inner exploration.

Using Sanskrit terms for asanas and other aspects of the practice is a matter of personal choice. You might feel that Sanskrit does not resonate well with your students (or with your employer or you), or you might feel that using Sanskrit lends to a deeper feeling of authenticity in your teachings as you anchor your expressions in the ancient and traditional language of yoga. If you choose to use Sanskrit, try also to give the English terms for the words. For example, say, "Preparing for Ardha Chandrasana, Half-Moon Pose, please...." Some Sanskrit terms have become so ubiquitous in yoga classes that they have now entered the English lexicon: *Chaturanga* (short for *Chaturanga Dandasana*) is surely more familiar to most students than its English translation, "Four-Limbed Staff Pose." As with other aspects of your teaching, play around with this to find what is most comfortable for you and your students.

BASIC ELEMENTS OF ASANA PRACTICE

Asana practice is a process for being present in the moment with an abiding sense of freedom and wholeness that brings about an experience of being fully alive, energized, and in bliss. As a practice of self-transformation, yoga asanas give us a set of tools for untying the binding knots that create patterns of holding and stagnation deep in our being. Joel Kramer (1980, 13) claims that this artful practice "lies in learning how to focus and generate energy into different parts of the body, in listening to the body's messages (feedback), and in surrendering to where the body leads you." On the one hand it is a practice involving physical precision, yet on the other, as Dona Holleman (1999, 22) explains, it has a "poetic side, where the body loses its sharp division line between it and the surrounding space, and the asana

becomes part of the unified field, the continuum of space/time in which we all have our being." The art of teaching the asana practice is one of guiding students into an expanding awareness of this process of doing yoga.

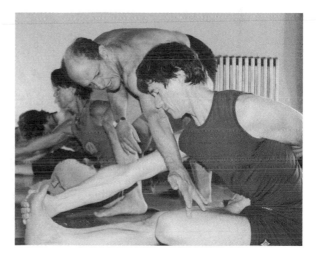

When thinking about asana, we can identify a variety of important essential elements: being present, relaxing, breathing, rooting, stabilizing, aligning, moving, and energetically engaging. But when expressed in an integrated practice—that is, when doing yoga—these elements are not separable but are part of the whole of practice. While the practice is one of movement into these qualities, we also begin with these qualities, gradually honing and refining them through the practice.

Being Present

In Aldous Huxley's utopian novel *Island* (1962), shipwrecked journalist Will Farnaby washes up on the fictional Palanese coast, a Westerner whose cluttered mind is far from aware of where he is, let alone "what is what." Scaling the isolated island's jungle-covered cliffs, the words "attention, attention" and "here and now, boys, here and now" echo from different directions. His adventure will eventually lead him to discover that the voice belongs to a particularly adept tropical bird chanting the mantras at the heart of Pala's tantra-Taoist-Buddhist-ecological culture.

As Ram Dass would later title a popular 1970s book, the idea to "be here now" is the starting point of asana practice, focusing one's attention fully and directly on what is happening in the moment—in this place, this body, this breath, this sensation.

Relaxing

The intensity of many styles of yoga asana practice can seem anything but relaxing because of the effort that is required to do certain asanas or asana sequences. This common dissociation of effort and ease, rather than their integration, arises primarily from the idea of relaxation being conflated with letting the body go completely limp. In the context of the asana practice, relaxation means letting go of nervous tension while maintaining the active engagement of whatever muscular and energetic action is required in maintaining the integrity of alignment. In releasing nervous tension, students can work strongly with willful determination while integrating effort and ease in a manner that allows the body to open in a stable way during asanas.

The integration of effort and ease in the expansion and deepening of bodily awareness takes practice. The key is in bringing awareness to the totality of the body, exploring what it takes to support the skeletal structure without straining. Encouraging students to use their even flow of ujjayi pranayama and bodily reactions such as pain and shaking as barometers of strain, you can guide students into the process of "playing the edge," discussed below. Because the tendency is to work the more superficial muscles most intensely, the deep muscles closest to and most capable of supporting the joints are not appropriately engaged. Using the breath to draw awareness more deeply into the body, students can begin to feel how they can activate the deep muscles while allowing the more superficial muscles to release unnecessary tension. Expanding their awareness from the activated deep muscles to the surface of their skin, students will begin to feel how they can play with varying degrees of engagement throughout their body, working as strongly as they can while being as relaxed as possible at the same time. Guide your students toward a feeling of expanding their body from the inside out, cultivating spaciousness, levity, and a sense of transparency that allows the free flow of energy.

Breathing

Breathing consciously is at once the most important part of asana practice and often the most elusive. The breath fuels and guides the asana practice yet tends to disappear from our awareness amid everything else that is happening, including the natural tendency to lose focus and allow attention to drift away from the here and now. We can see the emphasis on breath in asana practice in the Yoga Sutras immediately following Patanjali's definition of *asana* as "sthira sukham asanam," and in his use of the word *prayatna,* which is typically translated literally as "effort." But as Srivatsa Ramaswami (2000, 95–96) points out, prayatna is of three types, one of which, *jivana prayatna,* refers to "efforts made by the individual to maintain life and,

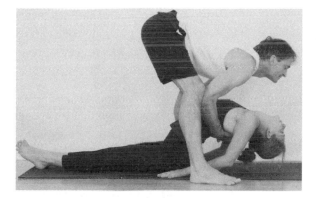

more especially, breathing." The point is to explore asana practice through the steadiness and ease of the breath, continuously connecting the breath with the body and mind.

Foundation: Grounding and Radiating with Lines of Energy

When casually standing or sitting, the tendency is to connect passively with the earth. The effect is that the body collapses into itself, each joint compressing as the body slumps and sags. But the moment you consciously root down into whatever is on the floor, the immediate effect is creation of space in the body. Referred to as the "rebounce effect" by Dona Holleman (1999, 26), this relationship between roots and extension is an expression of the "normal force"[1] explained by Isaac Newton's Third Law of Motion: for every action there is an equal and opposite reaction. To the extent that you apply effort through intentional muscular action—for example, pressing down more firmly through your feet and into the floor when standing—the "equal and opposite reaction" of energy drawing up the body occurs. Emphasizing the application of consciousness in the discovery of foundational elements in each asana, yoga teacher Chuck Miller has referred to this as the intention of seeking the origin of every action. In rooting down we naturally stimulate muscular engagement and manifest space through the joints, particularly through the spine, creating the foundation of structural stability and ease that is increasingly important as students move into more and more advanced asanas.[2] The specific point or points vary in the different asanas, but the practice of establishing and exploring from the basis of this foundation is consistent throughout all the asanas.

While maintaining this initial foundation, students can find further stability and ease in asanas by consciously applying what Joel Kramer (1980, 19) coined as "lines of energy."[3] Bringing conscious effort to the radiation of neuromuscular effort (or "current," in Kramer's terms) through the body creates lines of energy. By radiating out from the core to the periphery, these lines of energy expand your body from the inside out in every direction, creating spaciousness while maintaining the stability that is created by drawing the body's muscular support system to the skeletal structure.[4] Consciously running lines of energy through the body is a way of accentuating the principle of roots and extension. This technique can be variously applied by students in exploring the level of intensity that is appropriate in their personal practice, listening to the body-breath-mind for feedback that suggests when, where, and how intensely to move energy through their body. Remind students that it is not important how far they go in an asana; rather, keep them focused on *how* they go, cultivating steadiness and ease as they explore the relative intensity of asanas that are simultaneously grounded and expansive.

TABLE 6.1—**Roots and Extension**

FOUNDATION	PRINCIPLES AND VERBAL CUES	ASANA EXAMPLES
Hands	• When the palms are on the floor, instruct students to spread their fingers as wide as they comfortably can, their thumbs not quite so wide (about one-third less than maximum) in order to prevent injury in the thenar space between the thumb and index finger.[1] • Radiating out from the center of the palm through the knuckles and tips of each finger and thumb, students should root down firmly through all of their knuckles, the entire span of their palms, and through the entire length of each finger and thumb. • From this rootedness, ask students to create a feeling of drawing up energetically from the inner palm through the inner wrist and up through the arms and into the shoulders.[2] • It is important to root the knuckles of the index fingers and thumbs in order to balance the pressure across the entire span of the palms and create a balanced foundation for stability and space through the wrists.	Adho Mukha Svanasana (Down Dog) Adho Mukha Vrksasana (Handstand) Chaturanga Dandasana (Four-Limbed Staff Pose)
Feet	• Balance the weight equally through the "four corners" of each foot. • Root more firmly down into the inner edge of the balls of the feet to more fully awaken and lift the inner arches and ankles. • Spread the toes wide and press them down without clinching.	All standing asanas

FOUNDATION	PRINCIPLES AND VERBAL CUES	ASANA EXAMPLES
Sitting bones	• In all seated asanas, the primary initial action is to root down firmly into the sitting bones, emphasizing the front portion of the sitting bones rooting more firmly down as a means of cultivating a neutral pelvic tilt. • Do *not* pull the flesh of the buttocks away from the sitting bones.[3] • Create a subtle feeling of drawing the sitting bones toward each other to stimulate the light contraction of the transverse peroneus muscles and thereby awaken mula bandha. • Try to maintain the connection of the sitting bones into the floor when folding forward and/or twisting.	Tadasana (Mountain Pose) Paschimottanasana (Seated Forward Bend)
Legs	• When the legs are straight, run a strong line of energy from the tops of the thighbones down through the legs, ankles, and the center of the heels. Do this whether sitting or standing, whether with the legs together (as in Tadasana) or apart (as in Prasarita Padottanasana). • Create a feeling of drawing the musculature of the legs into the bones of the legs, while spiraling the inner thighs down (if sitting) or back (if standing in internally rotated standing asanas).	Dandasana (Staff Pose) Upavista Konasana (Wide-Angle Forward Bend)
Arms	• With the shoulder blades spiraling out away from the spine while rooted down against the back ribs, integrate the arms into the torso. • Extend strongly from the top of the arm bones down through the arms, elbows, and wrists into the hands and out through the fingertips. • Drawing the musculature of the arms evenly to the bone, energetically draw energy up through the arms.	Adho Mukha Svanasana (Down Dog) Adho Mukha Vrksasana (Handstand)
Head	• Maintaining the natural curvature of the cervical spine, press the top of the head (corona capitis) firmly into the floor without grinding the head down.	Sirsasana I (Headstand)

[1] Spreading the thumb as wide out as possible often strains the flexor tendon and first lumbrical muscle in the thenar space between the thumb and index finger.

[2] Holleman (1999, 44) offers a detailed discussion of hasta bandha.

[3] The all-too-common instruction to pull the flesh of the buttocks out does indeed create a stronger feeling of rooting the sitting bones, but in all forward bends this is at the expense of significantly greater risk of straining the hamstrings, the attachments of which are in the sitting bones (the ischial tuberosities). The hamstrings are most vulnerable to tearing at precisely these attachments. Keeping the flesh in its natural place will direct the stretch more into the bodies of the hamstrings without compromising the rooting of the sitting bones into the floor.

Aligning into Balanced Integration

In Chapter Seven we will look closely at the specific alignment principles for individual asanas. Here we will consider general principles that apply in guiding alignment in all asanas that are, as stressed throughout this book, not something that students assume mechanically but rather involve a mindful process of balanced integration. While you can teach your students technique and provide them with sound biomechanical alignment principles in the individual asanas along with kinesiological principles of movement, the quality of balanced integration is one that your students will begin to feel and develop through their personal practice. In guiding this process, be aware that the complexity and diversity of students' bodies requires refinements in which individual variation is often more important than the application of any universal principles of alignment. Rather than seeing this as a practice of deepening complexity, encourage it as a practice of refining simplicity in which students come into more subtle awareness of steadiness and ease that takes form around the integrity of their heart-centered intention and their breath.

Applying the concepts of grounding-radiating, roots-extension, and lines of energy discussed above, we can identify several actions in which the body is moving in opposite directions. This is an essential part of both foundation and refinement in the asanas, simultaneously creating space, easing pressure in the joints, and allowing the freer and more conscious movement of subtle energy. Oppositional movements, or dual actions, are guided through linked instructions that cue students into an alignment that creates balance, stability, and unification in the body. These oppositions, including front-back, upper-lower, inside-outside, left-right, and center-periphery,[5] are an essential element of every asana and movement, ensuring through these natural connections the integration of the entire body in each asana rather than experiencing the body as a set of fragmented parts. See Table 6.2, pages 132–133.

Supporting the process of cultivating unification in the body, your alignment instructions should begin with the outer form of the asana that addresses the biomechanical aspects of the pose as informed by your understanding of functional anatomy. These initial instructions give students the basic positioning of their outer body in the asana, creating the initial space in which they can then be cued in exploring qualities of inner alignment that create deeper harmony in their experience of body, breath, and mind.

Energetic Awareness

Stabilizing and balancing the body leads to a natural deepening of ease as students explore and discover a feeling of dynamic symmetry in their body-mind. Here we want to encourage students to sense how they can apply themselves with full energetic engagement while remaining as relaxed as possible. Practicing strongly yet simply and softly to stabilize the body increasingly brings about a sense of effortlessness amid the unique way that each individual asana presents itself to a student. Moving more and more into a sense of effortless ease, encourage students to tune in to the more subtle flow of energy through the whole of their body. Depending on the asana, you can cue your students to bring this awareness into different areas of the body where holding or tension tend to manifest, to different chakras, or to the overall experience of being as an expression of subtle energy itself.

Vinyasa: Moving into Synchronicity

Yoga asana practice becomes a practice of movement meditation when the continuous flow of body, breath, and mind are consciously synchronized, refined, and unified. This is the art of vinyasa, first introduced in the summary of the Vinyasa Flow style of Hatha yoga in Chapter Two. There we noted that the term *vinyasa* means "to place in a special way" (from *nyasa,* "to place," and the prefix *vi,* "in a special way"). This aspect of asana practice applies in every style and form of Hatha yoga, across the continuum of relatively "still" forms like Iyengar and yin yoga to "flow" forms like Ashtanga Vinyasa and Vinyasa Flow. It is expressed amid the relative stillness of a held asana as much as in a flowing movement from one asana to another.

This point can be somewhat confusing to students if only because yoga is also a practice of moving into stillness. However, in the context of asana practice, we are always moving, even when holding an asana: the breath is flowing, the heart is beating, indeed, all of the natural physiological processes of the human body are in motion, even if slowing. When students open their awareness to this reality of natural and conscious movement in the asana practice, they can create the space—mentally, physically, emotionally, and spiritually —that allows the body-mind to move more easily into a sense of stillness, thereby accentuating the deepening experience of yoga as a practice of spiritual awakening, unification, and bliss.

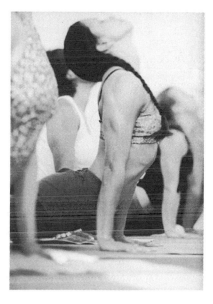

The essential quality of vinyasa in asana practice is precise synchronization of breath-body-mind within and between the asanas. Sustaining the flow of breath, conscious movement into and out of each asana is initiated with the inhale or exhale, the completion of each asana found with the completion of each cycle of breath, creating

TABLE 6.2—**Balanced Alignment Cues**

OPPOSITIONAL BALANCES	UNIFYING VERBAL CUES	ASANA EXAMPLES [1]
FRONT-BACK		
Feet	"Root down equally through your heels and the balls of your feet."	All standing asanas
Lower legs	"Draw your shins back while releasing your calves toward your heels."	All standing asanas
Knees	"Engage your quadriceps muscles, lifting your kneecaps while spreading the backs of your knees."	Tadasana
Thighs	"Press the tops of your thighs back while spreading evenly through your hamstrings."	Utthita Trikonasana
Pelvis	"Draw your pubic bone back and up while drawing your tailbone back and down."	Adho Mukha Svanasana
	"Lift the front of your hips away from your front leg while lightly drawing your lower belly and sacrum toward each other."	Virabhadrasana I
Spine	"Expand your lower back ribs while allowing your lower front ribs to soften in."	Virabhadrasana II
Shoulders	"Allow your shoulder blades to release down your back while spreading across your collarbones."	Tadasana
Neck/head	"Draw your chin very slightly forward, down, and in while spreading across the back of your neck."	Adho Mukha Svanasana
UPPER-LOWER		
Pada/mula bandha	"Rooting evenly through your feet while lifting your inner arches, spiral your inner thighs back while drawing your sitting bones toward each other and lifting steadily from the front floor of your pelvis with mula bandha."	All standing asanas
		All inversions
		All backbends
Feet/hips	"Root down from the tops of your femurs through your feet and into the earth while engaging pada bandha and drawing the muscular energy in your legs in and up."	Parsvottanasana
Pelvis/spine	"Maintaining a feeling of pelvic neutrality and mula bandha, energetically draw up tall through your spine."	Utkatasana
Shoulders/fingers	"Lightly hugging your shoulder blades to your back ribs, radiate out through your arms and fingertips."	Urdhva Hastasana

OPPOSITIONAL BALANCES	UNIFYING VERBAL CUES	ASANA EXAMPLES [1]
UPPER-LOWER		
Mula bandha/palate	"Aware of mula bandha, feel a sense of energy drawing up through your spine and lending a quality of light lifting and spreading of your palate."	Padmasana
Mula bandha/ corona capitis	"Staying with mula bandha, lengthen from the base of your spine out through the crown of your head."	Dandasana
Pada bandha/ corona capitis	"Connecting with the earth, feel the awakening of your feet and inner arches as a source of energy up through the midline of your body and out through the crown of your head."	Tadasana
INSIDE-OUTSIDE		
Feet	"While rooting the outer edge of your back foot, keep grounding through the ball of your foot."	Utthita Trikonasana
Ankles	"Bring the inner and outer anklebones level and centered between the foot and leg."	All standing asanas
Knees	"Relaxing through your hips and inner thighs, bend your knees and draw your feet together while maintaining a sense of even pressure through the inside and outside of your knees."	Baddha Konasana
Legs	"Cultivating pada bandha, spiral your inner thighs back while energetically drawing your shins toward each other."	Tadasana
Pelvis	"Spiraling your inner thighs back to create spaciousness in your sacrum, draw the outside of your hips in toward the core of your body, feeling an accentuated lift of your perineum."	Tadasana
		Dandasana
		Urdhva Dhanurasana
Spine	"Engaging mula bandha, visualize and consciously feel energy drawing into the core of your spine while radiating out from your spine through the sides of your torso."	All asanas
Shoulders	"Drawing your shoulder blades in against your back ribs, spiral your shoulder blades out away from your spine."	Adho Mukha Svanasana
Arms	"Spiraling your inner forearms toward the floor while rooting firmly across the entire span of your palms and out through your fingers, spiral your shoulder blades out away from your spine as if to wrap the triceps side of your arms out and down toward the floor."	Adho Mukha Svanasana

[1] These are representative, not exhaustive, examples. See Chapter Seven for details on each asana.

an unbroken "mandala" of asanas around the continuous rhythmic flow of the breath. As we will see later in this chapter, this leads to a clear pattern of verbal cues in guiding students in their practice as each movement cue is associated with a phase of the breath. We will return to breath-movement cues and transitions in the following section on instructing asanas.

The vinyasa process centers around the steady flow of ujjayi pranayama. Whether transitioning from one asana to another or exploring within the relative stillness of a held asana, guide students to adjust their body movement around the rhythm and integrity of their breath. Every breath is a vinyasa in and of itself. Consciously breathing throughout the practice, each inhale and exhale creates a new space for exploring the relationship between the breath and body, breath and mind, body and mind. Giving primacy to the breath, encourage students to adapt and adjust the movement of their body to allow the breath to flow smoothly and steadily, connecting breath to body-mind as asanas take form around the integrity of the breath.

While staying present in the moment throughout the asana practice, vinyasa also calls on what came before just as it anticipates whatever is next. Thus the vinyasa aspect of practice is one of relationship as the asanas are linked seamlessly together into a set of complete and coherent sequences combining a set of interrelated asanas. The vinyasa of one asana leads to the next, which leads to the next, creating an entire practice. The actual sequencing, informed by basic principles of vinyasa krama (see Chapter Ten), varies depending on the class, with combinations of sequences brought together to form a complete class.

INSTRUCTING ASANAS

The central irony and challenge of teaching yoga is that the essence and mechanisms of yoga asana practice are purely internal and largely invisible to you as a teacher. How a student feels in an asana is his or her principal source of instruction and refinement. What he or she does in an asana to explore that refinement ultimately relies on internal mechanisms of feeling, reflection, and action, including intention, attention, the breath, and the body with its many springs and levers of movement. Thus your role as a teacher is somewhat limited, relying as it does on your ability to give clear instructions about the breath, alignment, energetic actions, variations, modifications, use of props, risks, and techniques for finding greater ease and stability in each asana and transition. Since every student is different, your effectiveness depends on your ability to give both general guidance to a class and individualized suggestions that address the unique experiences of different students. Your ability to see and hear students in their practice—including challenges to their alignment, the qualities of their stability and ease, their attentiveness—and then to relate to them meaningfully and appropriately based on your perception and understanding are the keys to your effectiveness in instructing the asana practice.

Working with this reality, it is important to teach asanas sensitively and systematically. This begins with acknowledging your own personal abilities and limitations, then committing yourself to teaching what you know from experience. Before instructing an asana, you should know what you will teach and how you will teach it, including at least the basic alignment principles and energetic actions, stage-by-stage verbal cues that clearly guide students into and out of the asana, methods of demonstration, alternative forms of the asana, physical cues, and the use of props to support students in most safely and deeply exploring the asana. Your years of practice, intensive study, teacher training, apprenticing, and practice teaching now all come together, fully incorporated into your personal practice and transferred from there onto your teaching palette.

Before teaching an asana to your class, teach it to yourself first. Do the asana over and over, testing what you think you know and playing around with what you understand as its basic principles. Then do the same for a sequence of asanas, experimenting with the effects of different sequences and ways of transitioning. Put together the sequences into an entire class, then do the class on your own, giving yourself silent verbal cues throughout to develop and hone the narrative overlay to your class. Go through each of these steps teaching your friends or family, practicing again and again to refine your skills and knowledge. Reflect on what seems to flow easily and not so easily for you, gradually integrating more and more knowledge into your practice teaching. Focus more on the asanas you find most challenging in your own practice and those that seem most difficult to explain throughout your career as a teacher, continuously refining your knowledge and skills.

Positioning and Demonstration

Earlier in this chapter we discussed how to begin your class, including where to position yourself in the room when demonstrating asanas. Demonstration is a very important part of the instructional and learning process, particularly for your more visually oriented students. There are two basic types of demonstration:

- *In-the-flow demonstration:* Here you or an assistant will model what you are instructing as you are saying it, giving students a live example of what you are asking them to do as they are doing it. Ideally, you will mirror the class, facing them from a place where they all see you and vice versa, then demonstrating as if they are looking into a mirror (i.e., your left foot turns out when you say, "Please turn your right foot out."). This is an essential skill for all flow-type classes and one that is useful in all styles of Hatha yoga, allowing your students to see what you are asking them to do without interrupting their practice.

- *Gather-around demonstration:* Here you pause the flow of the class and ask students to gather around you or an assistant to observe an asana. This allows you to provide more detailed instruction and demonstration while students can more closely observe the various elements of an asana as you demonstrate and explain it to the class.

Generally, do in-the-flow demonstrations to cue the initial movement visually into each asana throughout the class. Depending on the nature of the class—primarily the steadiness of the flow and the students' level of proficiency with the asanas—you can devote more or less time to this initial visual cue. With more beginning classes that move more slowly, give slower demonstrations that more fully highlight the alignment and risk-reduction elements of the asana, even when in the flow of the practice. With more advanced classes, you might give the visual demonstration in the span of a single breath, instructing the class to stay with the asana as you begin to move around and observe students in their practice.

Try positioning yourself where everyone can most easily see you, initially on your mat, but throughout the class wherever your visual line with the most students is most open (see Chapter Five for a discussion of space and positioning). From the first asana, demonstrate exactly what you are asking your class to do. For example, say, "Stepping your feet together at the front of your mat, please draw your palms

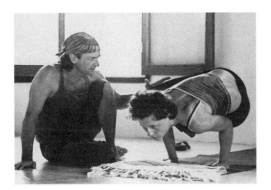

together at your heart." While saying these words, do exactly that in a slightly dramatic fashion that captures the students' attention and effectively conveys what you are asking them to do, matching verbal cues with your physical movements. As the class progresses into more complex asanas, continue to show how to move into each asana, emphasizing how the breath initiates and guides the movement of the body.

While workshops are the likeliest place you will give elaborate gather-around demonstrations, it benefits students when you pause the flow from time to time to focus on a single asana or small number of linked asanas.[6] When using the gather-around method, do the following:

- Position yourself in the middle of the room, and ask everyone to gather in to see you.

- Encourage the class to move around during the demonstration so that they can observe from different vantage points.

- Explain what you are about to do, and very briefly demonstrate the final pose or the short sequence while explaining what you are doing and noting any significant risks. For example, if demonstrating Bakasana (Crane Pose) from Sirsasana II (Tripod Headstand), come to all fours (discuss the wrists), place your head down on the floor (discuss placement and alignment of the head, neck, and shoulders), slide your feet in (discuss changes in the foundation and spine), extend your legs overhead into Sirsasana II (offer alternatives, including one leg, bent knees, both legs together), draw your knees to your shoulders (address core and lower back), elevate into Bakasana (highlight shifting the weight, pada bandha, and mula bandha), release your head back to the floor (reiterate neck alignment), return to Sirsasana II (address lower back and neck), and return to all fours or Balasana (Child's Pose).

- Repeat the same demonstration, this time pausing stage by stage to explain in detail the alignment, energetic actions, modifications, variations, and use of props for the asana. Speak as clearly as you can, staying with the essentials of the asana(s) and giving only three or four main points for each.

- Be particularly clear about the gradual and successive movements of the body while transitioning into the asana, holding it and transitioning out (all are addressed below).

- After the demonstration, ask for questions. Ask the students if anything was unclear to them. Further prompt questions by asking about specific aspects of the asana, including transitions in and out.

- When students return to their mats, guide them through the same sequence of steps while moving around the room to offer individualized guidance and support.

Transitioning into Asanas

Frequently reminding students to stay present, stay with their breath, and relax, begin your instruction of every asana by succinctly explaining its initial foundation. This includes the initial alignment of the body prior to coming into the asana, focusing on whatever is (a) most connected to the floor and (b) most immediately relevant to the spine and any associated risks. From the foundation, explain the other elements of the asana while guiding the class into it stage by stage. Depending on the style of Hatha yoga and the level and intention of the class, the methods of transition will vary to some degree. For example, in some styles such as Iyengar yoga, standing asanas are generally approached from Tadasana, while in flow-oriented classes such as Vinyasa Flow, most standing asanas are approached from Downward-Facing Dog Pose or directly from another standing asana.

Allowing ample time to guide your class clearly into each asana will help ensure that each student comprehends your instructions in both the mind and the body. Your exercising of patience and speaking with clarity will allow your students to feel more comfortable in gradually establishing the various elements of the asana. By encouraging more conscious transitioning into the asanas, students will more deeply appreciate the importance of paying attention to what they are doing and will move with more refined awareness. The effect of this more conscious transitioning will be the safer exploration and refinement of students' asana practices.

Refining Asanas: Individualizing Instruction

Asanas are always alive and evolving with every breath. As students tune in to what they feel in an asana, they have the opportunity to explore the deepening of their experience in it—stretching more or less, applying more or less effort, cultivating simpler balance, involving different parts of their bodies in varying ways, smoothing out the breath, consciously awakening and moving energy, opening their spiritual heart to more subtle awareness. In a student's personal practice, he or she might constantly be present to all these elements, practicing pratyahara and dharana.

As a teacher, you can encourage and guide this process of self-reflection and refinement by suggesting attentiveness to these elements of refinement along with giving specific suggestions for modification based on your observation. Indeed, your guidance on refinement, including modifications, began when you initially guided students into an asana, your verbal cues always deriving in part from what you are observing in the moment. Once students are in an asana, you will have plenty of new insight that lends to more specific guidance. This starts with keen, appreciative, systematic observation. Beginning from the initial setting of the foundation of the asana, your verbal cues will increasingly reflect your observation of the entire class and individual students as you teach to what you are observing.

You can now apply the observational skills discussed earlier in this chapter in the reality of an actual class. After guiding students into an asana, pause and notice what they are actually doing. The relative attentiveness, understanding, body intelligence, muscle strength and flexibility, bone structure, and other factors will result in often tremendous variation in how different students appear in the asana. Looking closely, what do you see? Look at the student from her foundation to her spine to her breath to her face to her limbs, observing from different angles to notice what might be more or less obvious from the front, back, and different sides. Does she appear stable? Relaxed? How is her breath flowing? Does her face appear relaxed or tense? Are her eyes soft and focused, or hard and shifting? Does she appear balanced? Is she making occasional large adjustments in position, or smaller adjustments synchronized with her breath? What is your overall impression? What do you first notice, especially in relationship to what is most at risk in the asana? What one or two simple modifications do you think will most benefit the student's sense of stability, ease, balance, and happiness in the asana? Has she followed the initial alignment instructions? Does it appear that she is consciously grounding and radiating? What parts of her body appear actively involved in the asana? Do you see where she might benefit from applying more or less effort to create more stability, ease, and space?

Based on your observations, give more specific instructions. Be clear in directing instructions to the entire class versus to an individual student or subset of students. For example, in Triangle Pose, some students will likely hyperextend the knee of their front leg. Instructing the entire class, you can say, "Rooting down strongly from the top of your leg and down through your feet, keep awakening the muscles in your legs, engaging your quadriceps and feeling your kneecap lifting." Addressing those with hyperextension in their knee, continue by saying, "If you tend to hyperextend your knee, try to microbend it and maintain that 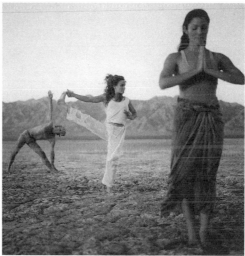 positioning while still trying to engage your quads." If you are addressing a single student with specific instructions, either go directly to that student to work with him or her (observe, give verbal cues, give hands-on cues, offer a prop) or say the person's name from a distance to ensure that it is clear the specific instruction is for that student only. Ideally, you will give more individualized verbal cues quietly to just that student.

When holding an asana for a relatively long duration, you can introduce a variety of instructions to cue a deeper refinement. In Chapter Seven we will cover specific alternatives you can offer to students in modifying asanas, including adaptations and use of props to accommodate physical limitations and injuries as well as exploration of more challenging variations. Here are a few examples, each of which assumes that the class is ready to go deeper and that individual student modifications have been addressed:

TABLE 6.3—**Examples of Deeper Refining Cues**

Tadasana (Mountain Pose)	"Maintaining pada bandha, feel the awakening of your inner thighs, slightly spiraling them back, and from there a feeling of lightly drawing your sitting bones toward each other, awakening a sense of mula bandha as you lift lightly and steadily from your perineum, energetically lifting from the floor of your pelvis up through your spine, expanding across your heart center and lengthening out through the crown of your head."
Uttanasana (Standing Forward Bend)	"While rooting through your feet and feeling the rebounding effect as your legs engage, feel your sitting bones extending up. Now try to create a feeling of pitching your pubic bone more back and up while stretching your belly button toward your heart, your heart toward the earth."
Urdhva Mukha Svanasana (Upward-Facing Dog Pose)	"Inhaling into Upward-Facing Dog, create a feeling of pulling your spine through toward your chest, lifting and spreading across your collarbones while drawing your shoulder blades down and in against your back ribs; exhaling, engage from your belly to lift your hips up and back to Downward-Facing Dog, your pubic bone leading the way."
Adho Mukha Svanasana (Downward-Facing Dog Pose)	"While pressing firmly and evenly down through your palms and fingers, try to engage your legs more fully, pressing the tops of your thighbones strongly back to cultivate more length through your spine."
Virabhadrasana I (Warrior I Pose)	"Keeping the outer edge of your back foot firmly rooting down, try to maintain a feeling of pelvic neutrality while spiraling the inner thigh of your back leg strongly back. Feel from that strong foundation more openness in your lower back, breath by breath consciously lengthening up through your spine. Try to keep your lower front ribs softening in to help maintain the natural curvature of your spine while stretching strongly up and back through your arms and fingertips."
Virabhadrasana II (Warrior II Pose)	"Without moving either of your feet, imagine your mat is covered with warm honey and ghee. How would you maintain your stability? Bring more awareness into your feet. Without actually moving them, create an energetic action of drawing your feet toward each other. Feel this more fully awaken the muscles in the inside of your legs, and from there feel a more natural and full awakening of mula bandha, all the while breathing and creating more and more space through your spine and across your heart center as you run lines of energy out through your fingertips and the crown of your head."
Ardha Chandrasana (Revolved Half-Moon Pose)	"Exploring wrapping, please either stay as you are, or, being attentive to keeping your left hip revolved on top of your right hip, change as little as possible in reaching back with your left hand to clasp your left foot. Honoring your intention and your lower back, explore either pulling that foot back away from your hip, or,

if you have the flexibility in your hips and shoulder, explore placing your hand on your foot in a Bhekasana (Frog Pose) position, then press your left foot toward your left hip. See if you can clamp your left hip with that same hand. If that is easy and you feel stable, begin to explore clasping that foot with both hands, and balance on just your standing leg."

Sirsasana I (Headstand I)	"Without gripping in your belly, feel the light, subtle engagement of your belly with each and every exhale, feeling with it a sense of more stability yet spaciousness through your pelvis and spine. Maintaining that awareness, stability, and spaciousness, begin to explore slowly lowering your legs halfway down toward the floor while running lines of energy out through your legs and through the balls of your feet. Go only so far down as you feel stable and free of strain. Try to hold for up to five breaths before slowly extending your legs back up overhead, all the while extending from the crown of your rooted head up through your spine and out through your feet."

Pacing and Holding Asanas

There is no correct pace for Hatha yoga classes. Nor is there a correct duration for holding or transitioning between individual asanas. Yet pace and duration are important considerations in the practice, giving character to a class and making it more or less accessible or challenging. While we ultimately want to develop a personal practice in which we follow our inner teacher in the yoga process, pace and duration are two of the central qualities of any class.

Many years ago, feeling the pressure of a time conflict, I raced through a Second Series Ashtanga Vinyasa practice in just over an hour, breathing quickly and holding some of the asanas for less than the traditional five breaths. Ordinarily I would take around two hours for the same set of asanas. The next day my teacher commented about the pace and suggested that I try doing a practice at the other extreme. I took more than three hours to do the same series of asanas, stretching my breath and sometimes holding the asanas longer than usual. The difference between the two practices was profound, planting another seed of playfulness in my practice that blossomed into a deeper commitment to exploring yoga with an open mind and intuitive body rather than always following preconceived prescriptions.

"Pace" refers to the temporal flow and intensity of a class, including the time and activity between asanas. In some Hatha yoga styles such as Ashtanga Vinyasa, the pace is partially given by a specific structure of the practice: each breath is connected to a movement in or out of an asana, most asanas are held for exactly five breaths, and many asanas are connected by a vinyasa sequence that involves pressing up from sitting and essentially moving through Tolasana and Lolasana to

Chaturanga, then to Upward-Facing Dog and Downward-Facing Dog before floating through usually to sitting in preparation for, or directly into, the next asana. This is a very intense, essentially nonstop practice of connecting ujjayi pranayama to movement within and between the asanas until resting in Savasana. In a restorative class, you might do as few as five or six asanas in ninety minutes, focusing on deep relaxation and integration. There are several factors to consider in pacing a class:

- *Basic considerations:* Start with basic elements—being present, staying with the breath, relaxing. Go slow enough to maintain the integrity of these elements. With newer students and in basic classes, further slow the pace to give more time for exploration, questions, and to allow students to feel the effects of each asana. It is OK if students in beginning classes take two or more breaths to complete a movement that might ordinarily be done with a single breath. In introductory classes, go even slower, frequently pausing to assess for understanding and encourage questions. With experienced students and flow-oriented classes, pace the class a little faster, yet slow enough to encourage attentiveness, expansive breathing, steadiness, and ease amid the greater physical exertion.

- *Class definition:* If a class is described on a schedule as "Level 1 Gentle Flow," this suggests a slower pace than one described as "Level 3 Power Yoga." The more basic class might also be scheduled for a shorter overall time period, perhaps an hour rather than ninety minutes to two hours.

- *Student ability:* With more experienced students, gradually maintain a steady pace free of breaks between asana sequences. Yet with even the most experienced students, you can create the space for deepening the practice inestimably by offering moments to pause, feel, reflect, renew intention, and feel the full integration of the experience. Note that a common misunderstanding among teachers and students alike is the notion that a fast pace is somehow more challenging and "advanced." Moving slowly and consciously with smooth and spacious ujjayi pranayama is actually more physically (and mentally and emotionally) challenging than the extremely fast-paced "yoga-robics" type classes. Encourage all students to make the steady flow of the breath more important than getting right into an asana; encourage them to move with their breath, not your words—and to take as many breaths as needed for them to transition safely and comfortably.

- *Class theme:* If it is the summer solstice and you are teaching a heart-opening intensive, this suggests keeping the class moving to help students stay warm as you offer sequences to open the quads, hip flexors, spinal erectors, and shoulder girdle. A winter solstice class focusing on heart-openers could move much more slowly, tapping into deep release more than internal warmth to prepare the body for expansive backbends.

- *Time constraints:* Many classes offered at gyms are scheduled for less than an hour. In this situation you can either teach fewer asanas or increase the tempo. These are good classes to offer "homework" assignments, encouraging students to do certain sequences on their own outside of class. Regardless of the time you have, ensure that the pace feels comfortable to you and your students. Always save at least five minutes for Savasana.

"Duration" refers to the length of time and energetic intensity with which asanas are held. As with pace, temporal duration is prescribed in some Hatha yoga styles, including Iyengar yoga, which often gives specific seconds or minutes for holding an asana. The effects of duration are inextricably intertwined with intentional actions in the held asana, including the relative degree of active or passive energetic engagement and where that energetic effort is consciously directed in the asana.[7] While duration itself is significant, what a student is actually doing while holding an asana—how one is playing the edge—is even more important. Another important variable is the extent to which the asana requires strength to hold, thus building strength when held longer.

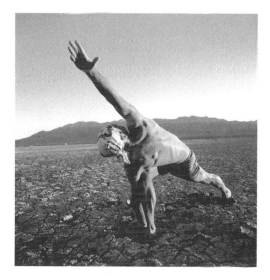

Passive stretching is what the name implies: the body is at rest, affected primarily by gravity, allowing the stretch receptors in the muscles to "quiet down" and the muscle to relax into elongation. While this method increases flexibility, it does not produce long-term changes in the viscoelastic properties of muscle as found in active or dynamic stretching. We also find in the scientific study of static stretching that there is considerable evidence that the effect on flexibility from static stretching is maximized at thirty seconds, with no further effect on flexibility when holding for sixty seconds.[8] However, there is no evidence—at least no scientific evidence—that holding static stretches for longer than one minute does not create other important effects, such as calming the nervous system and allowing stretch receptors to acclimate further to a stretched position. Anecdotal evidence—my own asana practice and observation of thousands of students over the years—suggests that deeper release occurs in muscles and noncontractile elements such as connective tissue and the fascial sheath with long passive holds, particularly when using the breath and consciousness to feel, visualize, and allow such release.

In active stretching, one set of muscles (agonists) are steadily and perhaps variously contracted to allow another set of muscles to relax and stretch. This is based on the principle of reciprocal innervation, in which contraction of the opposing antagonist muscle is neurologically inhibited by contraction of the agonist. For example, actively contracting the quadriceps muscles in Paschimottanasana (Seated Forward Bend) relaxes the hamstring muscles, allowing them to stretch more easily. This is not to be confused with ballistic or dynamic stretching, conventionally described as bouncing to force a stretch. Common in sports and gymnastics, ballistic stretching appears in the graceful, fluid, wavelike actions found in many asana transitions, particularly in flow styles of asana practice. Here the movement itself carries a limb into an extended range of motion when the muscle has not relaxed enough to enter it passively. Done excessively, this is a common cause of muscle strain and other injuries in yoga.

When holding asanas that require significant physical strength, longer duration will build that strength while requiring greater physical exertion. Guiding students to stay with the overarching asana principle of sthira sukham asanam, you can offer a more strength-building sequence or class by holding certain asanas—primarily standing and arm balance asanas, and others such as Navasana (Boat Pose) that require core abdominal engagement—for longer. Encouraging students to stay with their intention (within a space where they can genuinely feel it is perfectly acceptable to come out of an asana whenever they want), you can play with varying durations, observing students to determine when it appears time to transition to another asana. As a general rule, when you observe some students showing instability or coming out of a long-held asana, reaffirm the importance of honoring one's personal intention in the practice, encouraging students to stay in or come out based on how they feel, not how they compare. This is a good time to affirm that the "no pain, no gain" mentality that pervades Western fitness culture is a risky proposition that more typically results in injury rather than health, wellness, or self-transformation. A similarly questionable notion is found in much of yoga culture where "real yoga" is said to begin when one thinks one cannot hold an asana any longer. While it is important to self-assess when mental or emotional factors might lead us to avoid something that is challenging, the feedback of the body, heart, and mind is quite worth listening to and may make all the difference in cultivating a lifelong sustainable practice.

Holding asanas for relatively longer duration can allow deeper exploration of the practice. Depending on the asana and what is happening in one's body and life, long holds done with conscious breathing and subtle awareness of the movement of energy can release deeply held tension, bring awareness to dormant parts of the body, and stimulate insight into the inner dynamics of one's practice and life. When approaching feelings of discomfort in a long-held asana, there is an opportunity for students to discover anew the patterns and tendencies that manifest in their larger lives as obstacles to living with conscious openness and willful determination. Experiencing what one gravitates toward, resists, or finds enjoyable, frustrating, or perturbing in asanas can be a source of awakening to a clearer understanding of the deeper self. The more *tha* part of Hatha yoga the more calming and integrative part of class—is a wonderful time to go into this aspect of practice, especially in forward bends, hip openers, twists, and supported inversions such as Salamba Sirsasana I (Headstand I), Salamba Sarvangasana (Supported Shoulder-Stand), and Viparita Karani (Basic Inversion).

Particularly with beginning students, offer more dynamic movements in and out of an asana several times in rhythm with the breath.[9] Moving dynamically allows students to gradually feel the requirements and effects of an asana, contributing to their awareness of how to move in synchronization with the breath and how to use the breath as a tool connecting the body and mind. "A dynamic practice," Desikachar (1995, 29) says, "gives us greater possibilities for bringing breath to particular parts of the body and heightening the intensity of the effect." This, he intones, is beneficial to experienced practitioners who "often get caught in the habit of focusing their attention on fixing the posture somehow in static practice rather than really working in it and exploring its possibilities."

In creative flow classes, including Vinyasa Flow and its many branded expressions, there is an opportunity to be more playful as a teacher in exploring with your students the infinite possibilities for dynamic pacing and varied duration. Connected with the earth, flowing with the breath, the body expresses itself in flowing asanas that are expressions of spirit. It is here that you can introduce the "three friends: gravity, breath, and wave," as Vanda Scaravelli (1991, 24, 28) says, "that should be constantly with us."

Transitioning out of Asanas

The very idea of asana can exert a powerful effect on the awareness of teachers and students, especially when asanas are approached as something to be attained or mastered rather than as part of a process of self-discovery and transformation. One consequence is focusing so intently on getting into the deepest possible expression of an asana that little awareness is given to transitioning out. Considerable anecdotal evidence based on years of observation indicates that more students are injured coming out of an asana than either transitioning into it or holding and exploring it. As Desikachar (1995, 27) says, "it is not enough to climb the tree; we must be able to get back down too."

Guiding students out of asanas involves applying your understanding of what is at risk in the transitional movement and giving specific physical actions that students can apply in their own movement. Just as the extent of risk will vary depending on the asana and the students, your instructions should be tailored to address this varied situation. In most asana transitions this begins with bringing awareness back to the foundation of the asana and reestablishing a feeling of stable grounding. Encouraging students to keep the spine and other potentially vulnerable joints in mind, your verbal cues should guide them through sequential releasing actions in which the stable foundation of the asana is maintained. In most asanas this involves bringing greater effort into a specific line of energy that, when activated, relieves potential pressure on vulnerable joints. For example, in transitioning a class from Utthita Trikonasana back to standing upright, some students may experience stress in their lower back and/or neck. To cue actions to minimize these risks, you can say, "Completing your exhale, root down more firmly from the top of your back hip into your back foot. Maintaining that strong energetic action, inhaling, draw your torso back up to standing." In a variety of other standing asanas in which the torso is extended laterally or folded forward, you can use a similar cue along with emphasizing the natural engagement of the abdominal muscles as the breath flows out, then cueing the class to maintain the light engagement of their core while inhaling back up.

Many asana transitions involve moving part of the body toward the earth more than away, in which case the risk is in losing control and either straining a stabilizing muscle or falling to the floor. This includes many standing balance asanas, arm balances, and inversions. As appropriate for the level of experience among students in your class, give a visual demonstration of how to safely transition out of these asanas prior to guiding students into them. Once you have guided the class into the asana, give clear cues on transitioning out a few breaths prior to asking them to release out or down. When releasing from inverted asanas, encourage students not to suddenly spring fully upright, as this can cause light-headedness and fainting.

In all asana transitions, it is important to emphasize a gradual release connected with the breath, allowing students to feel what starts to happen as they initiate the transitional movement. This allows the gradual relaxation of muscles that were active in supporting the asana while bringing more awareness to the muscles being newly activated when releasing out. To the extent that the exiting transition is smooth and graceful, students can remain more attuned to the subtle energetic effects of the asana, which will then carry over more fully into the next asana.

The Integration of Asana

Each practice is a movement into deeper self-transformation. This movement occurs within each breath, each asana, each sequence, and extends across all the practices a person does in a lifetime. Cultivating a gradual, simple, stable, expanding awakening in this process of self-transformation revolves around continuously coming back to a sense of *samasthihi*—equanimity in body, breath, mind, and spirit. This gives the asana practice a quality of yoga chikitsa—literally "yoga therapy"—in which the body is restructured and a person's entire energetic being is refined.[10] This is an essential element of every class, one that requires you as a teacher to create the space, sequence the asanas, and guide the class in a way that helps endow students with a practical 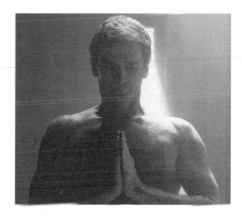 awareness of this transformation and integration in their bodies. Here are several ways to promote this integration of asana practice in classes and thereby maximize the benefits of each practice, building on what we have already covered in this section:

- *Create space for rest.* Toward the beginning of every class, remind students that it is important for them to feel a sense of steadiness and ease throughout the class while practicing near the edge of their ability. Give them explicit permission—even encouragement—to rest as they feel the need, creating a space in which they can calm their breath and energy before resuming their practice. At the conclusion of any particularly intense sequence of asanas, always offer an opportunity for rest.

- *Create space for renewed self-assessment.* Give brief or long pauses in the flow of the class in which you invite students to come back to their initial intention in the practice, to check in with how they are feeling, and to stay with their intention and sense of samasthihi as you resume the asanas.

- *Apply pratikriyasana (prati* meaning "against," and *kr* meaning "to do") to neutralize tension from asanas and establish balance in the body (see Chapter Ten).

- *Offer energetically balanced sequences.* When planning a class, give careful consideration to the energetic arc and waves of the asana sequences to achieve the intended energetic balance for that class.

- *Savasana.* A few minutes—five or more—in Savasana is absolutely essential for the full integration and completion of a practice. Lying down with effortless breath, surrendering to gravity, and allowing the body, breath, and mind to completely settle is the most important way to integrate the practice.

- *Create space for meditation.* While the entire practice is ideally a meditative experience, students can deepen this experience when you create the space in class for moving into a deeper sense of stillness. This can be done at the beginning of class, during the flow of asanas, or at the conclusion of the asana practice (before or after Savasana).

- *Moving off the mat.* Rising from one's mat, the next vinyasa starts with being conscious and present in the next transition—back out into the world. Encourage students to pay attention to how they are moving, breathing, thinking, and feeling. Consider concluding class with a moment of reflection with the palms and fingertips together at the heart and forehead to symbolize and feel a sense of connecting the head and the heart in setting intention in moving out into the rest of the day.

GENERAL PRINCIPLES IN GIVING PHYSICAL CUES AND ADJUSTMENTS

The role of touch varies widely across the many styles and traditions of Hatha yoga. Physical cues have a variety of benefits and are an essential aspect of most therapeutic approaches. They are used extensively in the Krishnamacharya lineage of Ashtanga Vinyasa, Iyengar, and Vinyasa Flow, and are virtually absent in Bikram and Power yoga. Precise touch can effectively convey an energetic action; clarify a verbal alignment cue; give students a feeling of support; bring awareness to an unconscious part of the body; stimulate the internal cultivation of spaciousness and release; assist in stabilizing or deepening an asana; assist in increasing range of motion; help you as the teacher to be more aware of a student's overall condition; and create a more trusting and open sense of connection between teacher and student.

The purpose of physical cues is to help students deepen their practice by establishing a more stable foundation, aligning their body safely and comfortably, and encouraging deeper release while staying connected to their breath as the principal source of guidance. Focusing on guiding students into a deeper practice, you will give assists that are clearly intended and specific. Your effectiveness in doing this is predicated on your skills and knowledge in seeing, understanding, and relating to students in asanas in a meaningful, sensitive, ethical, and individualized way.

The physical intimacy of human touch brings ethical and personal considerations to the forefront in giving hands-on cues and adjustments.[11] Every person comes to their experience of physical intimacy in different ways. An adjustment one person finds comfortable might be felt as invasive by someone else. What is welcome with a particular student one day might not be on another day. Rather than presuming that physical touch is welcome, always ask permission before touching a student, even with a longtime student to whom you have given innumerable adjustments in the past. Remembering that one of your primary roles as a yoga teacher is to create and maintain an emotionally and physically safe space for students, it is very important to simply ask, "Is this OK?" before or as you begin to touch.

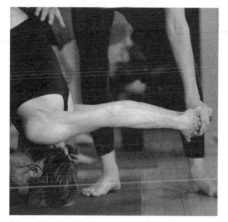

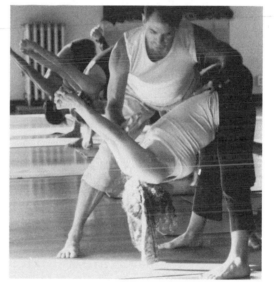

More proximal adjustments (as shown at right) minimize potential strain in the joints.

The yamas are a useful starting place in approaching physical cues, beginning with the intertwined values of ahimsa, not hurting, and satya, truthfulness. Respecting ahimsa in giving hands-on adjustments starts with being truthful with yourself about what you know and don't know, as well as your intention in touching. As with teaching in general, it is important to share and give from a place of truthful understanding. If you do not understand what is happening with a student in an asana, then you are not prepared to give that person a physical cue. By allowing the clarity of your intention in giving physical cues to arise from your knowledge and skill in seeing and relating to students in asanas, you will be more effective in giving appropriate cues that help your students to deepen their practice.

It is just as important to honor your own sense of safety and comfort when giving adjustments. Positioning yourself in a way that is stable and comfortable, then moving into the adjustment with a feeling of your own stability and ease will help ensure that you do not hurt yourself while helping students. This requires being especially attuned to your lower back, wrists, and parts of your body that are either strained or more susceptible to injury. Rather than adopting a specific stance for each and every adjustment, be open to playing around with how you position your own body to take care of yourself while giving active assistance to your students. The relative size of your body and those of your students will be a significant factor in your positioning. You may find yourself standing, kneeling, sitting down, or positioning yourself in other ways that allow you to work most stably and easily while staying attuned to your student.

Aparigraha, the yama meaning "not grasping," applies equally to your intention in giving an assist and to guiding your students in letting the asana naturally open up to them without forcing it. Sometimes teachers become attached to a certain preconception of what a student can or should be able to do in deepening an asana rather than staying attuned to observing how the asana seems to be presenting itself to the student. This can result in pushing students too far, with verbal and/or physical cues. Similarly, students are often attached to their own idea of how or how far to go and may ask for a more intense adjustment than their body is ready for at that moment. Navigating these tendencies depends on staying with your larger intention and purpose as a teacher and encouraging your students to stay with asana as a process of deepening self-awareness and self-transformation in which the "less is more" adage has much currency.

The intimate quality of touch can also stimulate reactions that bear on matters of bramacharya, the yama loosely translated as "right use of energy" and more literally as "sexual restraint." As Esther Myers has stressed, sexual feelings tend to arise naturally in students, teachers, or both, leading to or heightening existing feelings of attraction, transference, and projection. Myers (2002, 3) notes that "While most yoga teachers today are not choosing to be celibate, our ethical practice *as teachers* requires Bramacharya in relation to our students."[12] When this attitude is embedded in your intention, you will be able to approach any student with clarity expressed through your physical energy that unambiguously conveys compassionate caring free of any confusing thoughts or feelings. Should such thoughts or feelings arise in you, let that signify that it is time for you to step away and reexamine your intention and purpose in working closely with your students. Should you perceive such feelings arising in a student, which is not at all uncommon as dormant sexual energy is triggered or other feelings of emotional or physical awakening in the practice are projected onto you, consider creating more distance between you and the student and give only those adjustments that you are confident of being clearly understood by the student as professional support and not as an expression of personal interest or desire.

In a world where many people feel judged, yoga classes offer a space where students can feel fully accepted for who they are. Yet as teachers we carry a responsibility for honestly conveying to students our sincere best insights into what they are doing in their practice. This inevitably includes seeing value in the student doing something different from what that person is presently doing. For example, if a student's knee is splayed inward and projects out beyond her heel in Uttthita Parsvakonasana (Extended Side Angle Pose), you will see and appreciate the benefit of realigning her knee to be centered above her heel. Rather than communicating this as a "correction," try to find the language and voice that conveys the beauty of what she is doing along with the support you are offering in suggesting and even physically cueing the realignment. For example, you might say, "Good, keep rooting down into feet, and see how it feels to bring your foot further forward and align your knee just above your heel, which is a more stable position and better for your knee." You might give a light tactile cue encouraging her to press her knee slightly out to align it toward the center of her foot and simply add, "Beautiful. Stay with the breath."

In your practice of looking at and seeing students in a class, you will find that with increasing experience you will more easily scan the entire class as students are moving into an asana and notice which students might benefit most from your earliest individual contact. Offering verbal cues from what you see might be enough to address perceived or common alignment issues. In any asana you can find ways to help any student refine his or her positioning. In prioritizing your adjustments, go first to those students you observe most at risk of strain or injury and address those risks first. Focus specifically on the primary alignment principles and modifications that directly pertain to the perceived risk. Talk softly with the student in asking permission to touch and in offering verbal cues that relate directly to your hands-on cues. Depending on the duration of the asana (which you have the option of varying), try to stay with the student long enough for that person to begin integrating the new positioning into the full integrity of the asana.

After giving your attention to primary alignment principles that are related to what is most at risk, begin to address the refinement of the asana, giving primary focus to the breath and spine. Many students will compromise the integrity of their breath and spine in order to attain what they perceive to be the full or more advanced form of the asana. With clear, compassionate, and direct encouragement, use verbal and physical cues (and in many cases demonstration) to guide the student to a place where he or she can find the fullness of the breath and the more refined alignment and elongation of the spine. In working with a student to explore these refinements, give instructions that help that person to maintain the foundational anchoring of the asana rather than taking the shortcut of compromising the foundation in order to achieve a refinement. Shortcuts that "unplug" the foundation of the asana tend to become habitual tendencies in the practice that often lead to longer-term strain and injury.

Consider the following general principles in giving the physical cue or adjustment:

- Practice giving hands-on adjustments under the direct guidance of an experienced mentor teacher as part of your teacher training before giving adjustments to students in a class.
- Learn to feel how different bodies respond to your hands under varying conditions relating to gravity, resistance, and positioning.
- Stay grounded and attentive to your own stability and ease.
- Always ask permission to touch.
- Consider how you can use individualized verbal cues and/or further demonstration to achieve an effect prior to using physical touch. Give the student the opportunity to respond to your instructions before using your hands.
- Explain what you are looking for and doing as you begin to touch the student.
- Stay attuned to the student's breath, stability, and ease. Be particularly aware of how your physical contact with the student can disturb his or her foundation in the asana, especially with asanas involving physical balance.
- Be clear and specific in giving the cue or adjustment without attachment to a specific preconceived outcome. Students' bodies will respond in different ways. Go with their response in refining your interaction with them. Feel and adapt as you go.
- As you are giving the adjustment, again ask, "Is this OK?"
- Feel how the student's body is responding, including shifts in other parts of his or her body and signs of increased tension.
- Work as proximally as appropriate in adjusting a student in an asana, using only very light tactile cues when the touch is fully distal. Phrased another way, never give a strong adjustment distally, such as turning the hand to create external rotation of the arm.
- Do not apply pressure to vulnerable joints, organs, or injured areas.

- Find the natural handles on the body in any given pose.
- Consider asking the student to come partially or completely out of the asana if there are fundamental misalignments or other sources of instability or potential strain.
- Breathe with the student and synchronize your physical cues with the student's breath.
- Pay attention to and reinforce the foundation of the asana.
- Use physical cues to accentuate a student's sense of where to run lines of energy.
- When pushing, pulling, elongating, or rotating part of a student's body, make the movement in the same direction as the principal or refined lines of energy.
- Concentrate on what you are doing while staying attentive to the larger class.
- Gain considerable experience and find comfort and confidence with hands-on adjustments before using other parts of your body. As you gain more experience and expertise, try to work with different modalities and make different kinds of adjustments.
- Release physical contact gradually to ensure that the student is stable, especially in standing and balancing asanas.

Whether working with a new or experienced student, consider giving the student the space to explore asanas free of your individualized attention. New students can feel overwhelmed by the newness of basic positions, by ujjayi pranayama, and all the simple nuances of a class. Often the best approach to new students is to leave them largely on their own unless you see them doing something that could cause an injury, thereby giving them the opportunity to feel what it is like to be in the class and in their body in a new way. As students gain more experience and you give them more individual guidance, occasionally give them periods of several classes or even weeks where you attentively observe them from a distance while giving them the space to explore on their own. Be careful when working with more experienced students to be just as attentive to how their body is responding, and resist giving hard, aggressive adjustments even when asked.[13] With practice you will develop more subtle hands-on touch that conveys different types of information, including the qualities of touch shown in Table 6.4, on page 154. In Chapter Seven we will look at specific physical cues and adjustments for every asana, offering examples of the various ways you can use your hands, arms, feet, knees, hips, and chest.

TABLE 6.4—**Qualities of Touch**

QUALITY	EXAMPLE
Clarifying	Touching the quadriceps muscles to see if they are contracted in Adho Mukha Svanasana or the upper fibers of the gluteus maximus to see if they are relaxed in Urdhva Dhanurasana.
Awakening	Lightly touching the top of the head in Tadasana to encourage the line of energy out through the top of the head, pressing into the heel of the foot of the grounded leg in Supta Padangusthasana to encourage extension and energetic engagement through the leg and heel.
Stabilizing	Placing your hip lightly against a student's hip in Ardha Chandrasana or Vrksasana to help keep the student balanced while using your hands to offer other physical cues.
Emphasizing	A slight surface cue to encourage a specific movement, such as rotational and elongating cues to the outer rib cage in Utthita Parsvakonasana.
Moving	Repositioning part of the body in a significant way to achieve a change in basic alignment, such as lifting and shifting a student's lower hip to the midline of his or her mat in a supine twist.
Grounding	Pressing part of the body down to enhance the foundation of an asana, such as evenly pressing down on a student's hip bones in Paschimottanasana.
Comforting	Giving support, human contact, such as resting your hand on a student's shoulder to convey compassion.

MODIFICATIONS, VARIATIONS, AND THE USE OF PROPS

Everyone comes to yoga somewhat uniquely, with different genetics, body structure, strength, flexibility, intention, and other qualities that bear on the asana practice. One of B. K. S. Iyengar's many invaluable contributions to Hatha yoga is his
recognition that this beautiful tapestry of human diversity requires options in the
asana practice in order for it to be equally accessible and enjoyable to all students.[14]
These options start with offering students modified forms of asanas that are otherwise inaccessible in their full form of expression. In practicing modified asanas,
students can experience many if not most of the full asana's benefits while gradually exploring movement toward its deeper, fuller expression. It is here, again, that
we can usefully apply the yogic maxim that it is not about how far one goes in

asanas, but about how one goes. Coming back to our mantra of sthira sukham asanam—steadiness, ease, and presence of mind—we can more fully appreciate the wisdom and efficacy of modifying asanas to support students in exploring, refining, and deepening their practice.

Whereas modifications adapt the positioning of the asana to make it more accessible to students who would otherwise be unable to enjoy its benefits, variations go beyond the basic form of an asana to offer students new and different ways to experience the interconnections of body, breath, and mind. Variations are explored once a student has developed steadiness and ease in the basic form of an asana and can begin to move into more challenging extensions of the asana without compromising that steadiness and ease. Curiosity, a sense of adventure, ego-driven competitiveness, and other motivations often lead students to attempt variations that they are not ready to do. Part of your role as a teacher is to counsel students on when and what forms of variation might make sense for where they are in their practice.

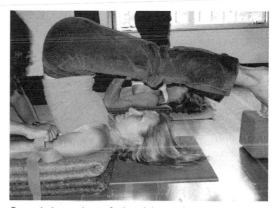

Props help students find stability and ease.

A prop, in B. K. S. Iyengar's (2001, 164) definition, is "any object that helps stretch, strengthen, relax, or improve the alignment of the body." Thus props include the teacher's body when used to offer support to a student. It also includes a yoga mat, the primary uses of which are (1) preventing the bones from grinding painfully into the floor and (2) keeping foundational parts of the body from slipping. Objects more commonly considered as props include blocks, bolsters, blankets, straps, walls, chairs, sandbags, and eye pillows, but the possible objects that can be used as props are limited primarily by a teacher's imagination. Introduced and given basic descriptions in Chapter Five, props and their specific uses in each asana are explored in greater detail in Chapter Seven. As with modifications of asanas that make them more accessible, with practice students may become increasingly less reliant on the prop, gradually opening to a place of stability and ease relatively or entirely free of props.

BRINGING IT ALL TOGETHER

The art and science of teaching yoga draws from multiple sources: yoga philosophy and history, theories and models of subtle energy and human anatomy, the practical realities of setting and context, the needs and intentions of students, your own values and intentions as a teacher, pedagogical principles and practical methods for giving clear and effective instruction. One of the joys of teaching yoga is in creatively mixing these elements in ways that help students discover and follow their inner teacher. As we now turn to the details of teaching asanas, pranayama, and meditation, keep coming back to this broad palette of ancient wisdom and contemporary insight as you develop and refine your knowledge and skills as a yoga teacher.

CHAPTER SEVEN

TEACHING ASANAS

For most students, the first attraction to asana is for healing physical or emotional pain, reducing stress, or gaining strength and flexibility. At the very least, the practice should support these intentions. As we saw in Chapter Six, to really do asana practice involves cultivating steadiness, ease, and an attentiveness that allows each asana to become as if it is so many different windows onto the nature of our mind and the condition of our heart. By cultivating a consistent openness to being fully tuned in, what at first was a more purely physical practice becomes a tool for calming the mind, settling the emotions, and awakening to an abiding sense of spirit. As teachers, we can best guide students along the asana path by encouraging these qualities in every practice, recognizing along the way the uniqueness of each student and the continuous evolution of the asanas themselves, with new forms and variations appearing with increasing frequency as the yoga movement grows. Here we will emphasize basic asanas as described and variously taught in the mainstream legacy of Krishnamacharya, which constitutes about ninety percent of yoga asana practices in the West today.[1] Numerous other books offer excellent descriptions of asanas, exhaustively and often repetitively explaining their benefits, risks, contraindications, anatomical alignment principles, energetic actions, lines of energy, modifications, variations, subtle energy aspects, and other qualities.[2] Rather than duplicating these works, here we will address the primary concerns of teachers by focusing specifically on supporting students in individual asanas and dynamic movements. Drawing from the foundational material presented in the previous chapters, we will address where to focus your visual attention, what to cue, how to give adjustments, and how to support modifications and variations as appropriate for individual students.

Each asana is categorized into an asana family: standing, core, arm balance, backbends, twists, forward bends, hip openers, and inversions. Note that many asanas can reasonably be placed in more than one family; in those cases, they are placed according to their primary effects or actions. Surya Namaskara draws from several families and is addressed in detail as a unique blended family of dynamic

movement. Common aspects of each family are presented before looking at its individual asanas. For detailed visual guidance in teaching these asanas to different
students, view the 108 videos available at www.markstephensyoga.com/teaching.html.

SURYA NAMASKARA: THE SUN SALUTATIONS

Sun Salutations are an excellent way to begin a practice. With modifications and
variations, nearly anyone can do them. In a group class, they help to unify the class
as everyone breathes and moves largely in unison. They warm and awaken the entire body, soften the muscles, open the joints, and stimulate the neurological, circulatory, and subtle energetic pathways, initiating conscious awareness and
synchronization of movement in the breath, body, mind, and spirit. There are numerous variations and adaptations of Surya Namaskara. In her book *Sun Yoga* (2001),
Janita Stenhouse describes twenty-five different variations of sun salutes. Here we
will focus on three forms: Classical Surya Namaskara as described by Erich Schiffmann, and Surya Namaskara A and B as taught in the Krishnamacharya lineage.
Within each form, there are many variations and modifications that enable teachers to accommodate the varying abilities, special needs, and conditions of different students.

TABLE 7.1A—**Twelve Asanas in the Surya Namaskara Family**

ASANAS	SALUTATION FORM
1. Tadasana (Mountain Pose)	Classical, A, B
2. Urdhva Hastasana (Upward Salute)	Classical, A
3. Uttanasana (Standing Forward Bend)	Classical, A, B
4. Ardha Uttanasana (Half Standing Forward Bend)	Classical, A, B
5. Anjaneyasana (Low Lunge)	Classical
6. Phalakasana (Plank Pose)	Classical (A/B option)
7. Chaturanga Dandasana (Four-Limbed Staff Pose)	A, B
8. Salabhasana B (Locust or "Easy Cobra")	Classical (A/B option)
9. Utkatasana (Chair Pose)	B
10. Urdhva Mukha Svanasana (Upward-Facing Dog Pose)	A, B
11. Adho Mukha Svanasana (Downward-Facing Dog Pose)	Classical, A, B
12. Virabhadrasana I (Warrior I Pose)	B

Classical Surya Namaskara

Classical Sun Salutations are an excellent way to begin any Hatha yoga practice. This integrated series of asanas sequentially highlights several essential physical qualities of asana practice:

- Roots, extension, and equanimity in Tadasana/Samasthihi.
- Spinal integrity and lengthening in Urdhva Hastasana.
- Calming stretch of the back body in Uttanasana.
- Grounded spinal extension and heart awakening in Ardha Uttanasana.
- Awakened stretching of the hip flexors, quadriceps, and shoulder girdle in Anjaneyasana.
- Strengthening of the arms, shoulders, core, and legs in Phalakasana.
- Strengthening the spinal erectors and hip extensors in a modified form of Salabhasana B.
- Strengthening and stretching of the entire body in Adho Mukha Svanasana.

The Classical Sun Salutations move fluidly through the following asanas, each of which is held for just the length of the natural pauses between breaths.

TABLE 7.1B — **Breath and Movement in Classical Sun Salutations**

INHALING	EXHALING
1. Reach the arms out and up from Samasthihi to Urdhva Hastasana;	2. Fold forward and down into Uttanasana;
3. Extend the spine and heart center forward into Ardha Uttanasana;	4. Step the right foot back, knee down to the floor, toes back;
5. Draw the torso and arms up into Anjaneyasana;	6. Swan-dive the palms to the floor;
7. Step back to Phalakasana;	8. Slowly release the knees — chest — chin sequentially to the floor;
9. Root into the palms and lift the chest to Salabhasana B (with feet rooting down);	10. Press to all fours or directly up and back to Adho Mukha Svanasana;
11. Step the right foot forward and rise into Anjaneyasana;	12. Swan-dive the palms to the floor;
13. Extend the spine and heart center forward into Ardha Uttanasana;	14. Fold into Uttanasana;
15. "Swan-dive" up to Urdhva Hastasana;	16. Grow taller while drawing the palms back to the heart, Samasthihi.

Tadasana to Urdhva Hastasana

- Begin by standing in Tadasana/Samasthihi, with the palms together in anjali mudra.
- For details on instructing Tadasana, see "Standing Asanas" below.
- Emphasize pada bandha and encourage students to maintain this energetic action whenever their feet are on the floor in a standing asana.
- Transitioning from Tadasana to Urdhva Hastasana, emphasize keeping the pelvis neutral (it will tend to tilt anteriorly) while softening the lower front ribs in and away from the skin to maintain a neutral spine. This will help students to feel and develop integrity of alignment in their lumbar-pelvic relationship and in their shoulder flexion while cultivating stability and ease in the spine.
- Always offer the option of gazing forward rather than up in Urdhva Hastasana as a means of protecting the neck.

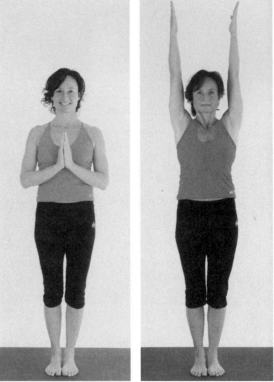

Samasthihi (left); Urdhva Hastasana (right)

Urdhva Hastasana to Uttanasana

- Offer the option of bending the knees to reduce stress on the hamstrings and lower back.
- As students find comfort in the hamstrings and lower back, encourage them to focus more on activating their feet, keeping their legs firm, knee caps lifted, spine long, shoulder blades drawing down their back, and heart center open as they fold forward.
- Most students will tend to shift their hips back while folding forward in order to maintain their balance and keep from falling forward. Encourage them to work on gradually keeping their legs vertical while folding forward by bringing their

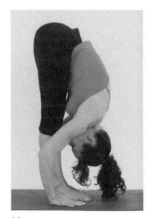

Uttanasana

weight forward into the balls of their feet while keeping their heels firmly rooted down.

- *Arm/Shoulder Option 1:* "Swan diving" is the easiest on the lower back and hamstrings, helps to maintain expansiveness across the heart center, and helps to open the shoulder girdle. This method can be contraindicated for students with unstable shoulders.

- *Arm/Shoulder Option 2:* Folding forward and down with the palms drawing through center—through anjali mudra—can foster a sense of heart-centered awareness. It is relatively easy on the lower back and hamstrings, but the chest tends to collapse.

- *Arm/Shoulder Option 3:* Folding forward and down with the arms fully extended overhead, this option requires considerable lower back, leg, and core strength. If lacking strength in these areas, this method of folding can strain the lower back and hamstrings.

Uttanasana to Ardha Uttanasana

- Emphasize lengthening the spine, drawing the shoulder blades down the back, and further expanding across the heart center.

- Offer and demonstrate the options of having the knees bent, coming up onto the fingertips, and/or placing the hands high up on the shins.

- All of these options help to fully extend the spine. As students develop the flexibility in the hamstrings and hips, cue them to keep their feet grounded and legs firm, thereby cultivating a more stable foundation from which to lengthen their spine.

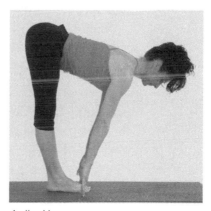

Ardha Uttanasana

Ardha Uttanasana to Anjaneyasana

- In stepping the right foot back and releasing the knee to the floor for Anjaneyasana, emphasize maintaining the length of the spine and openness of the heart center.

- Students whose knees are sensitive to pressure when placed on the floor can place padding under their grounded knee.

- With the first Anjaneyasana, consider offering students the following instructions to help break down and integrate the various actions in this asana:

- Partially straighten the front leg, place the hands on the hips, and create a slight posterior pelvic tilt to find pelvic neutrality.
- Slowly bend the front knee to deepen the lunge and the stretch of the hip flexors while continuing to cultivate pelvic neutrality.
- Play with slowly moving in and out of the full depth of the lunge, gradually releasing into a deeper stretch in the hips and groin.
- Once fully into the lunge, ask students to release their arms down by their sides, turn their palms out to externally rotate their arms, and then reach their arms overhead.

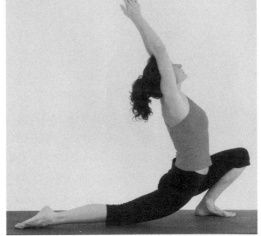

Anjaneyasana

- With their arms overhead, ask students to look down for a moment and lightly soften their lower front ribs in while maintaining pelvic neutrality, then try to reach their arms further back without letting their lower front ribs protrude out.
- The arms can be held shoulder-distance apart, and the head held level. Invite students who can keep their elbows straight to press their palms together overhead while lifting through their sides, chest, back, arms and fingertips. If it is OK with the neck, gaze at the thumbs.
- When flowing through the Sun Salutations, instruct students to inhale into Anjaneyasana; then with the exhale, swan-dive their palms to the floor.

Anjaneyasana to Phalakasana

- From Anjaneyasana, transition into Phalakasana.
- On the first time through this sequence, keep students in Phalakasana for several breaths while guiding them through the basic alignment principles and energetic actions.

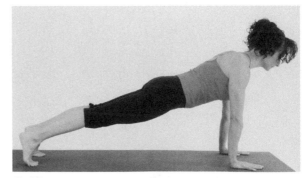

Phalakasana

- Many students will benefit from placing their knees on the floor when holding Phalakasana as they gradually develop the necessary strength in their arms, shoulders, core, and lower back to support their body comfortably in the full form of the asana.

- Use Phalakasana to teach the "Dandasana" qualities that will appear later in Chaturanga Dandasana: firm legs, heels pressing back, soft buttocks, inner thighs slightly rotating up, tailbone and pubic bone drawing slightly back, belly lightly engaged to support the middle body from sagging, shoulder blades drawing down the back with the lower tips drawing lightly into the back ribs, sternum extending forward, back of the neck long (or looking slightly forward if OK with the neck).

Phalakasana to Salabhasana B

- From Phalakasana, sequentially bring the knees, chest, and chin to the floor (Ashtanga Pranam) on the exhale, then inhale into modified Salabhasana B (Locust Pose), grounding the hips and feet firmly into the floor, energetically extending back through the legs and feet, spiraling the inner thighs up, and pressing the tailbone toward the heels.

- While students maintain this active engagement of their legs, guide them to press into their hands—placed beneath their shoulders—and lift their chest up while shrugging their shoulder blades down their back and looking slightly down to maintain ease in the neck.

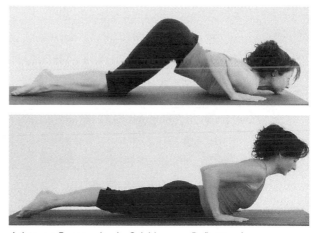

Ashtanga Pranam (top); Salabhasana B (bottom)

- The relative intensity of Salabhasana B can be heightened by rooting more firmly down into the palms while creating a feeling of energetically spiraling the palms outward. This will further depress the shoulder blades and expand the chest.

- Suggest energetically pulling back on the palms to gently deepen the backbend while keeping the hips rooted, legs strong, tailbone drawing toward the heels, and breath active.

- It is very important to distinguish this modified version of Salabhasana B from Bhujangasana (Cobra Pose). Bhujangasana is a deep backbend that should be explored as part of a backbending sequence, not in the steady flow of Surya Namaskara. Inhaling directly into full Bhujangasana and exhaling out does not allow students to give Bhujangasana the attention and energetic actions required to do it safely. Keeping the belly on the floor in Salabhasana B is a safe and gentle backbend that will strengthen the back muscles in the context of flowing movement.

Salabhasana B to Adho Mukha Svanasana

- In transitioning from Salabhasana B to Adho Mukha Svanasana, suggest and demonstrate the option of pressing up onto all fours along the way. Consider bringing the entire class to all fours to teach the fundamentals of the hands, arms, and pelvis that apply in Adho Mukha Svanasana, which is the easiest way to transition from Salabhasana B to Adho Mukha Svanasana: pressing up onto all fours, curling the toes under, then lifting the hips up and back while moving toward straightening the legs.

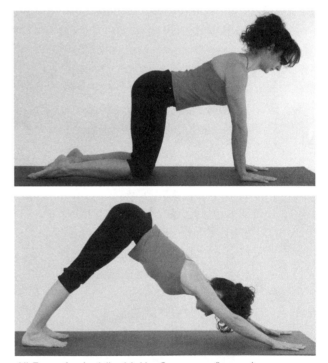

- This method should be encouraged for students with lower-back issues.

- Healthy students with sufficient arm, shoulder, and core strength and stability can explore lifting the hips directly up and back into Adho Mukha Svanasana, either stepping over one foot at a time (relatively

All Fours (top); Adho Mukha Svanasana (bottom)

easier) or rolling over the toes on both feet simultaneously (more challenging).

- Many newer, very tight, or weak students are not prepared to safely practice full Adho Mukha Svanasana; they can stay on all fours to continue the preparatory work or explore the pose with their hands up a wall.

FOCUS ON ADHO MUKHA SVANASANA

Following the basic principles of asana practice, instruct the building of full Adho Mukha Svanasana from the ground up and from what is at most risk of strain or injury: the wrists, shoulders, and hamstrings. We will look alternatively at the upper body (from the hands up) and lower body (from the feet up). Adho Mukha Svanasana is an excellent asana for learning and embodying the principle of roots and extension. Encourage students to press firmly down into the entire span of their hands and length of their fingers, paying close attention to rooting the knuckle of the index finger as a way of balancing pressure in the wrist joint. This rooting action should originate at the top of the arms. With it, ask students to feel the "rebounce" effect of this rooting action in the natural lengthening through their wrist, elbow, and shoulder joints. The fingers should be spread wide apart, the thumbs only about two-thirds of the way in order to protect the ligaments in the thenar space between the thumbs and index fingers. Generally, the middle fingers should be parallel and in line with the shoulders. Look to see if the student's arms are parallel; this will indicate if their hands are in line with their shoulders. The alignment of the wrists with the shoulders allows the proper external rotation of the shoulders, which activates and strengthens the teres minor and infraspinatus muscles (two of the four principal rotator cuff muscles), stabilizes the shoulder joint by drawing the scapula firmly against the back ribs, creates more space across the upper back and thereby allows the neck to relax more easily. If a student has difficulty straightening his or her arms, play with asking that person to turn his or her hands slightly out; if a student tends to hyperextend his or her elbows, have that person turn the palms slightly in.

Tight or weak shoulders create specific risks to the neck, back, elbows, wrists, and shoulders themselves in Adho Mukha Svanasana. In either case, moderate effort in this asana develops both strength and flexibility, opening the shoulders to full flexion while developing deeper, more balanced strength. The shoulder blades should be rooted against the back ribs while spreading the shoulder blades out away from the spine. Note that externally rotating the shoulders tends to cause the inner palms to lift. This can be countered by internally rotating the forearms.

The roots-and-extension principle applies equally to the lower body. Rooting into the balls of the feet will contribute to lifting the inner arches, which is one effect of pada bandha. This will help to stimulate the awakening of mula bandha (as discussed in Chapter Four). The feet should be placed hip-distance apart or wider, with the outer edges of the feet parallel. Firming the thighs and pressing the tops of the femur bones strongly back is a key action (along with rooted hands) in lengthening the spine in this asana. While firming the thighs, encourage students to slightly spiral the inner thighs back to soften pressure in the sacrum, all the while drawing the pubic bone back and up, the tailbone back and slightly down. The first few times in this asana in any given practice, it can feel good and help the body in gently opening to "bicycle" the legs, twisting and sashaying alternately into each hip and stretching long through the sides of the body while exploring the hamstrings, lower back, shoulders, ankles, and feet.

Very flexible students tend to hyperextend their knees in Adho Mukha Svanasana. Guide them to bend their knees slightly. Students with tight hips and hamstrings will find it difficult, painful, or impossible to straighten their legs. Encourage them to separate their feet wider apart (even as wide as their yoga mat) to ease the anterior rotation of the pelvis and the natural curvature of the lumbar spine. Let them know that it is OK to keep their knees bent while holding this asana, very gradually moving into deepening the flexibility of their hamstrings and hip extensors.

With regular practice, the neck will become sufficiently strong and supple to support holding the head between the upper arms (with the ears in line with the arms). Until that strength is developed, encourage students to let their neck relax and head hang. With each and every exhale, students will feel the light and natural engagement of their abdominal muscles. Encourage them to maintain that light and subtle engagement in their belly while inhaling, without gripping or bearing down in their belly. Keep bringing students' awareness back to balanced ujjayi pranayama, to roots-and-extension, to a steady gaze, and to the cultivation of steadiness and ease.

Adho Mukha Svanasana to Anjaneyasana

- After completion of an exhale, instruct students to step their right foot forward, releasing their left foot to the floor and extending their toes back, then inhaling into Anjaneyasana.
- With the following exhale, instruct swan-diving the palms to the floor, with the palms placed shoulder-distance apart. With the following inhale, the left foot steps forward next to the right foot while extending the spine and heart center forward into Ardha Uttanasana, then with the exhale folding down into Uttanasana.

- With the following inhale, instruct swan diving up to Urdhva Hastasana, and complete the sequence by exhaling the palms to the heart to Samasthihi. Offer and encourage the option of keeping the knees bent in this transition to reduce potential strain on the hamstrings and lower back.

Surya Namaskara A

Surya Namaskara A begins and ends the same as in the Classical Sun Salutations, with Samasthihi, Urdhva Hastasana, Uttanasana, and Ardha Uttanasana. It introduces four new elements to the Sun Salutations: Chaturanga Dandasana (Four-Limbed Staff Pose), Urdhva Mukha Svanasana (Upward-Facing Dog Pose), "floating," and holding Adho Mukha Svanasana for five or more breaths. In combination, these new elements make this sequence considerably more challenging and tapas-oriented than the Classical form.

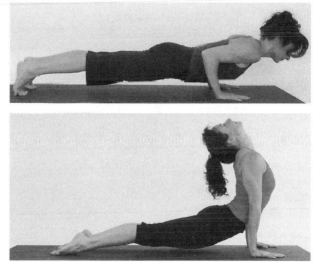

Chaturanga Dandasana (top); Urdhva Mukha Svanasana (bottom)

Teach as with the Classical Sun Salutations until arriving in Ardha Uttanasana. In instructing the first Surya Namaskara A, ask the entire class to step back from Ardha Uttanasana to Phalakasana (Plank Pose). Explain the various aspects of Phalakasana as described above for Classical Surya Namaskara. Emphasize that the *danda* (staff or stick) aspects of Phalakasana are essential in the transition down to Chaturanga Dandasana. When instructing the movement from Phalakasana to Chaturanga, emphasize the following five energetic actions: (1) active legs (firm thighs, inner thighs spiral up), (2) heel pressing back, (3) active core (belly drawing lightly to the spine with the exhale), (4) shoulder blades down the back, and (5) sternum toward the horizon. Suggest (and demonstrate) the option of lowering all the way down to the floor with "knees-chest-chin" as in Surya Namaskara C as an alternative to lowering to Chaturanga Dandasana. If a student is lowering with "knees-chest-chin," encourage him or her to stay with Salabhasana B rather than Urdhva Mukha Svanasana (Upward-Facing Dog Pose). As the elbows bend, they track directly behind the shoulders without squeezing into the sides or splaying out. While lowering down, encourage students to press firmly across the entire span of their palms and to keep the knuckles of their index fingers rooting down; these actions in the hands will help balance pressure in the wrists and thus reduce the incidence of repetitive stress in this vulnerable joint. The gaze is down so the neck is in its natural curvature, or over time and with practice, stability, and ease in the neck, the gaze is toward the horizon.

The flowing quality of the Sun Salutations often results in a very sloppy (and thus potentially injurious) Chaturanga Dandasana or the virtual disappearance of this asana altogether. Remind students that Chaturanga Dandasana is an asana that should be held for that brief natural pause in the breath between the exhale and the inhale that initiates movement into Urdhva Mukha Svanasana. In guiding students into Chaturanga, emphasize that the front of the shoulders should lower just to the level of the elbows while continuing to root the shoulder blades down the back and in against the back ribs for greater stability. This is the essential preparation for transitioning into Urdhva Mukha Svanasana (Upward-Facing Dog Pose), as described below. When the shoulders go lower than the elbows in Chaturanga, excessive pressure is placed on the labrum of the shoulder joint. This positioning also collapses the chest and leads to an Urdhva Mukha Svanasana in which the shoulders tend to scrunch up toward the ears, creating undue pressure in the neck and compromising the expansiveness of the heart center. If students lack the strength to keep their shoulders from going lower than their elbows when lowering to Chaturanga, tell them to keep their knees on the floor in this transition.

As students develop the strength to stably and comfortably lower into Chaturanga from Phalakasana, introduce them to the more fluid movement of floating from Ardha Uttanasana directly to Chaturanga Dandasana (or to the floor). Many students have learned to jump back to Phalakasana, which is problematic for two reasons: (1) the jarring impact on the lumbar spine, and (2) disruption of the synchronized connection of the breath to movement into Chaturanga (due to exhaling the breath completely out when jumping back). Teach the floating movement from Ardha Uttanasana by instructing students to bend their knees deeply enough to firmly root their palms into the floor while pulling their chest forward through the window of their arms on the inhale. Then guide students to bend their elbows while simultaneously jumping the feet back and extending the chest forward directly into Chaturanga (or to the floor). Encourage students to keep this movement simple; with time and practice, they might float up into Adho Mukha Vrksasana (Handstand) along the way to Chaturanga. When introducing the floating technique, hold Ardha Uttanasana for a few breaths while highlighting how the belly naturally engages when exhaling, stimulating the light uddiyana bandha that creates greater levity.

Urdhva Mukha Svanasana (Upward Facing Dog Pose) is an intense and pow-erfully awakening backbending asana. It is set up through the alignment qualities of Chaturanga Dandasana described above. Always offer students the option of Salabhasana B as an alternative in the following conditions: lower-back pain or insufficient arm, shoulder, or leg strength to suspend their body on the hands and feet. In first learning Urdhva Mukha Svanasana, it is helpful to first practice Salabhasana B, which strengthens the lower back and teaches the leg activation that is important in this asana. Emphasize active and aligned legs: the feet are extending back and pressing firmly down while legs are firm with the inner thighs spiraling up. Encourage students to press the tops of their feet firmly down and create a sense of extending their toes straight back. In rooting the feet down, the legs become more active. From this base in the feet, instruct students to pull their pelvis forward, away from their ankles, press their tailbone back toward their heels, and keep their buttocks soft while allowing the weight of the pelvis to provide traction on the lower back. Do not instruct squeezing the gluteal muscles, which causes the femurs to externally rotate and compresses the sacroiliac joint.

Guide students into the full expression of the asana by asking them to press firmly into their hands, lift their chest, and create a feeling of focusing the backbend in their heart center. Rooting firmly into the knuckles of the index fingers helps to ensure balanced pressure across the hands and wrist joints, thereby reducing the likelihood of strain in the wrists. Strong and balanced rooting of the hands also leads to greater extension of the arms and lifting and spreading of the chest, which is essential in creating the length in the spine required for deepening the backbend. The wrists should be aligned directly beneath the shoulders in Urdhva Mukha Svanasana. If the wrists are positioned forward of the shoulders, students will feel excessive pressure in their lower back; if positioned farther back than the shoulders, they will hyperextend their wrists. Where the shoulders end up relative to the wrists is determined by the movement of the feet in the transition from Chaturanga. Keeping the tiptoes fixed and rolling over them will bring the hips and shoulders farther forward; extending the feet back while pressing the arms straight will result in the shoulders being farther back. There is no correct method. Rather, the unique (and changing) geometry of each student's body—length of the arms, legs, feet, and torso, plus the degree of their backbending arc—determines how much to emphasize rolling over the toes versus extending the feet back. Demonstrating these alternatives, highlight the effect on the lower back, wrists, and overall integrity of Urdhva Mukha Svanasana.

Ask students to draw the curve of the backbend up their spine consciously and to create a sense of pulling the lower tips of their shoulder blades in and up as if into their heart center. Students with weak shoulders will tend to hang in their shoulders. This tends to strain the neck, close the heart center, compromise the breath, and exacerbate the tendency to dump into the lower back. Encourage these students to more actively press into their hands (wrists allowing) in order to better draw the shoulders down away from the ears. The head can be held level; with practice, ease, and stability, the final action of the asana can be releasing the head back. While pressing the palms firmly down, encourage students to energetically spiral the palms out to create more space across the heart center and pull the spine through toward the heart to deepen the backbend.

The transition from Urdhva Mukha Svanasana to Adho Mukha Svanasana is initiated with the exhalation. After feeling the fullness of Urdhva Mukha Svanasana at the crest of the inhale, cue students to feel their belly naturally engaging with their exhale, using the gradual engagement of their abdominal core to help lift their hips up and back. In an effort to find pelvic neutrality in Adho Mukha Svanasana, guide students to create a feeling of their pubic bone leading the way in pulling the hips up and back. Over time this movement involves rolling over the toes of both feet simultaneously. Newer students and those with tender toes or feet can "step" over first one foot and then the other. The arms should remain straight (but not hyperextended) and strong in this transition, with the shoulder blades spiraling out broadly away from the spine. Newer students and those whose strength is very challenged in this transition can bring their knees to the floor, tuck their toes under, and then press to Adho Mukha Svanasana. Experienced students with strong and stable shoulders can build additional strength by first lowering back to Chaturanga and then pressing back to Adho Mukha Svanasana.

Move from Adho Mukha Svanasana to Ardha Uttanasana by either walking the feet forward or "floating" the feet to the hands. Encourage new students and those with lower-back or wrist issues to walk forward. The floating technique is best introduced by asking students to practice springing from their legs as high as they can, keeping their arms and shoulders strong and stable, and landing where their feet started in Adho Mukha Svanasana. Repeating this exercise several times, encourage them to fully straighten their legs as soon as they spring off the floor, aiming to elevate their shoulders over the wrists, hips over their shoulders, and legs level with the floor in a pike position. Students will find greater ease and levity by keeping their palms rooted and arms strong; they will feel even more levity by completing the exhale and cultivating a very light uddiyana bandha just before launching their feet off the floor. After practicing this several times, instruct your students to once again spring as high as they can with the inhale, this time allowing their feet to release down to the floor as close to their hands as they can, with their torso already extended forward and spine long in Ardha Uttanasana at the crest of their inhale.

When exhaling down into Uttanasana in Surya Namaskara A or B, encourage students to place the back of the hands on the floor for just that moment of exhale as a means of counter-posing tension in the wrists that might arise from all the Chaturanga–Up Dog–Down Dog–floating movements. They can also draw their fingers into a light fist to further stretch the back of their wrists. From here the path back to Samasthihi is the same as in the Classical Sun Salutes. Over time, encourage students to build up to doing five continuous Surya Namaskara A cycles.

Surya Namaskara B

Surya Namaskara B introduces two more asanas to the Sun Salutation family: Utkatasana (Chair Pose) and Virabhadrasana I (Warrior I Pose). The sequence is initiated by a fluid movement from Samasthihi to Utkatasana (Chair Pose). In instructing the first Utkatasana, ask students to place their hands into the creases of the groin, push the femoral heads toward the heels, and then rotate their pelvis forward and back a few times to find where it feels like their spine is drawing naturally out of their pelvis. Maintaining this pelvic neutrality, instruct them to release their arms down by their sides, turn their palms strongly out, and feel their chest expanding as their shoulder blades draw down and in and against their back ribs. Cue the class to reach their arms out and up overhead with an inhale, keeping their shoulder blades rooting down as they stretch up through their chest and arms. Students can keep their arms shoulder-distance apart and their gaze slightly down or, with ease in the neck, toward the horizon. If they can keep their arms straight, invite them to draw their palms together and gaze up to their thumbs. Play around with guiding your classes from Samasthihi to Utkatasana and back to Samas-

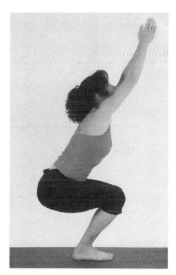

Utkatasana

thihi several times, emphasizing the connection of breath to movement, pada bandha to mula bandha, roots to extension up through the spine and arms. In the regular flow of Surya Namaskara B, transition from Utkatasana to Uttanasana by exhaling the legs straight while swan-diving forward and down. From Uttanasana, follow the same sequence from Surya Namaskara A to Adho Mukha Svanasana.

In transitioning from Adho Mukha Svanasana to Virabhadrasana I, there are two basic techniques. In traditional Ashtanga Vinyasa yoga, the left heel is turned in about halfway and rooted down before stepping the right foot forward. In many Vinyasa Flow classes, the right leg is first extended back and up while inhaling, then when exhaling the foot is drawn forward and placed next to the right hand. When using either method, consider first instructing Ashta Chandrasana (Crescent Pose) rather than Virabhadrasana I as a way of introducing high lunge poses and offering the space in which to gently awaken the hip flexors and groin while ensuring that students understand the important alignment principle of knee-over-heel. In further preparation for either the first Ashta Chandrasana or Virabhadrasana I, ask students to come high onto their fingertips, draw their shoulder blades down their back, and extend their sternum forward to draw more length through their spine and create more space around their neck.

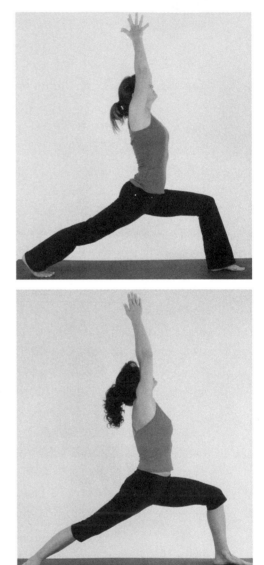

In either the Ashta Chandrasana or Virabhadrasana I, ask students to straighten their front leg all the way while drawing their torso all the way up into a vertical position, place their hands on their hips, and bring their pelvis to a place of neutrality while pressing the back leg straight and strong. If starting with Ashta Chandrasana, next cue students to draw their back heel in and down to the floor to establish the foundation there for Virabhadrasana I: cultivate pada bandha, rotate the back hip forward, the inner thigh of the back leg rotating back and the pelvis level. With the hands still on the hips, ask students to try to maintain as much pelvic neutrality as they can—space between their hip and front thigh—while slowing bending their front leg and consciously guiding their knee toward the little-toe side of the foot. It is very important to ensure that the front knee does not

Ashta Chandrasana (top); Virabhadrasana I (bottom)

travel out beyond the heel; allowing the knee to go farther forward places excessive pressure on the ACL. If a student feels pressure in the back knee or lower back when bending the front knee into Virabhadrasana I, guide that person to back out of the lunge or explore bending the knee less deeply. Keeping the back heel lifted straight up in the Ashta Chandrasana positioning will also reduce or eliminate the pressure in the back knee and lower back. In either asana, once students are up in the lunge position, ask them to release their arms down by their sides, turn their palms out to feel the external rotation of their arms at the shoulder joint, and then reach their arms out and up overhead while keeping the shoulder blades rooted down and in against their back ribs. Cue the class to look down for a moment and draw their lower front ribs slightly in, then try to maintain that positioning while bringing the gaze forward and the arms back. This will help students to develop neutral extension of the spine with greater shoulder flexion, which is intrinsically beneficial and helpful in creating the body intelligence for asanas such as Handstand. Encourage students who can keep their arms straight to draw their palms together overhead, and if it is OK with the neck, to gaze up to the tips of their thumbs.

To deepen the experience of Virabhadrasana I, emphasize the steady grounding of the feet, internal rotation of the back leg while pressing the shin firmly back to further ground the back heel, pada bandha in both feet, mula bandha, and steady energetic lifting through the spine, through the heart center, and out through the fingertips. Suggest lifting the lower rim of the ribs up and away from the upper rims of the hips to create more space and ease in the lower back. The breath should be steady and even, the eyes soft, the heart open. Virabhadrasana I is an excellent asana in which to teach multiple lines of energy, the relationship between roots and extension, and the balance of sthira and sukham. In the transition from Virabhadrasana I to Chaturanga Dandasana, encourage students to keep the movement simple, fluid, and connected to their breath. You will observe many students, especially advancing beginners, keeping one foot off the floor all the way into and even through Chaturanga Dandasana. This undermines the stable foundation of Chaturanga Dandasana; the integrity of Four-Limbed Staff Pose is lost to an asymmetrical three-limb variation that compromises the balanced movement into Urdhva Mukha Svanasana. Done repetitively, this can destabilize the sacroiliac joint and lead to potentially chronic lower-back problems. After repeating Virabhadrasana I on the other side, transition from Adho Mukha Svanasana to Ardha Uttanasana to Uttanasana to Utkatasana and back to Samasthihi, completing the sequence. In subsequent sequences, guide the class to flow continuously with the breath through this sequence of asanas. Over time, encourage students to build up to doing five continuous Surya Namaskara B cycles.

STANDING ASANAS

Standing asanas are the powerfully grounding foundation for all the other asanas. Standing on their feet, students begin to experience how a stable foundation creates support up through their legs, pelvis, spine, arms, and head. They also discover that a stable foundation is resilient, beginning with the activation of pada bandha in the feet.[3] Blending sthira and sukham in the standing asanas, students begin to find samasthihi (equal standing), which invokes an attitude and awareness of equanimity as they feel the connection of body, breath, mind, and spirit. In deepening this sense of equanimity, students develop an embodied awareness of how the lightness of being depends on being grounded, allowing them to move about in their yoga practice and daily life with greater ease and joy.

Standing asanas are divided into two categories: externally and internally rotated femurs. Externally rotated standing asanas generally stretch the inner groin and thighs while strengthening the external rotators and abductors. Internally rotated standing asanas generally strengthen the adductors and internal rotators while stretching the external rotators and abductors. Standing balance asanas strengthen the entire standing leg and the pelvic girdle while creating an opportunity to explore the instinctual fear of falling. Taken together, these asanas teach us about the integration of practice as we discover how the feet are connected to the legs, pelvis, spine, heart center, head, and arms—and ultimately to the breath and spirit. In teaching standing asanas, start with Samasthihi. Instruct from the ground up, as follows:

Feet and Ankles
- Give instructions for pada bandha and teach the importance of balancing the weight equally between the front, back, inside, and outside of each foot.

Legs and Pelvis
- With pada bandha active, instruct the contraction of the quadriceps along with the slight internal rotation of the femurs while pressing the femurs back, emphasizing how the internal rotation eases discovery of pelvic neutrality while broadening the space between the sitting bones.
- Note that most students tend to tilt their pelvis anteriorly, which compresses the lower back and can lead to disk problems. A practice of opening and

strengthening of the hip flexors, hip extensors, and abdominal core will help students move into stable pelvic neutrality.

- Guide students into feeling the connection between pada bandha and mula bandha, encouraging them to maintain mula bandha throughout their asana practice.

The Spine and Torso

- With pelvic neutrality, the spine will come into its natural curvature (neutral extension) in most students, unless there is significant muscular imbalance or a pathological condition such as scoliosis or kyphosis.
- Guide students into the light abdominal engagement that occurs naturally with complete exhalations, emphasizing how this helps to stabilize and lengthen the lumbar spine. The belly should be supple and stable.
- Cue the further lengthening of the spine by encouraging lifting the lower rim of the ribs up and away from the upper rim of the pelvis while allowing the floating ribs to soften naturally into the body.

The Shoulders and Heart Center

- Cue students to lift and broaden the sternum from inside while allowing the shoulder blades to draw lightly down and against the back ribs, further accentuating an expansive heart center while stabilizing the shoulders and creating ease in the neck.
- Instruct the broadening of the collarbones by first lifting the shoulders toward the ears, then drawing them back and down without losing the alignment in the lower- and mid-thoracic areas of the spine.

Neck and Head

- Refine the positioning of the neck and head by instructing students to feel the positioning of their ears in line with their shoulders, then to draw the chin very slightly forward and down, lengthening the back of the neck while lifting through the throat.
- Finally, cue opening the crown of the head to the sky.

Standing Asanas—Externally Rotated Femur(s)

VRKSASANA

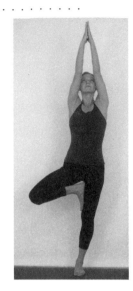

Primary Risks
Knees: flexion of bent knee, hyperextension or pressure on standing knee.

Guiding Students into the Asana
Start in Tadasana; use the wall for support; heel of lifted leg placed below the knee if unable to place it above; keep hands on hips or at heart; lightly cue even hips, pelvic neutrality, and abduction of lifted leg.

What to Look For and Emphasize
Stability in the standing leg, lifted heel above knee, even hips, neutral pelvis, neutral spine, steady gaze, steady breath. Release slowly.

UTTHITA HASTA PADANGUSTHASANA B

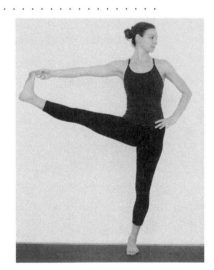

Primary Risks
Stability of standing knee, hamstrings of lifted leg, lower back.

Guiding Students into the Asana
Use the wall for support. Start as for Utthita Hasta Padangusthasana A, then as with Vrksasana. Encourage students to be more interested in keeping their standing leg stable, hips level, and pelvis neutral than getting their lifted leg out to the side. Offer the option of using a strap around the foot of the lifted leg, or clasp that knee and keep it bent when abducting the thigh.

What to Look For and Emphasize
Grounding down through the standing leg, feel more space through the standing hip, the spine, and out through the top of the head; expanding across the chest, explore looking over the shoulder to the opposite side of the lifted leg while extending that leg out on abduction. Steady breath and gaze.

VIRABHADRASANA II

Primary Risks
Front knee if misaligned, back knee if hyperextended, shoulders if impingement, lower back if pelvis not neutral.

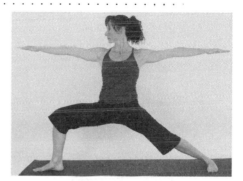

Guiding Students into the Asana
Start in a wide Prasarita stance, turning the right foot out, the left foot slightly in, slowing bending the right knee while guiding it toward the little-toe side of the foot; if the knee goes beyond the heel, crawl the toes farther forward for a longer stance. If starting from Virabhadrasana I, emphasize keeping front knee alignment while rotating the other hip back.

What to Look For and Emphasize
Front knee aligned directly above heel (it will tend to splay in); front sitting bone drawing under; hips level; pelvis neutral; back leg firm, arch lifted; shoulder blades down back; energy up through spine and out from heart through the fingertips. Press through the feet to release.

UTTHITA PARSVAKONASANA

Primary Risks
Same as Virabhadrasana II; also neck when looking up, upper shoulder if unstable or impinging.

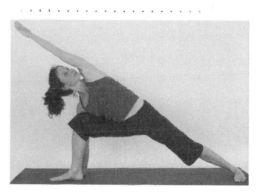

Guiding Students into the Asana
From Virabhadrasana II, keep the feet grounded and reach out through the right arm and side, initially placing the elbow on the knee; drawing the shoulder blades down the back, revolve the torso open, reach the left arm down the back leg, turn the palm up to feel external rotation of the arm, then reach the arm overhead; over time, bring the lower fingertips or palm to a block or the floor to the inside of the front foot, and over time to the outside of the foot.

What to Look For and Emphasize
Minimize lateral flexion of the spine while rotating the torso open; strong line of energy from grounded back foot through extended fingertips; press elbow or

shoulder against knee isometrically to keep knee aligned and leverage rotation of the torso; gaze to upper fingertips or relax the neck and look across the room or to the floor.

UTTHITA TRIKONASANA

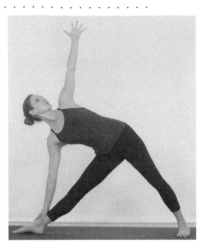

Primary Risks
Neck, knees if hyperextended, lower back.

Guiding Students into the Asana
Start with the feet separated the length of one leg, turn the right foot out ninety degrees, the left slightly in. Shift the hips to the left, pressing the right sitting bone toward the left while reaching out to the right through the spine and arm to the point of maximum extension, then release the hand onto the lower leg or ankle. Offer the option of looking down to make it easier on the neck. Suggest initially bringing the hand higher up the shin to ease the lengthening and slight rotation of the spine.

What to Look For and Emphasize
Straight, strong legs without hyperextending the knees; front leg kneecap lifted and pointed forward; minimize lateral flexion of spine; torso turned to the side wall and aligned directly over the leg; neck long; radiate out from heart center through both arms and fingertips.

ARDHA CHANDRASANA

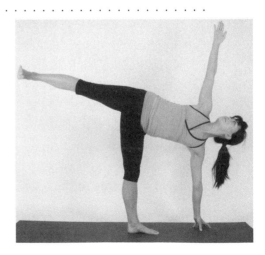

Primary Risks
Standing knee if unstable or hyperextended, standing hip if upper hip is rotated forward, neck.

Guiding Students into the Asana
Use the wall for balance; transition in stages from Utthita Trikonasana by bending the front knee, placing the fingertips about a foot in from the front foot (on the floor or a block), slide the back foot closer to the front foot until fully

weighting the front foot and hand, then begin slowly to straighten the front leg while keeping the back hip rotated fully open.

What to Look For and Emphasize

Maintain external rotation of the hips while transitioning; keep the standing foot from turning in; extend the lifted leg straight back from the hip; radiate out from the belly through the legs and spine, and from the heart center radiate out through the fingertips.

Standing Asanas—Internally Rotated Femur(s)

See the section on Surya Namaskara for the following internally rotated standing asanas: Tadasana/Samasthihi, Utkatasana, Anjaneyasana, Ashta Chandrasana, Virabhadrasana I.

PARIVRTTA PARSVAKONASANA

Primary Risks

Knee and ankle of back leg, front knee, lower back, neck.

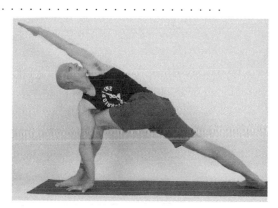

Guiding Students into the Asana

Start with the right foot forward in Ashta Chandrasana, or more challengingly, in Virabhadrasana I. Place the left hand on the left hip to help stabilize the hip in that position. Emphasize the importance of this positioning and the alignment of the front knee over the heel. Reach the right arm straight up to help lengthen through the right side of the torso, then stretch forward while twisting to the left, placing the left elbow on the right knee for a "prayer" positioning, or, if students have greater rotational flexibility and open hips, draw the shoulder across the knee and the hands to the floor outside of the left foot. Finally, stretch the left arm overhead, externally rotating the arm while rotating the torso to the left.

What to Look For and Emphasize

Emphasize alignment of the front knee above the front heel and the left hip directly back from that knee as in Virabhadrasana I. Keeping the back heel lifted in the Ashta Chandrasana positioning offers a more accessible preparatory approach. Keep the back leg strongly engaged. If in the full form of the asana with the back heel down, commit to rooting the outer edge of that foot to help rotate that hip forward.

PRASARITA PADOTTANASANA A, B, C, AND D

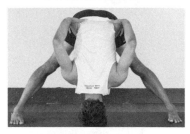

Primary Risks
Hamstrings and lower back, shoulders in variation C.

Guiding Students into the Asana
Start with the feet separated the length of one leg, outer edges of the feet parallel. The knees can be bent to relieve the hamstrings and lower back. In variation A, slide wrists back under elbows and create the feeling of sliding hands forward to lengthen spine, drawing shoulder blades down against the back ribs. In B, keep the hands on the hips to encourage anterior rotation of the pelvis while drawing elbows toward each other to expand the chest. In C, keep the shoulder blades rooted down against the back ribs while stretching the arm over head and expanding across the chest (if shoulders are tight, use a strap between the hands). In D, clasp and pull up on the big toes while renewing pada bandha, stretching the elbows away from each other while shrugging the shoulder blades down the back.

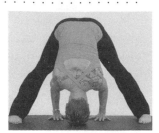

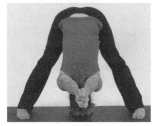

What to Look For and Emphasize
Straight, strong legs; slight internal rotation of the femurs to ease anterior rotation of the pelvis, drawing the pubic bone back and up while stretching the belly button and sternum toward the floor; try to bring the weight forward into the balls of the feet while grounding the fronts of the heels, hips directly over the heels; relax the neck.

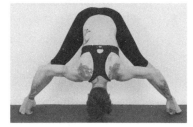

Prasarita Padottanasana A, B, C, and D (top to bottom)

PARSVOTTANASANA

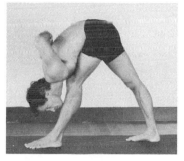

Primary Risks
Hamstrings and lower back, wrists and elbows if palms in reverse prayer.

Guiding Students into the Asana
Start with a Prasarita stance, initially with the feet separated the length of one leg, then bring the feet a few inches closer together. With the hands on the hips, turn the right foot out ninety degrees, then lift and replace the left foot on the floor, positioning it more or less parallel to the right, as much or as little as it takes to square the hips toward the front of the mat while still feeling a stretch in the left groin; extend the arms out, then draw them into reverse prayer or an alternate clasp. Rooting through the legs and feet, lift through the spine, opening across the heart center, then slowly rotate the pelvis anteriorly to extend the sternum forward and eventually toward the toes. As an alternative, bring the hands forward to a wall or down onto a chair or blocks.

What to Look For and Emphasize
Palms together behind the back in reverse prayer position (or clasp wrists or elbows); keep both legs straight and strong; keep the hip even and level by pressing down through the right leg and foot, drawing the right hip back, and rooting the back heel firmly down, internally rotating the thigh of the back leg; rotate the pelvis anteriorly, the pubic bone drawing back and up while stretching the belly button and sternum toward the floor.

PARIVRTTA TRIKONASANA

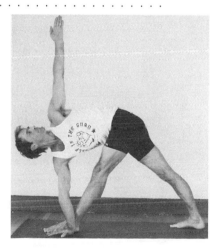

Primary Risks
Hamstrings, lower back, neck.

Guiding Students into the Asana
Most students will shift their hips in an attempt to bring their hand to the floor or to turn their torso farther to the right, which tends to bring the twist more into the lower back rather than into the thoracic spine; encourage students to make the stable positioning of their hips and legs more interesting than placement

of their hand or rotation of their torso. Start with the left fingertips high on a block (or wall or chair), and the right hand on hip to encourage the hip back and torso to revolve open. In extending the right arm up, remind students to keep that arm from going back beyond the plane of their shoulders. If the neck is strained, drop the head.

What to Look For and Emphasize

The legs and hips are identical to the upright starting position for Parsvottanasana. With the right leg forward, bring the right hand to the right hip to keep the hip positioned there, reach the left arm up and rotate the pelvis forward, bringing the right hand to the floor (or a block or chair) to the inside (over time to the outside) of the right foot, rotating the torso open to the right while maintaining the positioning of the legs and hips. Draw the shoulder blades down the back and radiate out from the heart center through the arms and fingertips.

VIRABHADRASANA III

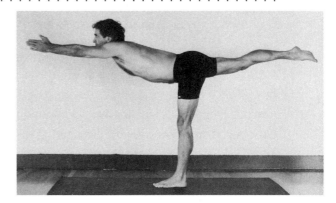

Primary Risks

Hamstrings and knee of standing leg, lower back, shoulders and neck.

Guiding Students into the Asana

This asana is most easily learned with the hands on a wall. Explore transitioning into it from Ashta Chandrasana, springing lightly forward onto the front foot and leg and back into Ashta Chandrasana, eventually keeping the weight on the front foot and exploring the slow, steady straightening of the front leg while lifting the back leg eventually level with the hips; offer the option of having the arms back by the sides to make it easier on the lower back, or out like an airplane for easier balance. Do not lock the knee of the standing leg.

What to Look For and Emphasize

Firm the thigh of the standing leg, keeping the ankle stable and kneecap pointing forward; keep the hips level and internally rotate the femur of the lifted leg; lengthen through the side of the torso and chest; in the full asana, reach the arms forward, eventually pressing the palms together and gazing to the thumbs.

PARIVRTTA ARDHA CHANDRASANA

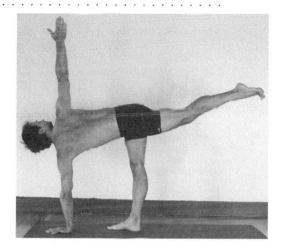

Primary Risks
Hamstrings and knee of standing leg, lower back, shoulders and neck.

Guiding Students into the Asana
As with Parivrtta Trikonasana, many students tend to compromise the stable positioning of the legs and hips in order to create the feeling or appearance of a deeper twist; cue keeping the hips level and the back leg lifted and energized, then twist from there. As with Parivrtta Trikonasana, in extending the right arm up, remind students to keep that arm from going back beyond the plane of their shoulders. If the neck is strained, drop the head.

What to Look For and Emphasize
The legs and hips are identical to their positioning in Virabhadrasana III. Standing on the right leg, bring the left hand (initially the fingertips) to a block or the floor directly under the left shoulder, and consider the option of placing the right hand on the right hip as offered in Parivrtta Trikonasana; rotating the torso to the right, eventually reach the right arm up.

GARUDASANA

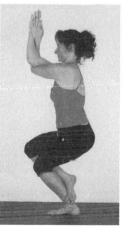

Primary Risks
Knees if ligaments strained, shoulders if impingement.

Guiding Students into the Asana
Use the wall for support. Teach in stages: bend the knees slightly, reaching the arms out with elbows bent down and the chest expanding; lift and cross the right ankle on the left knee, flexing the foot to stabilize the right knee, or, if possible, draw the knee all the way across the left knee and hook the right foot behind the left ankle or calf; reach out through the arms, then cross the left elbow over the right, drawing the forearms up and palms together (or try to clasp the right thumb), keeping the breath and gaze steady.

What to Look For and Emphasize

Try to lift the elbows level with the shoulders while drawing the shoulder blades down the back and pressing the hands away from the face; deepen the stretch between the shoulder blades by pressing the elbows and palms more firmly together. Try to bend the knees more deeply while lifting the spine and chest.

PADANGUSTHASANA AND PADAHASTHASANA

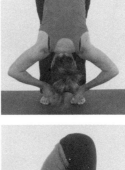

Primary Risks

Hamstrings and lower back.

Guiding Students into the Asana

With pada bandha in both feet, for Padangusthasana, fold forward as for Uttanasana, then clasp and pull up on the big toes while stretching the chest forward as for Ardha Uttanasana, then fold down, stretching the elbows away from each other and shrugging the shoulder blades down the back. For Padahasthasana, offer the same cues except with placement of the palms under the feet, toes to the wrists and fingertips to the heels.

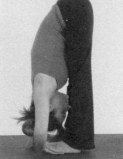

What to Look For and Emphasize

Start as for Uttanasana. Radiate down through the legs to ground the feet firmly and activate the legs; internally rotate the femurs, pitch the pubic bone back and up, and stretch the sternum toward the floor. Try to bring the weight forward while grounding the heels. Lengthen the spine from the strength and action in the legs.

UTTHITA HASTA PADANGUSTHASANA A

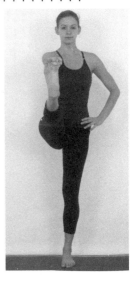

Primary Risks

Stability of standing knee, hamstrings of lifted leg, lower back.

Guiding Students into the Asana

Use the wall for support. Start as for Utthita Hasta Padangusthasana A, then as with Vrksasana. Encourage students to be more interested in keeping their standing leg stable, hips level, and pelvis neutral than getting their lifted leg out to the side. Offer the option of using a strap around the foot of the lifted leg, or clasp that knee and keep it bent when abducting the thigh.

What to Look For and Emphasize

Grounding down through the standing leg, feel more space through the standing hip, the spine, and out through the top of the head; expanding across the chest, explore looking over the shoulder to the opposite side of the lifted leg while extending that leg out on abduction. Steady breath and gaze.

ARDHA BADDHA PADMOTTANASANA

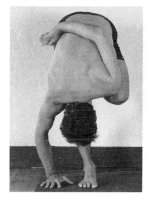

Primary Risks

Knee of lotus leg, stability of standing knee, hamstrings, lower back.

Guiding Students into the Asana

From Tadasana, lift the right knee, cradle the lower leg, and draw the right heel toward the left hip (ASIS), then release through the inner right groin to allow the right knee to release down into a half-lotus position. Draw the right hand around behind the back to clasp the lotus foot. Reach the left arm straight up, then slowly fold forward and down as for Uttanasana. Inhaling, lift as for Ardha Uttanasana, then exhaling fold back down and hold for five to eight breaths. To come up, inhaling, lift to the Ardha positioning, stay to exhale and feel the belly draw to the spine, then use that support inhaling back up to standing.

What to Look For and Emphasize

Keep the standing leg strong and steady, bending the knee to take it easier on the hamstrings and lower back. Be very sensitive to the lotus knee, especially while folding forward, as this increases the potential twisting of the knee.

CORE REFINEMENT

In popular fitness culture, the ideal core is often symbolized by "six-pack abs," the most superficial of the abdominal core muscles discussed in Chapter Four. Yet when so overdeveloped and tight, this rectus abdominus muscle is a source of tension and spinal problems, compromising the grace and ease, poise and elegance, comfort and stability that come from a refined core. As Ana Forrest has long emphasized, we want to relieve emotional and physical constipation and restriction, to release deep guttural anxiety, not seal it in. Reminding students that yoga is largely about creating space, we want to guide students into cultivating a strong yet supple core, learning along the way to radiate outward while drawing awareness deep into the core of the body. As the core is strengthened, opened, and refined, it becomes a source of balance, stability, ease, and levity.

Taking an expanded view of the core, offer students a visual that extends from the medial arches of the feet, up the inseams of the legs to the floor of the pelvis, up through the spine and out through the crown of the head. Throughout the asana practice, encourage students to draw energetically in toward this expanded core while radiating out from it to create space. Refer to pada bandha and mula bandha as key energetic actions for awakening this energetic awareness. This in itself will help to strengthen and refine the muscles that are at the heart of core refinement and make the more specific core asana practices more accessible and simple.

Here we will focus on asanas to strengthen muscles in the front body that give support to the lower torso in its relationship to the pelvis and spine. (Contraction backbends and a variety of dynamic movements in and out of asanas will strengthen the muscles giving support from the back body.) These asanas are contraindicated for pregnant students and should be approached very gingerly by students with lower-back issues.

JATHARA PARIVARTANASANA

Primary Risks
Lower back, neck.

Guiding Students into the Asana
The basic form of this asana can be either a held twist (Supta Parivartanasana) or an abdominal core strengthening movement. With the arms extended out like a cross and palms pressing down, alternately move the legs (or bent knees) back and forth to the left and right while gazing in the opposite direction of the legs, keeping the knees or legs from touching the floor. Inhaling, extend the legs over; exhaling, draw them back up to center.

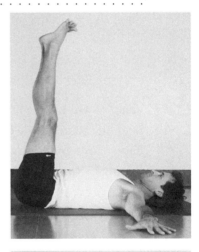

What to Look For and Emphasize
Press the shoulders and palms firmly down while moving the legs, going only so far in the rotation as feels comfortable on the lower back.

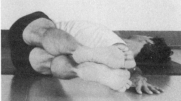

YOGIC BICYCLES

Primary Risks
Lower back.

Guiding Students into the Asana

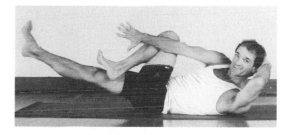

From Apanasana, interlace the fingers and cup the head in the hands. With the exhalation, curl the torso up, drawing the elbows toward the knees while extending the right leg straight out about one foot off the floor and extending the right arm out over the right leg. Complete the exhale while drawing the right arm across the left knee and drawing the elbows together. Inhaling, release down, drawing the knees toward the chest and head and elbows to the floor. Repeat on the other side, continuing for one to three minutes.

What to Look For and Emphasize
Emphasize moving slowly and working as low, deep, and broadly through the belly as possible. Encourage students to be more interested in moving slowly yet steadily rather than seeing how many they can do with a timed sequence. Move with the breath.

PELVIC TILTS

Primary Risks
Lower back, neck.

Guiding Students into the Asana

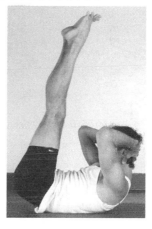

From Apanasana, extend the legs straight up, interlace the fingers, and cup the head in the hands. Keeping the legs vertical, on the exhalation draw the elbows toward the knees without changing the position of the legs. Keeping the upper back and shoulders lifted, with each exhale very slowly and smoothly curl the tailbone up, releasing it down as the breath flows out. Repeat five to twenty-five times.

What to Look For and Emphasize
Students tend to focus on jerking the tailbone up. Encourage them to be more interested in slow and smooth movement than in maximizing the pelvic tilt. Emphasize keeping the legs vertical rather than drawing them toward the elbows.

PARIPURNA NAVASANA AND ARDHA NAVASANA

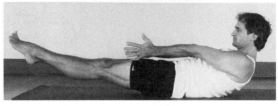

Primary Risks
Lower back, groin.

Guiding Students into the Asana
From Dandasana, slide one heel back toward the hip on the same side, clasping that knee to leverage the anterior rotation of the pelvis while sitting taller, then draw in the other heel, clasping behind both knees while leaning slightly back. Maintaining the weight on the front of the sitting bones, slowly lift the feet off the floor, eventually straightening the legs and bringing the toes level with the eyes without slumping in the spine. Gradually hold less strongly with the hands, eventually extending the arms forward.

What to Look For and Emphasize
Emphasize pelvic neutrality in relation to the spine and a spacious heart center. If able to straighten the legs, press out through the balls of the feet, spreading the toes and internally spiraling the thighs. For Ardha Navasana, release the lower back to the floor, palms to the heart in anjali mudra, knees either in (easier) or straight legs about one foot off the floor. Add kapalabhati pranayama to intensify.

TOLASANA

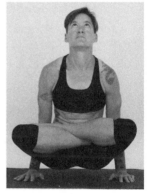

Primary Risks
Knees, wrists.

Guiding Students into the Asana
From Padmasana or Sukhasana (the simple cross-legged sitting position), place the hands on the floor by the hips. Gazing up, with the exhalation press the hands down to lift off the floor (or try!) and hold while breathing.

What to Look For and Emphasize
Focus on lifting straight up off the floor. To add intensity, do kapalabhati pranayama.

LOLASANA

Primary Risks
Wrists.

Guiding Students into the Asana
From Vajrasana, cross the ankles and place the hands
on the floor by the thighs. Gazing up, with the exhalation press the hands down while arching the spine
up, drawing the knees toward the chest and eventually the heels toward the tailbone.

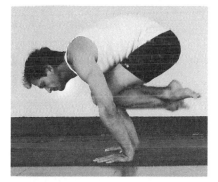

What to Look For and Emphasize
With practice, move fluidly from Dandasana to Tolasana to Lolasana to Chaturanga
Dandasana. More advanced students can transition from Lolasana to Adho Mukha
Vrksasana.

ARM BALANCES

Balancing the entire body on the hands requires absolute focus, bringing students
deeper into a sense of dharana in their asana practice. Arm balances also bring students closer to a deeply held and perfectly rational fear of falling, a fear that is inextricably interwoven with the ego and the desire at least to appear in control. This
makes arm balances the perfect asana family for cultivating self-confidence and
humility (Sparrowe 2003). Because most students will find at least some arm balances very challenging, these asanas are also a wonderful place to explore the practice with a sense of humor and playfulness. As with any asanas, patience and practice
makes them more accessible and sustainable, while impatience almost invariably
leads to frustration or injury.

Students should practice Phalakasana, Chaturanga Dandasana, and Adho
Mukha Svanasana for at least one year to strengthen the wrists, arms, and shoulders in preparation for bringing more weight onto their hands. The wrists are at
greatest risk in all arm balances. Students with acute wrist issues, including carpal
tunnel syndrome, should not do full arm balances, and students with even mildly
strained wrists are advised to minimize pressure on the wrists and use a wedged
hand prop until they are free of pain. Whether interspersing arm balances throughout a practice or teaching them as a cluster of asanas, it is important to offer students the wrist therapy exercises described in Chapter Eleven. Students should have
sufficient wrist extension to place their palms flat on the floor and move their

forearms perpendicular to the floor without strain or pain. Students with weak, unstable, or impinged shoulders are advised to do the healthy shoulder program described in Chapter Eleven until developing sufficient stability and flexibility in the shoulder girdle to hold Adho Mukha Svanasana for two minutes free of pain before attempting more shoulder-intense arm balances. Limited shoulder flexion is also the primary cause of a banana shape to the spine in Adho Mukha Vrksasana and Pincha Mayurasana.

Along with strength and stability in the wrists, arms, and shoulders, arm balances require and awaken the abdominal core muscles. As discussed in Chapter Ten, abdominal work prior to arm balances helps students create a feeling of lifting and radiating out from their core. Yet arm balances also require suppleness in the core, not gripping or bearing down. Finding this balance between active engagement and spreading through the core is one of the key elements to balancing the body on the hands. This is most evident in Adho Mukha Vrksasana, where strong core muscles stabilize the center of the body, but where tight core muscles, especially in the psoas and rectus abdominus muscles, limit full extension of the hips and spine in relation to the pelvis, exacerbating the banana shape in a student's spine.

In introducing arm balances, start with simple preparatory practices as described later for each asana. Offer students an opportunity to practice each arm balance two to three times. Ask them to pay close attention to what happens in each attempt: Where did they feel their weight? Where is their gaze? How is the breath flowing? What caused or led them to come out of the asana? What are they thinking about? What are they feeling? Encourage students to keep reflecting on what happens each time they try the asanas, gradually refining what they are doing to make the asanas simpler, stabler, and more fun.

BAKASANA

Primary Risks
Wrists and shoulders.

Guiding Students into the Asana
Bring students into a squat with the heels lifted and knees wide apart. Stretch the arms as far forward as possible, lengthening through the spine, shoulders, and arms, then slide the hands back under the shoulders while drawing the elbows outside the shins,

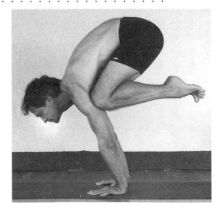

thereby placing the knees as high onto the arms or shoulders as possible. Squeezing the knees into the arms or shoulders, press firmly into the hands and feet while lifting from the belly to elevate the hips as high as possible. Lean forward to bring the weight more into the hands, then begin to explore lifting the left and right feet alternately off the floor, eventually drawing both feet up together to the buttocks and straightening the arms. Place a stack of blankets under the face to reduce fear.

What to Look For and Emphasize

Rooting firmly into the palms, with each exhalation renew the lifting of the belly toward the spine while drawing the pubic bone back and up. Keep the gaze steadily focused on a point directly beneath the head. If stable, teach floating directly to Chaturanga Dandasana: creating a feeling of reaching the sternum toward the horizon, root more firmly through the hands, and with an exhale, extend the feet directly back while bending the elbows to arrive in Chaturanga.

PARSVA BAKASANA

Primary Risks

Wrists, shoulders, lower back, neck.

Guiding Students into the Asana

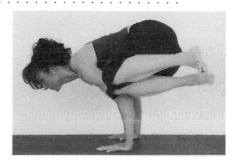

Begin squatting as for Bakasana, come up high on the fingertips, straighten the legs halfway, twist from the torso, turn both knees to the left, and squat back down; then stretch the left arm up, press the knees further back, and reach the left arm across the right knee (drawing the belly up and across the thigh), then place the left hand on the floor with both hands placed as though for Chaturanga Dandasana. Rooting through the hands while lifting the sternum, begin tipping lightly forward on the tiptoes to bring the weight fully onto the hands, bending the elbows while reaching the sternum forward and keeping the ankles together as they lift off the floor.

What to Look For and Emphasize

Keep rooting through the palms, keeping the elbows in line with the shoulders, knees even, breath and gaze steady. When stable, transition into Dwi or Eka Pada Koundinyasana.

DWI PADA KOUNDINYASANA

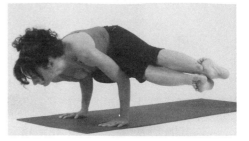

Primary Risks
Wrists, shoulders, lower back, neck.

Guiding Students into the Asana
From Parsva Bakasana, extend both legs straight out the side, keeping the knees and ankles close together.

What to Look For and Emphasize
Keep rooting through the palms, keeping the elbows in line with the shoulders, knees even, breath and gaze steady. Press out strongly through the balls of the feet, spreading the toes wide apart. When stable, transition into Eka Pada Koundinyasana.

BHUJAPIDASANA

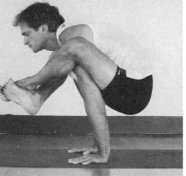

Primary Risks
Wrists, shoulders, lower back.

Guiding Students into the Asana
From Adho Mukha Svanasana, leap-frog the feet around the hands; slide the hands as far back as possible while keeping the wrists and palms rooted, positioning the knees against the shoulders. Squeezing the knees firmly into the upper arms or shoulders, release the hips slightly toward the floor to lift the feet off the floor more easily, then try to cross the ankles.

What to Look For and Emphasize
If the knees are positioned at the shoulders, try to draw the heels to the buttocks and the top of the head to the floor, holding for five breaths or longer before transitioning back up.

TITTIBHASANA

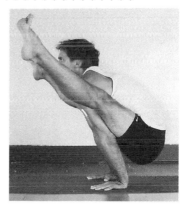

Primary Risks

Wrists, shoulders, elbows if hyperextended, lower back, hamstrings.

Guiding Students into the Asana

From Bhujapidasana, slowly extend the legs straight, spreading the toes and radiating out through the balls of the feet.

What to Look For and Emphasize

Be very sensitive to the wrists, rooting more firmly through the knuckles of the index fingers. Intermediate students can try to transition to Bakasana, lifting the hips while drawing heels out, back, and up.

ADHO MUKHA VRKSASANA

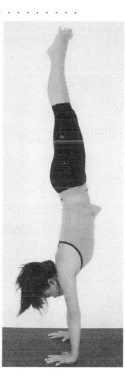

Primary Risks

Wrists, shoulders.

Guiding Students into the Asana

Introduce at a wall in three stages: (1) in an L shape (like Down Dog) with the hands on the wall and feet on the floor, alternately extending one leg up while maintaining all the qualities of Down Dog in the upper body; (2) in an L-shape with the hands on the floor under the shoulders and feet on the wall where the hands just were, alternately extending one leg straight up; and (3) in Adho Mukha Svanasana with the fingertips five inches from the wall. Extend one leg back and up, keeping it straight and strong; begin springing off the other foot while swinging the lifted leg up. The moment the springing leg is sprung, make it straight and strong, and draw it up next to the other leg overhead.

What to Look For and Emphasize

Pressing down firmly through the hands as in Adho Mukha Svanasana, first flex the feet and extend up through the legs and heels, then point and press out through the balls of the feet. While drawing longer through the core of the body, wrap the shoulder blades broadly as in Down Dog, lightly engage the belly to support the torso and pelvis, keep the floating ribs in away from the skin while pressing the tailbone and pubis up, activate mula bandha, spiral the femurs internally, and breathe.

PINCHA MAYURASANA

Primary Risks
Wrists, shoulders, lower back, neck.

Guiding Students into the Asana
Use the same steps as described for introducing Adho Mukha Vrksasana, except the forearms are placed on the wall or floor. If students' forearms splay, place a block between the index fingers and
a strap just above the elbows. In stage 3, press the shoulders as far
back from the wrists as possible. Maintain this positioning when
scissor-kicking the legs up overhead.

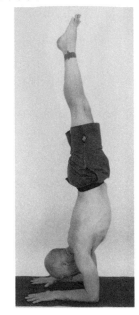

What to Look For and Emphasize
Once in Pincha Mayurasana, press firmly through the palms and
elbows, drawing the shoulders away from the wrists while pressing
the tailbone toward the feet and toward the ceiling. Internally rotate the femurs.

ASTAVAKRASANA

Primary Risks
Wrists, shoulders, lower back, neck.

Guiding Students into the Asana
In Dandasana, slide the right foot in, clasping
the knee to leverage the anterior rotation of

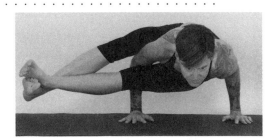

the pelvis and extension of the spine. Then: (1) clasp the right foot and move it
around in a figure 8 in front of the chest; (2) cradle the lower right leg between the
elbows, flex the right foot, and "rock the cradle"; (3) draw the right knee over the
right shoulder while reaching the right arm forward, placing the right palm next
to the right hip, left palm by the left hip; (4) lift the left leg off the floor, then with
an exhale press through the hands to lift the hips off the floor; (5) cross the right
ankle over the left ankle and extend the legs straight out to the left; (6) bend the
elbows until the shoulders are level with them.

What to Look For and Emphasize
Keep rooting the palms, lifting the hips, pressing out through the balls of the feet,
squeezing the knees toward each other, drawing the sternum forward and gazing

either down (easier on the neck) or to the horizon. Explore transitioning to Eka Pada Koundinyasana by (1) straightening the arms, (2) lifting the hips, (3) unhooking the feet, (4) threading the left foot and leg back between the arms, and (5) scissoring the legs apart. From there, float to Chaturanga.

EKA PADA KOUNDINYASANA

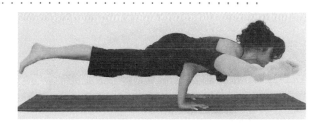

Primary Risks
Wrists, shoulders, hamstrings, lower back, groin.

Guiding Students into the Asana
From Parsva Bakasana, scissor the legs apart, with the top leg extended back while cantilevering the chest forward to balance.

What to Look For and Emphasize
Feed the legs, pressing out through the balls of the feet. Gaze forward, and with an exhale use light uddiyana bandha, floating to Chaturanga.

GALAVASANA

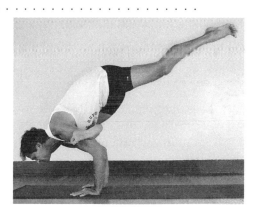

Primary Risks
Wrists, shoulders, knee and hip of crossed leg, lower back.

Guiding Students into the Asana
Teach in steps: (1) from Tadasana, bend the knees, then lift and cross the right ankle onto the left knee, strongly flexing the right foot; (2) draw the palms together at the heart center; (3) bring the palms to the floor under the shoulders, hooking the flexed right foot around the left shoulder while placing the left knee on the left shoulder; (4) pressing the palms, lean the weight forward; (5) extend the left leg back and up.

What to Look For and Emphasize
While rooting through the hands, draw the sternum forward and press out through the extended left leg. Either float to Chaturanga or transition into Sirsasana II in preparation for transitioning directly to the other side of the asana.

UTTANA PRASITHASANA

Primary Risks
Wrists, hip of lower leg, shoulders, lower back.

Guiding Students into the Asana
Come to step 2 of Galavasana Prep, then: (1) use the left hand to stabilize the right ankle on the left knee; (2) stretch the right arm up to lengthen through the right side; (3) twist the torso and draw the right

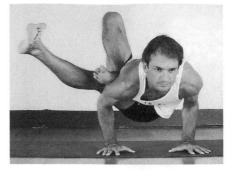

elbow to the left arch, pressing the palms together to leverage the twist; (4) draw the right shoulder to the arch and release the right hand to the floor outside the left ankle; (5) place the left hand on the floor shoulder-distance from the right hand; (6) lean the weight to the left while bending the elbows, extending the left leg to the left and off the floor and reaching the chest forward.

What to Look For and Emphasize
Instruct students to try to bring their shoulders level with each other. Energize out through the extended leg. Float to Chaturanga.

VASISTHASANA

Primary Risks
Wrist and shoulder of grounded arm, hamstrings of lifted leg, neck.

Guiding Students into the Asana
From Phalakasana, roll onto the outer edge of the left foot while drawing the right hand to the right hip. Placing the right ankle on top of the left ankle, flex both feet, and press the lower hip up. Rooting from the left shoulder through the left hand, explore either (a) sliding the right foot up the inner left thigh (like Vrksasana) or (b)

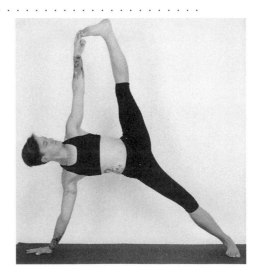

clasping the left big toe and extending the left leg straight up.

What to Look For and Emphasize
Keep the left hand and outer edge of the left foot firmly rooted. When lifting the right knee or leg, try to keep the right hip from moving either forward or back. Gaze up to the big toe, across toward the wall, or down to the floor.

URDHVA KUKKUTASANA

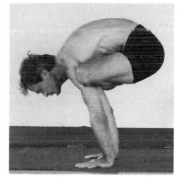

Primary Risks
Wrists, shoulders, knees, lower back, neck.

Guiding Students into the Asana
There are two ways in: (1) from Padmasana, press through
the hands while standing on the knees, then with an exhale
slide the knees up the arms; (2) from Sirsasana II, fold the
legs into Padmasana position, lower the knees to shoulders,
and press the hands to straighten the arms.

What to Look For and Emphasize
Maintain pada bandha, mula bandha, and light uddiyana bandha. Gaze straight
down. Transition to Chaturanga or to Sirsasana II (and from there, explore Parsva
Kukkutasana by twisting across as in Parsva Bakasana).

BACKBENDS

With deep stretching across the entire front of the body, especially through the
heart center, belly, and groin, backbends stimulate a passionate response among
students. The passion tends to go toward either unbridled effort or fearful withdrawal, offering students another opportunity for cultivating equanimity amid
these emotional poles. The primary physical purpose of backbends is to open to
the full movement of breath and energy in the front of the body, not to go into the
most gloriously deep backbend. You can guide students into finding a sense of sustainable effort in playing the edge in their backbend practice by emphasizing the
heart-opening qualities of this practice: feeling compassion toward one's self in
feeling one's way toward the edge, opening to a sense of innate inner harmony as
a source of aparigraha, sensing a healing presence within the breath that reinforces
a sense of assessment rather than judgment, and recognizing pure love in the heart
as the glue that holds everything together in the unending process of change. Encourage backbends as a practice of equanimity, not attainment, and purification
for the purpose of freedom, not perfection, focusing on opening the heart. Several
technical aspects of backbends will help ensure students practice them safely:

- *Rotate the thighs internally.* This action is most effectively instructed and felt
  using a block between the thighs in Tadasana, then in Setu Bandha Sarvan -
  gasana, and drawing the block back (in Tadasana) or down (in Setu Bandha
  Sarvangasana). Apply pada bandha to accentuate this action.

- *Never squeeze the buttocks.* Instead, soften the upper (more horizontal) fibers of the gluteus maximus, which, if contacting, will externally rotate and abduct the thighs, thereby putting undue pressure on the sacroiliac joint at the base of the spine.

- *Posteriorly tilt the pelvis.* This action will draw more length into the lumbar spine, reduce pressure on the lower intervertebral disks, and help share the backbend up the spine. Further cue this by asking students to bring the anterior superior iliac spine (ASIS bones) toward their lower front ribs.

- *Create length through the spine to allow greater spinal extension.* After relaxing along the spine, elongate the spine as much as possible before creating extension.

- *Focus the backbend in the thoracic spine.* The attachment of ribs (and muscles) to the spine, combined with the structure of the thoracic vertebrae, limits the extension of the spine and leads to excessive bending in the lumbar and cervical spine segments.

- *Add extension of the cervical spine last.* Allow the cervical spine to remain neutral or bring it into extension only after maximizing the backbend through the thoracic spine.

- *Draw the lower tips of the shoulder blades in and up toward the heart.* This deepens the thoracic center of the backbend and further opens the heart center.

- *Lift the sternum up.* This adds more expansiveness to the heart center.

- *Keep the breath steady and soft.* Breathe as if through the heart and into areas of tension.

These technical qualities apply in contraction, traction, and leverage backbends, each of which has important distinctions and actions:

- *Contraction backbends:* The back muscles (primarily spinal erectors and multifidi) concentrically contract to overcome gravity (e.g., lifting up into Salabhasana A).

- *Traction backbends:* Muscles in the front of the body eccentrically contract to overcome gravity (e.g., lowering back into Ustrasana).

- *Leverage backbends:* The arms and/or legs press against an unmovable object (floor, wall, or another part of the body) to stretch the front of the body (e.g., Urdhva Dhanurasana).

Within each of these categories of backbends, the humerus can either be in extension (e.g., in Salabhasana A, Ustrasana, or Setu Bandha Sarvangasana) or flexion (Salabhasana C, Kapotasana, or Viparita Dandasana), these positions requiring different areas of engagement and release through the shoulder girdle (see Chapter Ten for sequences that support these movements):

- *Shoulder extension backbends:* Extension of the arms requires the scapulae to be stabilized by the rhomboids, lower trapezius, and serratus anterior muscles while the pectoralis major and minor must release.
- *Shoulder flexion backbends:* Flexion requires the rhomboids, latissimi dorsi, pectoralis major, and triceps to release.

SALABHASANA A, B, AND C

Primary Risks
Lower back, neck, shoulders in C.

Guiding Students into the Asana
See Surya Namaskara for B and basic elements of all three asanas.

What to Look For and Emphasize
In variation A, keep the backs of the hands pressing firmly into the floor to leverage the lifting of the chest and the feeling of bringing the thoracic spine forward into the heart center. In variation C, emphasize keeping the shoulder blades rooted down against the back ribs while spiraling them broadly out as in Adho Mukha Svanasana.

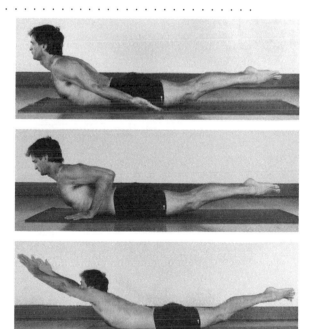

Salabhasana A, B, and C

NARAVIRALASANA

Primary Risks
Lower back, neck.

Guiding Students into the Asana
Lying prone, prop up onto the forearms, aligning the elbows under the

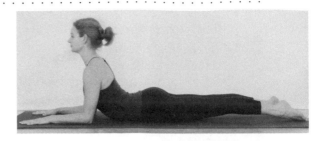

shoulders and the forearms and hands forward and parallel. Activate the legs as for
Salabhasana preparation, rooting the hips and feet, internally rotating the femurs
and pressing the sacrum toward the heels. Rooting the forearms while energetically pulling them back and inward, expand the chest while depressing the shoulder blades and pulling the spine in toward the heart. Over time, lift the head and
gaze forward.

What to Look For and Emphasize
This is a deceptively deep backbend that can strain the lower back and neck. Reinforce the active engagement of the legs and posterior tilt of the pelvis to maintain space in the lower back. Encourage students to look down to take it easier on
the neck.

BHUJANGASANA

Primary Risks
Lower back, neck if hyperextended.

Guiding Students into the Asana
Lying prone with the forehead on the
floor, place the palms down by the shoulders and shrug the shoulder blades down

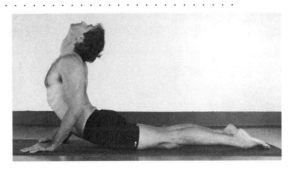

the back. Awaken the legs as in Salabhasana, internally rotate the thighs, and press
the tailbone toward the heels. Lift the chest as high as possible without using the
hands, then pressing the hands down, lift the chest slightly higher with each inhale, staying there with the exhale and drawing the spine forward toward the heart.
Continue in this manner, moving breath by breath to the deepest backbend while
remaining comfortable.

What to Look For and Emphasize

In pressing the palms down, energetically spiral them out (without actually moving them), feeling from this action how the elbows draw slightly in, the chest expands, and the lower tips of the shoulder blades draw in toward to heart.

URDHVA MUKHA SVANASANA

See Surya Namaskara for details on instruction.

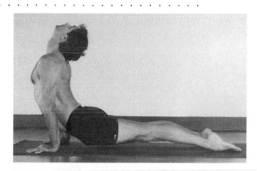

BHEKASANA

Primary Risks

Knees, lower back, shoulders, neck.

Guiding Students into the Asana

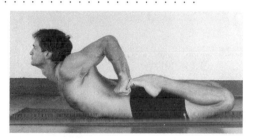

Start as for Salabhasana. Place the forearms on the floor with the elbows under the shoulders (Sphinx Pose). Explore one side at a time, first clasping the right foot with the right hand and drawing the right heel toward the outside of the right hip. In this effort, try to rotate the elbow up and to position the hand on the foot with the fingers pointing the same direction as the toes. Try to rotate the right shoulder forward to square the shoulders toward the front of the mat. If sufficiently flexible, do this with both hands and feet simultaneously.

What to Look For and Emphasize

Rooting the hips down and pressing the tailbone back, press the feet toward the floor while lifting the chest (be very sensitive to the knees and lower back). Try to draw the shoulder blades down the back, lower tips of the shoulder blades pressing toward the heart. Gaze down to take it easier on the neck, or forward.

DHANURASANA

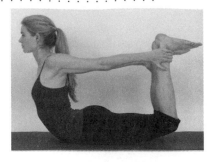

Primary Risks
Lower back, knees, neck if hyperextended, shoulders.

Guiding Students into the Asana
Lying prone, bend the knees and reach back to clasp the ankles. Flex the feet to activate pada bandha and stabilize the knees. Rooting down through the hips, pull on the ankles to leverage the chest and legs up off the floor, pressing the tailbone back while drawing the spine through toward the heart and spreading across the collarbones.

What to Look For and Emphasize
Try to rock back farther onto the thighs to lift the chest higher, then press the feet back up. Focus the backbend in the mid-thoracic spine. If the neck is stable, release the head back toward the feet.

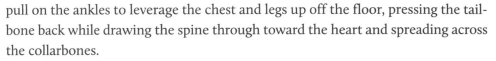

USTRASANA

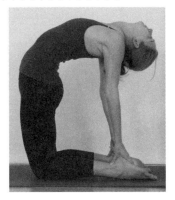

Primary Risks
Lower back, neck.

Guiding Students into the Asana
Standing on the knees with the toes curled under (or feet straight back for a deeper backbend) and knees hip-distance apart, place the hands on the hips to press the tailbone down, hips forward, and leverage the lifting of the sternum, creating a feeling of lifting the spine up into the heart. Rooting down through the legs and feet, press the hips forward and the tailbone down while drawing the hands to the heels or ankles (or to blocks).

What to Look For and Emphasize
Pressing from the hips through the knees, from the shoulders into the hands, and down through the feet, use these lever points to draw a deeper curve into the thoracic spine while pressing the tailbone down and under and lifting the sternum to the sky.

LAGHU VAJRASANA

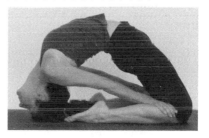

Primary Risks
Lower back, groin, knees, neck.

Guiding Students into the Asana
Maintaining all the elements of Ustrasana, bring the
hands forward toward or to the knees. Inhaling, release
backwards, drawing the head toward the floor only as far as the student can, while
exhaling, comfortably lift back up to Ustrasana, repeating five times and holding
the asana for five to eight breaths on the last drop-back.

What to Look For and Emphasize
Maintain the firm rooting of the feet and knees while elongating the spine, being
attentive to space and ease in the lower back and neck. Keep the sternum lifting
up and the breath steady. Gaze to the third eye.

KAPOTASANA

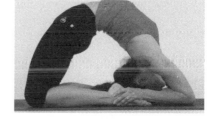

Primary Risks
Lower back, neck, shoulders.

Guiding Students into the Asana
From standing on the knees, draw the palms together
at the heart. Rooting and expanding as for Ustrasana,
slowly release back as practiced with Laghu Vajrasana, drawing the crown of the
head to the floor. Bring the elbows to the floor and clasp the feet (eventually the
knees) with the hands. After five to eight breaths, place the palms on the floor where
the elbows were placed, straighten the arms and hold for five to eight breaths.
Inhale to come up.

What to Look For and Emphasize
Try to maintain the firm rooting of the elbows, feet, and knees, expanding the front
of the body while maintaining space and ease in the lower back.

SUPTA VIRASANA

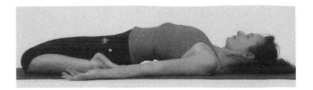

Primary Risks
Lower back, knees, neck if hyperextended.

Guiding Students into the Asana
From Virasana, explore in steps: (1) place the hands a few inches behind the hips, lift the hips slightly to tuck the tailbone under, then sit back down while lifting and expanding across the chest; (2) recline onto the elbows and repeat the actions in step 1; (3) recline onto the back and repeat the actions in step 1.

What to Look For and Emphasize
Keep the knees pressing to the floor, thighs rotating internally, tailbone tucking under. For more intensity, draw one knee in toward the shoulder on the same side. Explore drawing the arms overhead and clasping the elbows.

SETU BANDHA SARVANGASANA

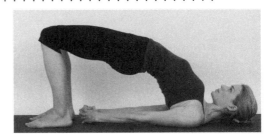

Primary Risks
Lower back, neck, knees.

Guiding Students into the Asana
Lying supine, slide the feet in close to the buttocks, hip-distance apart and parallel. With completion of the exhale, feel the lower back press toward the floor and the tailbone curl up. With the inhale, press through the feet (strong pada bandha) to lift the hips up with a feeling of the inner thighs spiraling down, the tailbone leading the way to keep space in the lower back. Interlace the fingers under the back and shrug the shoulders slightly under, just enough to draw any pressure off the neck.

What to Look For and Emphasize
Maintaining pada bandha and the internal rotation of the femurs, press down more firmly through the feet to lift the hips. Pressing down through the shoulders, elbows, and wrists, press the tips of the shoulder blades in toward the heart while lifting the sternum toward the chin and spreading broadly across the upper back and collarbones. To release, lift the heel, reach the arms overhead, and slowly roll down one vertebra at a time.

URDHVA DHANURASANA

Primary Risks

Lower back, wrists, shoulders, neck, groin. If a student is unable to straighten his or her arms in this asana, the forceful effort to do so will strain the wrists and shoulders while further tightening the muscles that need to release to open more naturally into it.

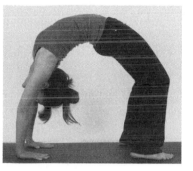

Guiding Students into the Asana

Start as for Seta Bandha Sarvangasana with the feet close to the hips; place the palms on the floor by and in line with the shoulders. Position the elbows to point straight up by externally rotating the shoulders; if unable to do this, play with separating the hands a little wider and turning the fingertips slightly out to ease the external rotation, creating a feeling of sliding the palms back to root the shoulder blades against the back ribs. With an inhale, press onto the top of the head with the hips lifted off the floor and reaffirm the positioning of the elbows and shoulders. With an inhalation, press the arms straight.

What to Look For and Emphasize

Maintain pada bandha, active legs, internal rotation of the femurs, and anterior rotation of the pelvis. Press evenly down through the hands, actively externally rotating the arms and expanding across the upper back and chest. Over time, deepen the asana by bringing the hands toward the feet. If the wrists are strained or the elbows slightly bent, explore placing the hands on blocks set against the wall at a 45-degree angle.

VIPARITA DANDASANA

Primary Risks

Lower back, shoulders, neck.

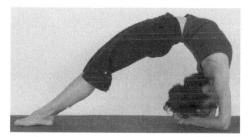

Guiding Students into the Asana

Start with the preparatory step of Urdhva Dhanurasana where the crown of the head is on the floor, draw the elbows to the floor shoulder-distance apart, and interlace the fingers around the head as in Sirsasana I. Pressing firmly down through the forearms, lift the head off the floor, extend the legs straight, draw the feet together, and energize down through the legs and feet.

What to Look For and Emphasize
Rooting through the forearms and feet, strongly internally rotate the thighs, press the tailbone toward the heels, and expand across the chest.

EKA PADA VIPARITA DANDASANA

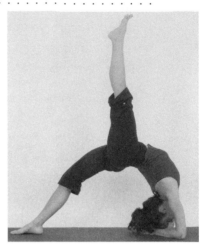

Primary Risks
Lower back, shoulders, neck.

Guiding Students into the Asana
In Viparita Dandasana, root more firmly down into the left foot. Slowly draw the right knee straight up, then explore straightening the right leg vertically.

What to Look For and Emphasize
Maintaining stable rooting in the standing foot and active internal rotation of the standing leg are essential for stability.

EKA PADA RAJ KAPOTASANA

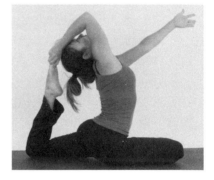

Primary Risks
Front knee, lower back.

Guiding Students into the Asana
From Adho Mukha Svanasana, bring the right knee just outside the right hand while releasing the left hip and leg to the floor. Prop the left sitting bone as high as necessary to ensure that (a) the sitting bone is firmly supported, (b) the hips are even, and (c) there is no pressure on the inside of the right knee. To explore as a hip opener, fold forward. For the backbend, keeping the sitting bone grounded and hips even, clasp the left foot with the left hand, and either (1) draw the heel toward the hip, (2) draw the elbow around the foot and draw the right arm overhead to clasp the hands, or (3) draw both arms over the head to clasp the foot and release the top of the head into the arch of the foot.

What to Look For and Emphasize
Keeping the hips even and grounded is essential in this asana in order to protect the lower back and front knee. In the backbend, rotate the hip of the bent leg

forward, spiraling the straight leg internally to reduce pressure on the sacrum. Press the tailbone down while lifting the chest and drawing the elbows toward each other, creating a feeling of lifting the lower tips of the shoulder blades up into the heart while lifting and spreading the heart open toward the sky.

NATARAJASANA

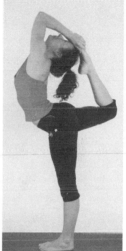

Primary Risks
Lower back, hamstrings and knee of the standing leg, shoulders if unstable or impinging.

Guiding Students into the Asana
From Tadasana, flex the right knee to draw the right foot up toward the right hip. Clasping the right foot with the right hand, rotate the right elbow in and up while extending the right leg back and up from the hip. Lift the left arm overhead, bend the left elbow, and clasp the right foot.

What to Look For and Emphasize
Maintain pada bandha in the standing foot to help stabilize the foot and ankle joint. Keep the standing leg straight and strong while aware of the tendency to lock the standing knee. Try to keep the pelvis level to create a symmetrical foundation for the full extension of the spine. Pressing the tailbone back and down, expand the chest, pressing the lower tips of the shoulder blades forward and up to open the heart center. If stable and at ease, release the crown of the head toward the arch of the foot and draw the elbows together. Breathe!

PURSVOTTANASANA

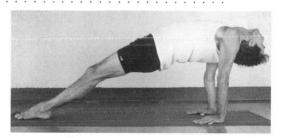

Primary Risks
Wrists, lower back, neck.

Guiding Students into the Asana
From Dandasana, place the hands on the floor about one foot behind the hips with the fingertips pointed forward toward the hips. On an inhale, press through the hands and feet to lift the hips as high as possible. As an alternative, lift up with the feet drawn in closer to the hips (Table Top Pose).

What to Look For and Emphasize

Try to press the balls of the feet firmly down, internally rotate the thighs, press the tailbone toward the heels, and expand across the chest by pressing the tips of the shoulder blades up into the chest. Honor the neck in allowing the head to drop back.

MATSYASANA

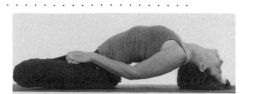

Primary Risks

Knees and neck.

Guiding Students into the Asana

From Pindasana, slowly release the spine to the floor, clasping and pulling on the feet to leverage the chest up and the crown of the head to the floor.

What to Look For and Emphasize

Press the knees toward the floor while pulling on the feet to deepen the arch through the spine. Transition directly to Uttana Padasana.

UTTANA PADASANA

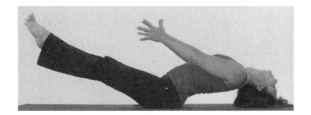

Primary Risks

Neck, lower back.

Guiding Students into the Asana

Lying supine, prop up onto the elbows with the fingertips slightly under the buttocks, pressing down through the elbows to press the chest up. Be sensitive to the neck in releasing the head back. For the full asana, lift the legs about a foot off the floor, keeping them straight and strong, release the top of the head to the floor, and draw the palms together over the legs at the same angle as the legs.

What to Look For and Emphasize

Internally rotate the thighs, press the tailbone toward the heels, draw the tips of the shoulder blades up into the chest, energize out through the arms and fingertips, and gaze to the tip of the nose.

SETU BANDHASANA

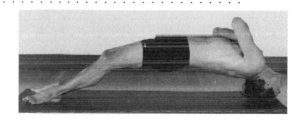

Primary Risks
Neck, lower back.

Guiding Students into the Asana
Lying supine, slide the feet in about one-third of the way toward the hips, drawing the heel together while turning the feet out like Charlie Chaplin's tramp character, rooting down through the elbows while arching the spine and expanding the chest. With an inhalation, press down more firmly through the feet to lift the hips off the floor and the top of the head onto the floor. If the neck feels stable and comfortable, cross the arms onto the chest.

What to Look For and Emphasize
There should be no pain or sharp intensity in the neck. Only introduce it to students with considerable strength, stability, and ease in the neck. Release by first bringing the elbows back to the floor.

SEATED AND SUPINE TWISTS

Twists delightfully penetrate deep into the body's core, stimulating and tonifying internal organs (particularly the kidneys and liver) while creating suppleness and freedom in the spine and opening the chest, shoulders, neck, and hips. Active supine twists (such as Jathara Parivartanasana) strengthen the abdominal obliques, which are the most important group in many asanas involving rotational movement (such as Parsvakonasana or Astavakrasana). Regular twisting helps maintain the normal length and resilience of the spine's soft tissues and the health of the vertebral disks and facet joints of the spine, restoring the spine's natural range of motion.[1] In a beautiful poetic irony, we find that in twisting our body more and more into a pretzel, we more easily unwind the accumulated physical and emotional tension contained in the body. As discussed in Chapter Ten, twists are excellent for neutralizing the spine after deep backbends and forward bends. Use these general guidelines in guiding students in twists:

- Breathing deeply, rooting down, and lengthening up are the keys to deeper twisting.
- When twisting, the vertebrae are naturally drawn closer together, compressing the rib cage and lungs, which makes it more difficult to fully inhale and slowly exhale. While emphasizing roots and extension, give even more emphasis to deepening the inhale and slowing the exhale.

- As with other asanas, the key to lengthening is rooting, especially in seated twists. Instruct students to firmly root down through their sitting bones and pelvis in all seated twists in order to maintain length and stability in the lower back.

- If one foot is on the floor as in Ardha Matsyendrasana, cue students to press it down as though standing on it to accentuate the roots-extension relationship.

- Whether seated or supine, guide students to bring more elongation through the spine with each inhale, creating more space to allow a deeper twist as the breath flows out.

- Encouraging students to explore this process dynamically, cue them to back slightly out of the twist with each inhale, thereby finding more ease in lengthening and further rotation on the following exhale, continuing in this way until releasing out of the twist.

- In asymmetrical seated twists, ask students to try to keep their sitting bones even and pelvis neutral; the tendency is for the sitting bone and the side of the pelvis that one is twisting toward to shift back, which creates the illusion of a deeper twist while tending to draw the twist more into the lumbar spine, and for the pelvis to slump back.

- In supine twists, invite students to be more interested in keeping their shoulder on the floor rather than getting the knee to the floor on the opposite side; this will help to keep the twist more in the thoracic spine rather than in the lower back.

- The neck can be held evenly or added to the twist if comfortable; students can add space and comfort to the neck when twisting by drawing the shoulder blades down the back and spreading across the collarbones.

- In all twists, guide students to initiate movement from the mid-thoracic spine, creating the twist up and down the spine from there.

- Counsel caution and comfort in leveraging twists (e.g., pressing the elbow or shoulder against the knee in Marichyasana C).

- Twist evenly on both sides. If a student is seated on an elevated prop, arrange the prop to be the same thickness under each sitting bone, thereby promoting the development of equal sitting amid the challenge of drawing the higher sitting bone down.

ARDHA MATSYENDRASANA

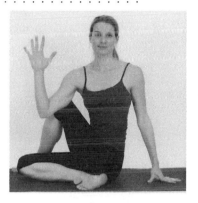

Primary Risks
Lower back, knees, neck.

Guiding Students into the Asana
From Dandasana, slide the feet in halfway and draw the
right heel back and under toward the outside of the left
hip, then place the left foot on the floor just outside the
right knee. Clasp the knee with both hands to leverage
the anterior rotation of the pelvis and lengthening of the
spine while pressing down through the sitting bones and left foot. Stretch the right
arm up to lengthen through the spine and shoulder, then rotate the mid-torso to
the left, either clasping the left knee, drawing the right elbow or shoulder across
the left knee to leverage the twist, or reaching the right arm along the outside of
the lower left leg and clasping the inner left foot.

What to Look For and Emphasize
Keep the sitting bones down, and press the right foot down as though trying to
stand on it. With each inhale, back slightly out of the twist to more easily elongate
the spine, twisting further with each exhale. Keep the shoulder blades drawing
down the back, heart center spacious, and breath steady. Gaze to the left. Advanced
students can transition out through Eka Pada Koundinyasana B to Chaturanga.

MARICHYASANA C

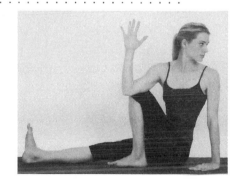

Primary Risks
Lower back, neck, bent knee.

Guiding Students into the Asana
From Dandasana, bring the right heel to the right
sitting bone with the knee lifted. Place the right
hand on the floor by the right hip, stretch up
through the spine and left shoulder and arm, then
rotate the torso to the right while drawing the left elbow of the shoulder across the
right knee, pressing against the knee to leverage the twist. With more flexibility,
reach the left arm around the right thigh and shin to clasp the right wrist behind
the back.

What to Look For and Emphasize

Ground down through the sitting bones and extend out through the strongly engaged left leg. With each inhale, back slightly out of the twist to more easily elongate the spine, twisting further with each exhale. Keep the shoulder blades drawing down the back, heart center spacious, and breath steady. Gaze to the left. Advanced students can transition out through Eka Pada Bakasana to Chaturanga.

BHARADVAJRASANA

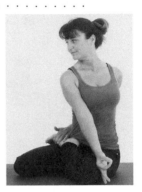

Primary Risks

Knees, lower back, neck.

Guiding Students into the Asana

For A: From Dandasana, leaning to the left, bend both knees to draw both heels back to the right, keeping the left ankle under the right thigh. For B: Start as for A, except draw the right heel close to the right hip in Virasana positioning and draw the left foot into half-lotus. Twisting to the left, reach the left hand behind the back and clasp a piece of clothing, the right inner thigh, or the lotus foot while clasping the left knee with the right hand. In B, try to place the left palm on the floor under the left knee and pointing toward the left heel.

What to Look For and Emphasize

Rooting the sitting bones, elongate the spine with each inhale, using the hand clasps to leverage the twist with each exhale. Create a feeling of drawing the upper spine in toward the heart center, drawing the shoulder blades down the back and spreading the collarbones. While twisting the torso to the left, turn the head to the right, drawing the chin slightly down toward the right shoulder.

SUPTA PARIVARTANASANA

Primary Risks

Lower back, neck.

Guiding Students into the Asana

The basic form of this asana can be either a held twist or the abdominal core strengthening movement of Jathara Parivartanasana. In the held twist, lay supine, knees in toward

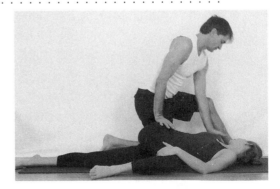

the chest as in Apanasana, arms out, palms down. Gazing over the right hand, release the knee to the left. Alternately, keep the left leg straight out onto the floor and draw the right knee across. For core strengthening, move the knees (or straight legs) back and forth to the left and right while gazing in the opposite direction, keeping the knees or legs from touching the floor.

What to Look For and Emphasize

The bent-knee position is easier on the lower back. In the held twist, encourage students to be more interested in keeping their shoulder on the floor than getting the knee to the floor, thereby twisting in the thoracic spine, not the lower back. In the core practice, press the shoulders and palms firmly down while moving the legs, inhaling the legs over, exhaling back to center.

PARIVRTTA JANU SIRSASANA

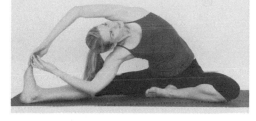

Primary Risks

Bent knee, lower back, hamstrings of straight leg, neck, shoulders.

Guiding Students into the Asana

From Dandasana, extend the right leg out as for Upavista Konasana, and draw the left heel in as for Baddha Konasana. Ground the sitting bones, sit tall, firm the right thigh, twist to the left, and lean to the right, moving in stages: (1) right elbow to right knee, left arm down toward left hip in external rotation, then reach the left arm overhead; (2) right elbow or shoulder to the floor, still rotating the torso open while reaching the left arm over the head to clasp the right foot.

What to Look For and Emphasize

If it troubles the neck looking up, either drop the head down or create a headrest with the right hand. Focus on lengthening the spine while in lateral flexion. Make it a side-stretch, not a forward bend. If it is easy to clasp the right foot with both hands, use the right hand to press the left thigh out and down, deepening the stretch.

FORWARD BENDS AND HIP OPENERS

Here we are looking at nonstanding forward bends and hip openers, which are often considered separately from each other. However, all forward bends stretch some muscles in or around the pelvis, and most hip openers involved flexion of the spine (e.g., Gomukhasana and Baddha Konasana). (Some hip openers are done with the spine neutral or in extension, such as Bharadvajrasana and Supta Virasana, respectively.) Thus, it makes sense to look at these asanas together while highlighting the elements that make the forward-bending or hip-opening aspects of them more significant. Since some of these asanas are more purely forward bends or hip openers, we will first briefly consider the qualities found in their separate families before exploring their blending.

Forward bends are deeply calming asanas that draw us into the inner mysteries and dynamics of our lives. The classic forward bend, Paschimottanasana, translates from Sanskrit as "west stretching pose," signifying the sunset of a practice traditionally done facing the rising sun. Other forward bends like Balasana are deeply nurturing; we are in this position during nine months of gestation and naturally return to this fetal position to nurture or protect ourselves. In stimulating the pelvic and abdominal organs, the subtle energetic effects of forward bends are concentrated in the lower chakras, often revealing base emotions held deep in the body. Holding forward bends for at least a few minutes while refining the flow of the breath allows students to safely explore these feelings.

In folding forward we stretch and expose the vulnerable backside of our bodies, most of which we will never directly see. Just as there is often heightened fear in dropping back into the unknown in backbends such as Laghu Vajrasana, we tend to hold on with the backside muscles when folding forward. To fully release into forward bends, we must let go of an entire chain of muscles that start in the plantar fascia of the feet and move through the Achilles tendons, gastrocnemius, and soleus in the lower legs, hamstrings and some adductors on the backs and insides of the thighs, gluteus maximus, piriformis and quadratus lumborum around the back of the pelvis and into the lower back, and then the muscles across the entire back, primarily the spinal erectors and multifidi (Aldous 2004, 65). This release requires patience as the backside gradually releases and allows the graciousness of the forward bend to manifest; when pursued aggressively, injury to the hamstrings or lower back is likely. Students with disk injuries should practice forward bends with great caution, staying with asanas in which they can focus the stretch in the hamstrings and hips, not the lower back (Dandasana and Supta Padangusthasana). Guide students into forward bends as follows:

- Before folding forward, draw awareness to the breath and through the breath to the entire length of the spine, focusing on relaxing and elongating the spine.
- In all seated forward bends, make the grounding of the sitting bones the primary action. This is best conveyed in Dandasana; rooting down through the

sitting bones naturally awakens lines of energy up through the spine and out through the legs, creating the foundation for a safe and deep forward fold.

- Assess students' posture when they are sitting in Dandasana; if they are unable to attain pelvic neutrality (with the sacrum tilted slightly forward), they should sit sufficiently high on a firm prop to ease into that neutrality and work there to elongate the spine.
- Initiate and maximize the forward fold through the anterior rotation of the pelvis while maximizing the neutral extension of the spine. For many students, this will mean remaining in an upright position when exploring most seated forward bends.
- Supine forward bends such as Apanasana and Supta Padangusthasana are easiest on the lower back and hamstrings.
- In seated forward bends in which one or both legs are straight (e.g., Dandasana or Paschimottanasana), internally rotate the thighs while pressing them down to ease the anterior rotation of the pelvis and thereby maintain space in the lower back.

While most standing asanas and forward bends stretch the muscles in and around the pelvis, the purer family of hip openers is found in seated, supine, or prone positions. When stable and open, the hips are the key to our mobility in the world. Yet habitual sitting in chairs and participation in intense athletic activity can combine with genetics to make the hips one of the tightest parts of the body, resulting in limited range of motion and, potentially, strain in the lower back. Open hips are one of the key elements to practicing safe and deep backbends, forward bends, and in sitting comfortably in meditation. We can develop and maintain a healthy range of motion in the hips through a balanced practice that addresses each of the associated muscles, with a variety of benefits to show up in standing, backbending, and forward bending asanas:

- *Hip flexors:* When the primary hip flexors—iliopsoas and rectus femoris—are tight, the pelvis is pulled into anterior rotation and the lower back tends to develop a lordosis. Tight hip flexors also limit backbends. While the standing asanas Anjaneyasana and Virabhadrasana are very effective in stretching these muscles, so are classic hip openers like Supta Virasana and Eka Pada Raj Kapotasana Prep.
- *Hip extensors:* Tight hip extensors pull the sitting bones toward the backs of the knees, potentially flattening the lower back and leading to kyphosis in the thoracic spine. Tight hip extensors—especially the hamstrings and lower

gluteus maximus fibers—limit forward bending; they are most directly stretched in straight-leg forward bends.

- *Hip abductors:* Tight abductors—especially gluteus medius—are a prime cause of the front knee splaying out in standing lunge asanas (along with weak adductors), the nemesis of students attempting to cross their knees in Garudasana and Gomukhasana and a source of pressure on the sacroiliac joint. Again, the asanas in which their tightness most limits the range of motion also most stretch them, especially Gomukhasana.

- *Hip adductors:* Tight adductors (along with weak abductors) cause the front knee to splay inward in standing lunge asanas and make it more difficult to bring the legs apart in a variety of standing, arm balance, and seated asanas. (Relatively short femoral heads and/or iliofemoral ligaments will also limit range of motion often thought to be caused by tight adductors.) Upavista Konasana and Baddha Konasana are the classic asanas for opening the adductors.

- *Internal rotators:* Tightness in the internal rotators can cause the knees to splay toward each other when standing in Tadasana and limit opening into poses like Padmasana and Virabhadrasana II. Closely associated with the adductors, Upavista Konasana and Baddha Konasana are effective for stretching these muscles.

- *External rotators:* The most powerful muscles in the body, glutei maximi are the primary external rotator of the femurs. When tight or overused—as is the case with many dancers—the knees and feet tend to turn out, causing misalignment in many standing asanas and placing pressure on the sacroiliac joint. Gomukhasana and Jathara Parivartanasana effectively stretch these muscles.

APANASANA

Primary Risks
Lower back, groin.

Guiding Students into the Asana
Lying on the back, draw the knees gently in toward the chest. Inhaling, release the knees slightly away from the chest; exhaling, hug them in.

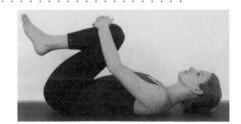

What to Look For and Emphasize

As simple as this appears, still counsel students to take it easy on the lower back. Play with rocking side to side or moving the knees around in circles to explore releasing tension in the lower back.

BALASANA

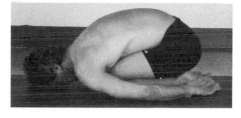

Primary Risks

Lower back, knees.

Guiding Students into the Asana

From all fours, release the hips back towards and to the heels, draping the arms onto the floor along the sides of the legs. Bringing the knees wider apart creates an easier release through the hips, easing pressure in the lower back. Placing a blanket behind the knees reduces pressure in the knees.

What to Look For and Emphasize

If the hips are more than a few inches above the heels, offer a blanket to be placed behind the knees. Among the most relaxing asanas, Balasana is a place of rest and inner calm. Encourage students to stay with the breath while completely letting go and relaxing deep inside.

SUPTA PADANGUSTHASANA

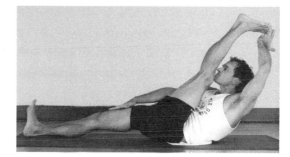

Primary Risks

Hamstrings.

Guiding Students into the Asana

Lying supine with the feet drawn in, as for Setu Bandha Sarvangasana, clasp the right foot and straighten the right leg (use a strap if needed). Move toward straightening the left leg onto the floor, pressing out through the heel while internally rotating the thigh and keeping the knee and toes pointing up. With an exhalation, bring the chin toward the shin while keep both legs straight and strong.

What to Look For and Emphasize

Try to rotate the pubis forward and down while lifting the sternum away from the belly. Transition to the B variation by releasing the back to the floor, turning the head to the left and slowly extending the left leg out to the left in abduction. Be more interested in keeping the left buttock on the floor than getting the right leg farther over.

ANANDA BALASANA

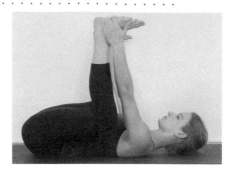

Primary Risks
Lower back, inner groins.

Guiding Students into the Asana
From Apanasana, clasp the feet and draw the knees toward the floor while keeping the sacrum on the floor and the heel aligned over the knees.

What to Look For and Emphasize
Some tight students will be unable to clasp their feet without lifting their upper back and pelvis off the floor. Encourage them to keep their knees bent.

DANDASANA

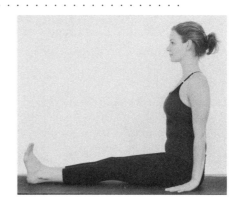

Primary Risks
Hamstrings and lower back.

Guiding Students into the Asana
This is the foundational asana for all other seated forward bends. The primary action of *all* seated forward bends is the firm rooting of the sitting bones. Do not pull the flesh away from the sitting bones, as this will overexpose the hamstring attachments at their most vulnerable place. Sit tall with the legs extended forward, pelvis neutral. If the sacrum tilts back, sit on a bolster to attain pelvic neutrality and neutral spinal extension.

What to Look For and Emphasize
Root the sitting bones, flex the feet, firm the thighs without hyperextending the knees, internally rotate the thighs, pubic bone down and sacrum slightly in, elongate the spine, shoulder blades down the back, palms rooting, chest spacious, head to the sky.

PASCHIMOTTANASANA

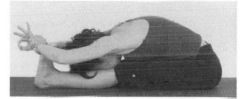

Primary Risks
Hamstrings and lower back.

Guiding Students into the Asana
Sitting tall in Dandasana, bring the hands toward the feet as far as possible without bending the spine. Clasp there (or a strap around the feet) to leverage the activation of the legs, lengthening of the spine, and anterior rotation of the pelvis. Draw the torso forward over the legs by rotating the pelvis forward. Stretch the elbows out away from each other, drawing the shoulder blades down the back.

What to Look For and Emphasize
Renew the firm grounding of the sitting bones. With each inhale, lengthen the spine; with each exhale, release the torso forward. Be more interested in drawing the heart center up and forward than getting the face to the legs. Keep the legs active, patiently allowing the back of the body to release.

JANU SIRSASANA

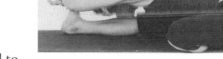

Primary Risks
Hamstrings and lower back, bent knee.

Guiding Students into the Asana
Sitting tall in Dandasana, draw the left heel to
the inner right thigh close to the pelvis with the knee resting on the floor or a block. Keeping the sitting bones even and firmly grounded, turn the torso slightly to point the sternum toward the right foot. In folding forward, proceed as for Paschimottanasana while lifting the belly and drawing it slightly toward the right thigh.

What to Look For and Emphasize
Renew the firm grounding of the sitting bones and firming of the left quadriceps. With each inhale, lift the chest slightly to more fully extend the spine. With each exhale, settle more deeply into the asana.

MARICHYASANA A

Primary Risks
Hamstrings, lower back.

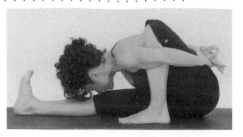

Guiding Students into the Asana
Sitting tall in Dandasana, draw the right heel in
toward the right sitting bone. Place the left hand
on the floor by the left hip and lean the torso slightly to the left while stretching
the right arm up. Hinging from the hips, slowly stretch the torso and right arm forward, and wrap the right arm low around the right shin while drawing the left hand
around behind the back to clasp the right wrist. Inhaling, lift the spine and chest;
exhaling, fold forward.

What to Look For and Emphasize
Renew the firm grounding of the sitting bones and firming of the left quadriceps. Press down into the right foot as though trying to stand up on it. With each
inhale, lift the chest slightly to more fully extend the spine. With each exhale, settle more deeply into the asana.

UPAVISTA KONASANA

Primary Risks
Hamstrings, lower back.

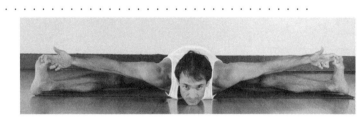

**Guiding Students
into the Asana**
From Dandasana, extend both legs out in abduction. Prop as needed to find pelvic
neutrality. Point the toes and kneecaps straight up while firming the thighs, elongating the spine, and spreading across the heart center. Press the hands into the
floor behind the hips to help rotate the pelvis forward. If able to sit tall on the
sitting bones with the hands off the floor, reach the arms forward and use the hands
on the floor to help draw the torso forward.

What to Look For and Emphasize
Keeping the sitting bones rooted, legs active, kneecaps pointing up, move with the
breath to fold forward through the anterior rotation of the pelvis, eventually bringing the chest to the floor and clasping the feet. Be more interested in a long spine
and open heart than folding down. Gaze either down or to the horizon.

KURMASANA

Primary Risks
Hamstrings, lower back, shoulders.

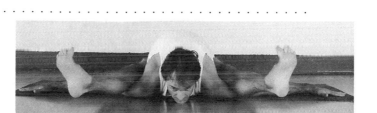

Guiding Students into the Asana
From Upavista Konasana, bring the legs slightly closer together, lifting the knees to create space for extending the arms straight out under the knees. Try to bring the legs closer together, eventually to the shoulders. Grounding the sitting bones, press the legs straight, toes spreading, gaze forward to the horizon.

What to Look For and Emphasize
Focus on grounding the sitting bones and extending through the legs and spine. Eventually cross the legs over behind the back and press up to Dwi Pada Sirsasana, transitioning out through Tittibhasana, Bakasana, and Chaturanga Dandasana.

HANUMANASANA

Primary Risks
Hamstrings, groin, lower back.

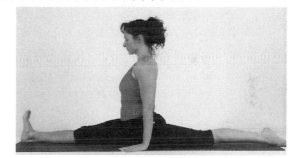

Guiding Students into the Asana
From Anjaneyasana, place the hands on the floor and shift the hips back above the rear knee while straightening the front leg. Stay here for one to two minutes. Keeping the hips even with the front of the mat, slowly slide the heel of the front leg forward while extending the rear leg. Since most students are unable to release fully into this asana, offer blocks to place (1) under the sitting bone of the front leg and/or (2) on both sides of the hips for hand support.

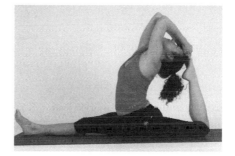

It is important to position the hips even with the front of the mat while the sitting bone of the front leg is firmly grounded, thereby creating a symmetrical foundation for spinal extension and reducing the risk of lower-back strain.

What to Look For and Emphasize

Once stably positioned with the spine upright, increasingly flex the front foot, engaging the quadriceps muscles and releasing the hamstrings. To the extent that the hips are even with the front of the mat, the back leg will more easily extend straight back from the hip. Emphasize internal rotation of the back leg, especially if exploring the backbend variation.

BADDHA KONASANA

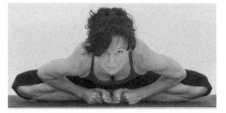

Primary Risks
Knees and lower back.

Guiding Students into the Asana
From the preparatory position for Upavista Konasana, bend the knees to bring the feet together. Reduce knee strain by placing a block under the knee(s). Press the hands into the floor behind the hips to help rotate the pelvis forward. If able to sit tall on the sitting bones with the hands off the floor, clasp and open the feet like a book, pressing the heels together while stretching the knees out toward the floor. Rotate the pelvis forward to draw the heart center toward the horizon. As a variation, invite students to play around with extending their arms fully forward, palms pressing down, using this alternative positioning to leverage the lifting of their heart center, elongation of their spine, and deeper forward rotation of their hips.

What to Look For and Emphasize
Keeping the sitting bones rooted, heels pressing together, shoulder blades down the back, heart center open, move with the breath to lengthen the spine while folding forward from the hips. Use the elbows to press the thighs back, knees out, and chest forward. Create a feeling of bringing the belly button toward the toes, sternum to the horizon. Cueing this action will encourage students to minimize the rounding of their back and reduce potential strain in the lower back and neck. If students report pain in the inner knee or groin, encourage them to place blocks under their knees.

VIRASANA

Primary Risks
Knees, ankles, lower back.

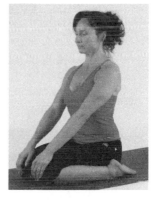

Guiding Students into the Asana
Standing on the knees with the feet extended back, press the thumbs into the middle of the calf muscles behind the knees. Slide the thumbs down the middle of the muscles, spreading them out from the center while drawing the sitting bones to the floor between the heels (or onto a block or bolster). Clasp the knees, root the sitting bones, internally rotate the femurs, and anteriorly rotate the pelvis to neutral while drawing tall through the spine, shoulder blades down the back, and chest spacious.

What to Look For and Emphasize
Keeping the sitting bones rooted, with each exhale, renew the light lifting of the perineum, cultivating mula bandha while energizing up through the spine. Allow the head to float on top of the spine, breathing deeply and steadily. This is an excellent asana for all pranayama practices.

TIRIANG MUKHA EKA PADA PASCHIMOTTANASANA

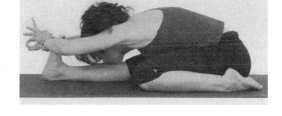

Primary Risks
Lower back, bent knee, hamstrings of straight leg.

Guiding Students into the Asana
From Dandasana, fold the right leg into the Virasana position. Try to root the sitting bones equally. Fold forward as for Janu Sirsasana.

What to Look For and Emphasize
Try to root the right sitting bone more firmly, internally rotating the right thigh while rotating the pelvis forward as the source of the forward fold.

KROUNCHASANA

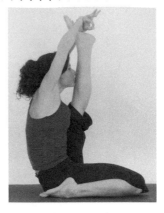

Primary Risks
Knee of bent leg, hamstrings of straight leg, lower back.

Guiding Students into the Asana
Sitting tall in the preparatory position for Tiriang Mukha Eka Pada Paschimottanasana, clasp the left foot with both hands, extend the left leg up, and draw the sternum toward the left foot. If necessary, use a strap around the left foot to keep the leg straight with lifting it up.

What to Look For and Emphasize
Resist the tendency to collapse into slumpasana by being more interested in rotating the pelvis forward, lengthening the spine, and lifting the chest. Draw the shoulders down away from the ears while lengthening from the pubis to the chin.

GOMUKHASANA

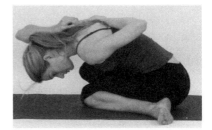

Primary Risks
Knees, shoulders, lower back.

Guiding Students into the Asana
Prepare as for Ardha Matsyendrasana, then draw the upper knee across the top of the lower knee with the heels close to the hips. If unable to fully cross the knees, come onto all fours to cross them; have a block waiting under the sitting bones before sitting back down. With the right knee on top, reach the left arm overhead, bending the elbow to draw the hand down the back while drawing the right arm back and reaching up to clasp the left fingers (use a strap if needed). Rooting the sitting bones, inhaling, lift the spine and chest; exhaling, fold forward.

What to Look For and Emphasize
As with all seated forward bends, keep the sitting bones grounded while lengthening the spine and folding forward. Be sensitive to the knees, lower back, and shoulders. Keep the heart center open and the breath steady. Switch sides by either simply recrossing the legs, spinning 360 degrees, or pressing in Salamba Sirsasana II and recrossing the legs overhead.

ARDHA BADDHA PADMA PASCHIMOTTANASANA

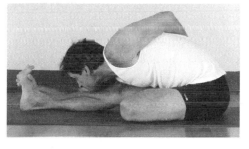

Primary Risks
Bent knee, lower back, hamstrings of straight leg.

Guiding Students into the Asana
From Dandasana, draw one leg into half-lotus position. Wrap the arm from that side of the body behind the back to clasp the lotus foot. Rooting the sitting bones and keeping the extended leg active and internally rotating, inhaling, lift the spine and heart center; exhaling, fold forward.

What to Look For and Emphasize
If the bent knee is off the floor, encourage the student to stay upright until the hip opens. Look for and cue a sense of symmetry amid the asymmetry of the asana.

PADMASANA

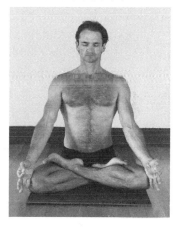

Primary Risks
Knees, hips, groin.

Guiding Students into the Asana
Explore Padmasana by releasing the hips, never straining the knees. Ground the sitting bones and sit tall. From a simple cross-legged position, clasp the right heel and draw it toward the left hip. Relaxing in the right hip and inner thigh and groin, externally rotate the femur to release the right knee toward the floor. Proceed in the same way with the other leg.

What to Look For and Emphasize
Ground through the sitting bones; keep cultivating pelvic neutrality, neutral spinal extension, and a spacious heart center. Never force the knees down. With the hands on the knees, gaze to the tip of the nose or to a point on the floor.

BADDHA PADMASANA

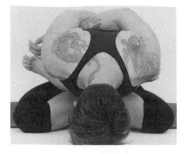

Primary Risks
Knees, shoulders, lower back.

Guiding Students into the Asana
From Padmasana, reach the arms behind the back to clasp the feet. If unable to clasp the feet, clasp the elbows or forearms. Inhaling, extend the spine; exhaling, fold forward.

What to Look For and Emphasize
Try to stay for ten slow breaths, using this asana to refine the breath and move into a deeper and quieter space inside.

ARKANA DANDASANA

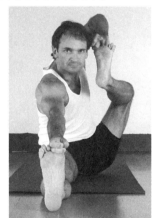

Primary Risks
Lower back.

Guiding Students into the Asana
Preparing as for Marichyasana A with one foot drawn in close to the sitting bone, clasp both big toes while rooting the sitting bones and lifting the spine. Slowly lift the foot of the bent leg and draw it back toward the ear.

What to Look For and Emphasize
Emphasize the Dandasana elements: active extended leg, anterior rotation of the pelvis, extended spine, open heart center, steady breath.

EKA PADA SIRSASANA TO CHAKORASANA VINYASA

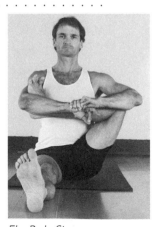

Primary Risks
Knee of bent leg, lower back, neck, hamstrings when folded forward.

Guiding Students into the Asana
In Dandasana, slide the right foot in, clasping the knee to leverage the anterior rotation of the pelvis and extension of the spine. Do the first three preparatory steps described for Astavakrasana before drawing the lower right leg behind the right shoulder and across the back. Sit tall with the palms in anjali mudra be-

Eka Pada Sirsasana prep

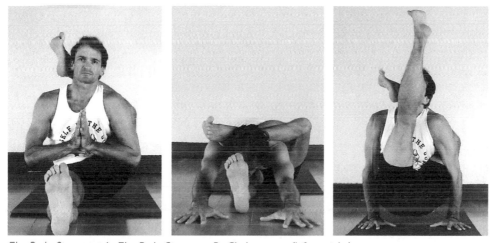

Eka Pada Sirsasana A, Eka Pada Sirsasana B, Chakorasana (left to right)

fore folding forward as described for Janu Sirsasana. Drawing the torso back up, press the hands down, and straighten the arms to lift the hips off the floor, drawing the extended leg up to the chin into Chakorasana.

What to Look For and Emphasize
Forcing this asana will strain the right knee, neck, and lower back. Keep the right foot strongly flexed to stabilize the knee. Use the lifting of the torso, elongation of the spine, and spreading of the collarbones to deepen the hip opening. Transitioning out, lift to Chakorasana and float to Chaturanga Dandasana.

AGNISTAMBHASANA

Primary Risks
Knees, lower back.

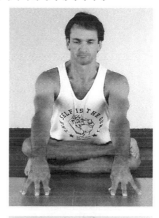

Guiding Students into the Asana
From a simple cross-legged position, place the hands on the floor behind the hips and lean back while sliding the heels forward to bring the shins parallel. Gradually rotate the pelvis forward to sit up taller. Once able to sit up with the hands free, stack the shins like logs with the ankles and knees atop each other on opposite sides. Fold forward.

What to Look For and Emphasize
Keeping the feet strongly flexed while engaging the muscles and ligaments around the knees, helping to protect the knees and accentuate the stretch in the hips.

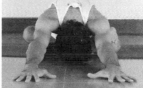

INVERSIONS

When we go upside down, the world appears to be inverted. Here even the simplest of movements can be confusing as we experience this opposite and unfamiliar relationship to gravity. This shift in perspective and neuromuscular awareness creates an opportunity to further expand our sense of being in the world while reversing the effects of gravity in the body. The brain is flushed with nourishing blood, the mind clears, the nerves quiet down, and everything seems to become more still yet awake, offering a graceful invitation to meditation. With practice, even what is at first the most challenging inversion—Salamba Sirsasana (Headstand)—becomes as stable its opposite, Tadasana, allowing students to remain in this asana for several minutes at a time. Whether in Salamba Sirsasana or Salamba Sarvangasana (Supported Shoulder-Stand), students develop more nuanced muscular coordination that adds stability and ease to a variety of other asanas, including in fluid movements into and out of Adho Mukha Vrksasana.

INVERSIONS AND MENSTRUATION

There is some debate over whether women should practice full inversions when menstruating. Some schools of thought assert that inversions reverse the flow of menses, maintaining that this retrograde menstruation can cause endometriosis. However, there is no medical evidence showing that inversion causes retrograde menstruation or any other disruption to the natural flow of blood. If there were such evidence, then even Adho Mukha Svanasana would be contraindicated when menstruating, and one would have to question even the effects of lying on the belly versus the back since the uterus and vagina are turned in opposite relationship to gravity. Looking further into the question of menstruation in relationship to gravity, the NASA Medical Division has found no changes in menstrual flow among women in zero-gravity environments, pointing to intravaginal peristaltic muscular contraction, not a relationship to gravity, as the cause of normal menstrual egress. In advising students on this question, longtime yoga teacher Barbara Benagh (2003) says that since "no studies or research make a compelling argument to avoid inversions during menstruation, and since menstruation affects each woman differently and can vary from cycle to cycle, I am of the opinion that each woman is responsible for her own decision."[5]

The greatest physical risk in inversions is to the neck (this does not apply to Viparita Karani). It is very important to give students clear and methodical guidance in setting up for inversions in a way that minimizes this risk. Students with cervical spine issues are advised not to practice any asanas that further strain their neck. Here we will look at setting up for the two most commonly taught inversions, Salamba Sirsasana I and Salamba Sarvangasana, before discussing other inversions. For Salamba Sirsasana I (Headstand):

- If students are new to this asana, have them practice it next to a wall.
- Instruct two basic roots: the forearms and top (crown) of the head, starting with the positioning of the arms with the elbows shoulder-distance apart.
- Begin with the knees and forearms on the floor. In interlacing the fingers, instruct students to keep the palms wide open and their fingers sufficiently loose to be able to firmly root down from the ulnar side of the wrists to the elbows.
- The top of the head should be placed directly down on the floor with the back of the head braced lightly against the base of the thumbs.
- Ask students to slowly straighten their legs while pressing firmly down through their forearms and drawing their shoulder blades down against their back ribs, their shoulders drawing away from their wrists.
- Maintaining this position, guide students to walk their feet in toward their elbows until bringing their hips as high as possible over their shoulders; encourage students to keep the spine long in this transition. Encourage steady ujjayi pranayama and dristana.
- Rooting down more firmly through the elbows, ask students to try to draw their knees in toward the chest and the heels toward their hips, and then to rotate the pelvis up and slowly extend the legs straight up toward the sky.
- Once upside down, bring awareness back to the roots in the forearms, cue students to create a feeling of pulling the elbows toward each other without actually moving them; this will broaden the shoulders, activate the latissimus dorsi muscles, and add stability.
- Now accentuate the other source of rooting: press the top of the head fairly firmly down, thereby triggering the roots-and-extension effect, activating the spinal erector and multifidi muscles close to the spine. This will relieve pressure in the neck, elongate the entire spine, and create a feeling of grounded levity.

- Finally, instruct students to bring their ankles together, strongly flex their feet (toes toward their shins), and energetically extend out through their heels before pointing their feet and spreading their toes like lotus petals.
- In releasing from Sirsasana, the easiest method is to bend the knees and draw them toward the chest, slowly lowering into Balasana.

In practicing Salamba Sarvangasana, most students' necks will press into the floor. Over time, with openness and strength in the upper back, shoulders, arms, and chest, their neck will not press into the floor. Until that develops, instruct students to set up a platform using folded blankets, then lay down with their shoulders in about three inches from the edge of the blankets. Once their legs are brought overhead, their shoulders should remain on the platform, their neck free, and their head on the floor. From there, instruct as follows:

- With the arms down by the sides, exhale, pressing into the palms and slowly drawing the legs overhead into Halasana (Plow Pose).
- If the feet do not reach the floor, either support the hips with the hands and elbows in Half-Shoulder Stand, or come down and practice with a chair or wall overhead for the feet.
- With the feet on the floor overhead, interlace the fingers behind the back and slightly shrug the shoulders under to bring the weight of the body more onto the shoulders and off the neck.
- Press the feet firmly down into the floor to activate the legs, pressing the tops of the femurs up to help rotate the pelvis anteriorly and thereby draw more length through the lumbar spine. If possible, do this with the feet pointed in plantar flexion; if necessary, keep the toes curled under and consider placing them on a block, chair, or wall.
- Now place the hands on the back as close to the floor as possible, supporting the back, and slowly extend the legs up toward the sky (the easiest method is with the knees bent and using one leg at a time, then over time with straight legs moving up together).

Students who are not practicing Salamba Sirsasana I or Salamba Sarvangasana can receive most of the benefits of full inversion in Viparita Karani ("the action or doing of reversing, turning upside down"), perhaps the most calming and deeply restorative asana, described below along with the other inversions. This is an excellent asana for all students, especially following a vigorous practice, stressful day, or when feeling energetically down.

VIPARITA KARANI

Primary Risks
Hamstrings, lower back.

Guiding Students into the Asana

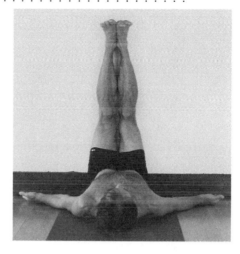

Sitting sideways next to a wall, slowly recline onto the back while swiveling the hips toward the wall and extending the legs up the wall. If tight hamstrings do not allow the legs to extend up with the buttocks touching the wall, slide the hips out away from the wall. Place a folded blanket under the lower back to create more ease through the lower back and sacrum. Relax.

What to Look For and Emphasize
The palms can rest on the belly and heart, or drape the arms onto the floor, palms turned up. The legs can be held together with a strap and a sandbag placed on the feet for stability. Play with positioning the legs as for Baddha Konasana or Upavista Konasana.

HALASANA

Primary Risks
Neck, lower back, hamstrings.

Guiding Students into the Asana

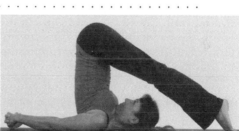

Lying supine, press the palms down, and with an exhale, bring the feet overhead to the floor (or to a block, chair, or wall). Interlace the fingers behind the back and slightly shrug the shoulders under to draw weight more onto the shoulders. If there is pressure on the neck or upper spine, prop onto a folded blanket. Press the feet firmly down (if possible, pointed back) to engage and press the thighs up, drawing the pubic bone away from the belly in lengthening the spine.

What to Look For and Emphasize
Keep the arms and feet firmly grounding. Draw the collarbones down while spreading across the chest and pressing the spine through toward the heart. Keep pressing the sitting bones up, lengthening through the spine.

SALAMBA SARVANGASANA

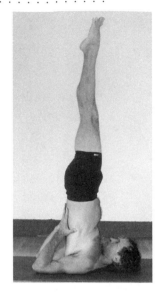

Primary Risks
Neck, lower back, shoulders.

Guiding Students into the Asana
See Inversions, pages 228–230.

What to Look For and Emphasize
See Inversions, pages 228–230. Either release to Halasana or Karnapidasana, or explore folding the legs into Padmasana position and balance with the hands to the knees with straight arms in Urdhva Padmasana before releasing into Pindasana.

KARNAPIDASANA

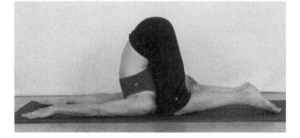

Primary Risks
Neck, lower back.

Guiding Students into the Asana
From Halasana, release the knees toward or to the ears while pressing the arms down into the floor.

What to Look For and Emphasize
Squeeze the knees into the ears, listening to the breath from inside. Keep the breath full.

URDHVA PADMASANA

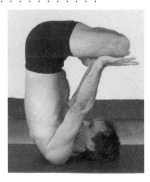

Primary Risks
Knees, neck, lower back.

Guiding Students into the Asana
In Salamba Sarvangasana, draw the legs into Padmasana, using one hand at a time to assist if necessary. Stretch the lotus knees

straight up, then extend an arm straight up and bring the knee on that side to the hand, then place the other hand and knee together.

What to Look For and Emphasize
Focus on rooting the shoulders, expanding the chest, extending the spine, and holding steady while breathing smoothly and spaciously. Engage mula bandha and gaze to the nose or belly.

PINDASANA

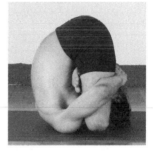

Primary Risks
Knees, neck, lower back.

Guiding Students into the Asana
From Urdhva Padmasana, draw the lotus to the heart, wrapping the arms across the legs and hugging the lotus more closely to the heart.

What to Look For and Emphasize
As with Karnapidasana, explore quieting inside while refining the breath.

SALAMBA SIRSASANA I

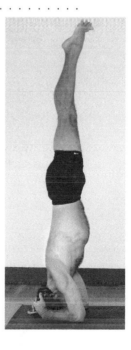

Primary Risks
Neck, lower back, shoulders.

Guiding Students into the Asana
See Inversions, pages 228–230.

What to Look For and Emphasize
See Inversions, pages 228–230.

SALAMBA SIRSASANA II

Primary Risks
Neck, wrists, lower back.

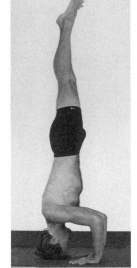

Guiding Students into the Asana
From all fours, place the top of the head and the palms on the floor with the wrists and head forming the points of a triangle. Keep the wrists under and in line with the shoulders while drawing the shoulder blades firmly down against the back ribs. Curl the toes under, straighten the legs, and slowly bring the feet toward the elbows to elevate the hips over the shoulders. Pressing firmly down through the head and hands, extend the legs overhead.

What to Look For and Emphasize
As in Salamba Sirsasana I, root the top of the head to elongate the spine. Keep the elbows from splaying out while keeping the shoulder blades firmly against the back ribs. Activate the legs as in Salamba Sirsasana I. With stability and ease, explore using this asana as the base for transitioning into and out of Bakasana and other arm balances.

SAVASANA

Savasana (from *sava*, "corpse") is the ultimate asana for reintegration after practicing other asanas and pranayama. Ask students to lay onto their backs and spread out as comfortably as possible with their arms draped onto the floor and palms facing up. If they feel any discomfort in their lower back, suggest placing a rolled blanket under their knees. Lift the chest a little to let the shoulder blades relax slightly toward each other, then lay back down with more spaciousness across the heart center. Take one last deep inhale, then with the exhale, let everything go, starting with allowing the breath to flow however it naturally will. Give minimal guidance in cuing students to scan and release tension all through their body. There is finally no need for the muscles to do anything at all. Encourage students simply to watch what is happening. Suggest a sense of all the muscles and bones letting go

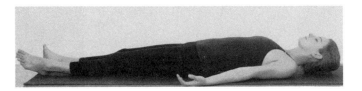

of each other, a sense of detachment all through the body. Similarly, as naturally as thoughts come and go, encourage letting the thoughts flow, interested without being attached, becoming stiller, quieter, and clearer—breath by effortless breath. Stay in Savasana for at least five minutes. If students must leave class early, encourage them to rest in Savasana before leaving. Gently awaken the class from Savasana with a soft voice, bringing awareness back to the breath. Suggest feeling the simple rising and falling of the chest and belly, cuing the class to gradually breathe more deeply and consciously, using the breath to reawaken awareness in the body-mind while changing as little as possible. Suggest bringing small movements into the fingers, hands, toes, and feet. With a deep inhalation, suggest stretching the arms overhead before rolling onto the right side, curling up, and nurturing one's self for a few breaths before slowly coming up to sitting. Now is an ideal time to meditate.

CHAPTER EIGHT

TEACHING PRANAYAMA

Breathe in experience,
breathe out poetry.
—*Muriel Rukeyser*

Breathing consciously is one of the most important parts of Hatha yoga and, for most students, often the most elusive. The breath nourishes and guides the asana practice. It is the source of energetic awakening throughout the body. Through conscious breathing we open in the asana practice to learning more about ourselves, cultivating wholeness in body, mind, and spirit. Yet the breath often disappears from awareness amid everything else that is happening in the asana practice. Slipping from awareness, the breath usually fades. Students tend to lose focus, their attention drifting or leaping away from the here and now.[1] As the breath fades, students lose subtle awareness of how energy is flowing in their bodies, of the subtlety of sensation in the body, of the unification of body-mind, of refinement in the practice. Maintaining attention to the breath can be especially difficult for new students trying to move their bodies into new and often awkward positions while in an unfamiliar place and situation. Even as students progress in their asana practice, their breathing practice typically lags behind. As asanas become more challenging, limited breathing skills limit the deep source of stability and ease found through full and conscious breathing. It is thus essential for teachers to guide students in basic yogic breathing—ujjayi pranayama—and to introduce students to more refined breathing techniques found in the larger art of pranayama.

Pranayama is among the most mystified aspects of yoga. Different schools of yoga describe even its most basic form, ujjayi, in different and conflicting ways. Is it "prana-yama," which most agree translates as "breath control" or "control of the life force"? Or is it "prana-ayama," which suggests the near opposite: "breath liberation" or "expansion of the life force"?[2] Even when demystified by some teachings and teachers, including such authoritative sources as the Hatha Yoga Pradipika and B. K. S. Iyengar, it gains intrigue when students are cautioned that "until the postures are perfected, do not attempt pranayama."[3]

This chapter unravels the discovery, development, practices, and teaching of pranayama. We will look briefly at the ancient teachings for insight into the original intentions and techniques of different pranayama practices. We will visit the modern science of respiration for further understanding of the anatomy and physiology of breathing. With this background, we will explore the art of teaching pranayama, starting with helping students rediscover their natural breath. Staying with our emphasis on Hatha yoga, we will explore teaching basic pranayama as part of contemporary asana practices and explore how to teach several more refined pranayama techniques that further balance energy in the body-mind and lead to a deeper sense of integration and overall well-being.

THE DISCOVERY AND DEVELOPMENT OF PRANAYAMA

Reflecting on the discovery process of ancient yogis, Dona Holleman (1999, 266–268) reasons that pranayama was first developed by ancient yogis through close observation of the natural cycles of breath in the laboratory of their bodies. When simply observing the breath, we first notice the body's rhythmic movement with each cycle of breath. As we tune in more closely, we discover that slower breathing is more relaxing, faster breathing more energizing. Holleman claims that this awareness led to kapalabhati ("skull-cleansing") pranayama, in which intense rhythmic breathing energizes the body, leading to another discovery: increased energy

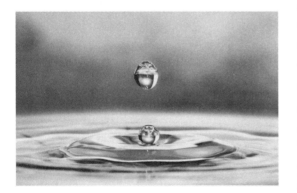

can be brought from the "long, snaky circles of the intestines that whorl around themselves, that promote heat" up through the spinal column to the "winding passages" of the brain where chemical (and perhaps alchemical) changes in the brain transformed one's perception and sense of being. Exploring natural breathing more closely, we notice the natural pauses between the breaths that, when expanded—especially when empty of breath— lead to the sensation of pranic energy rising up along the spine. Done consciously, this is the practice of *kumbhaka,* or breath retention. Yet sometimes the energy gets blocked rather than rising all the way up. The ancient yogis called these blockages chakras, or wheels of energy. Nadi shodhana pranayama, alternate nostril breathing, balances the flow of prana up through the ida and pingala nadis (energy channels) that rise along and cross the spine at each major chakra, which, when made conscious, allows the upward flow of prana.

While the breath is the principal vehicle for cultivating prana, pranayama is more than a set of breathing practices: it is a tool for "expanding our usually small reservoir of prana by lengthening, directing, and regulating the movement of the breath and then limiting or restraining the increased pranic energy in the body-mind" (Rosen 2002, 19). This practice of tapping the breath as a tool for cultivating prana—and with it self-awareness and self-transformation—is found as early as the ancient Vedas, particularly in the Rig Veda from more than four thousand years ago. It is given its first detailed discussion in the Prasna Upanishad, where its all-pervasive and life-sustaining nature is likened to the sun. (See Chapter Three for more on prana.) We first find the emphasis on breath in asana practice in the Yoga Sutras immediately following Patanjali's definition of *asana* as sthira sukham asanam in his use of the word *prayatna,* which is typically translated as "effort." Srivatsa Ramaswami (2000, 95–96) points out that prayatna is of three types, one of which, jivana prayatna, refers to "efforts made by the individual to maintain life and, more especially, breathing." As we breathe, so we feel, and in breathing more freely and fully, we feel more freely and fully. Although asanas in contemporary Hatha yoga are far more evolved and complex than in Patanjali's time, the point is to explore asanas with and through the steadiness and ease of the breath, continuously connecting the breath with the body-mind.

The Yoga Sutras tell us that mastering asana precedes breath control, which requires a still body and a calm mind. Many leading teachers abide by this advice. "Attain steadiness and stillness in asanas before introducing breathing techniques," says B. K. S. Iyengar (1985, 10). "When pranayama and asanas are done together," he stresses, "see that the perfect posture is not disturbed. Until the postures are perfected, do not attempt pranayama." In this traditional perspective, asana practice is seen as developing the physical and mental basis for safely and fully experiencing the benefits of pranayama. Just as asanas should never be forced or imposed, pranayama is best practiced once asanas have removed "the symptoms that arise from obstacles in the personality" (Yoga Sutras I.31)—suffering, depression, restlessness, and irregular breathing—that impede the flow of prana. Only then, it is said, can the practice of pranayama regulate that flow of prana throughout the body.

The approach taken here departs from this traditional path. As long as students practice sthira sukham asanam, there is no danger in exploring pranayama (the important exceptions are noted in Table 8.1). Pranayama enhances respiratory function, improves the circulatory system, and thereby improves digestion and

elimination. When the respiratory system is functioning at its best, the natural purification systems of the physical body function better as well. Combined with asana
practice, pranayama allows students to move energy more easily and thoroughly
through the body, especially as the lungs, muscles, and nerves of respiration are refined. Learning to breathe consciously and efficiently, students can relax more
deeply, loosening their grip over unnecessary tension in the body and organs of
perception. With deeper relaxation and clearer awareness, students find an easier path to concentration, equanimity, and serenity. In this way, pranayama can
help all students have a healthier life right now while giving them additional tools
for deepening and refining their asana and meditation practices.

THE MODERN SCIENCE OF RESPIRATION

While yogis in ancient India were pioneering pranayama as a somatic spiritual practice, the Greeks as early as the seventh century BCE were searching for knowledge
about respiration, while Egyptian and Babylonian scientists were developing practical knowledge about the overall physiology of human beings (Taylor 1949). The
scientist-philosopher Anaximenes of Miletus (born circa 570 BCE) was close to the
Indians and Chinese in his belief that the essence of all things was air, or *pneuma*
(literally, "breath"). He said, "As our soul, being air, sustains us, so pneuma and
air pervade the whole world" (Singer 1957).[4] Yet alchemical and spiritual traditions
giving sacred reverence to the breath often kept scientists at the threshold of discoveries about the nature of respiration. Only in the late eighteenth century CE
would Antoine Lavoisier, the father of modern chemistry, develop the concept of
oxidation that is at the scientific heart of breathing. With this discovery, Lavoisier
and others laid the foundation for the detailed study of the natural respiratory exchange of oxygen and carbon dioxide that is essential to life.

The breath flows in relationship to a basic physiological reality: our cells and
tissues need oxygen. Once they are oxidized, they need to flush out the resulting
carbon dioxide. In the respiratory process, oxygen is delivered to cells via arterial
blood from the lungs and heart, while carbon dioxide is returned to the heart and
lungs as deoxygenated venous blood. Capillary membranes in the lungs called alveoli exchange these gases. This exchange, which we experience as breathing, happens about twelve to fifteen times per minute, or around twenty thousand times
per day, with variations in rate depending on the health of the person's system, activity and emotional levels, and other factors. The mechanics of this exchange were
long misunderstood as resulting from the pumping actions of the heart and lungs.
While the heart and lungs are essential in the respiratory process, they are in

physiological service to the breath, not the physiological source of the breath. The mechanisms of breathing were first properly explained by Galenus around 170 CE and in much greater detail only in the sixteenth century by Leonardo da Vinci, who understood that when more space is made available in the lungs by the expansion of the thorax, the weight of the atmosphere forces air in through the trachea to fill the expanded space (French 2003; Keele 1952). As we will see, this discovery is directly relevant to guiding students in pranayama.

Modern science recognizes the same phases of breath highlighted by the ancient yogis: inhalation, exhalation, and the cessation of breathing, called apnea, which occurs naturally after each inhalation and exhalation. The volume, rate, sound, intensity, areas of relative physical movement or holding, and degree of passivity or activity can vary; the unique combination of these qualities gives us our experience of breathing. Each of these qualities can also be voluntarily affected, giving us the foundation for pranayama practices.

While we can sense and cultivate a feeling of the entire body breathing (or, depending on your perspective, being breathed), the primary functional organs of respiration are the two lungs, where blood and air are precisely mixed in support of the body's overall physiological functioning. Each lung has approximately 1,500 miles of airways and 300 million alveoli, the cellular structures where the exchange of oxygen and carbon dioxide occurs. The alveoli are rich in elastin fibers that give the lungs pulmonary elasticity, which is the primary cause of most exhalations. The lungs are enveloped in a two-layer pleural membrane that adheres to the ribs and diaphragm, allowing movement and supporting the lungs in place. Air moves in and out of the lungs through a system of airway passages, starting with the nose or mouth. The nose is the more refined and refining organ for filtering air into the body and conditioning, purifying, and humidifying the air. The olfactory and other nerves in the nose allow subtle sensitivity to the flow of breath, considerably more so than with air flowing through the mouth. While most pranayama practices are done through the nose, the mouth offers a shorter and more direct pathway to the lungs and thus greater ease in inhaling and exhaling large quantities of air (as we will see in exploring *bastrika* pranayama and sitali pranayama); complete exhalations through the mouth also stretch the diaphragm more.

There are two basic types of breathing that involve different ways of moving the lungs: costal (sometimes called "rib breathing") and diaphragmatic (sometimes called "belly breathing"). In costal breathing, the rib cage opens with the inhalation and closes with the exhalation. In diaphragmatic breathing, the belly expands with inhalation and contracts with exhalation. While neither type is "correct," they fit different circumstances and can be combined to create variations that more or less support certain activities, movements, or energetic intentions. Diaphragmatic breathing is responsible for about seventy-five percent of our respiratory effort.

How fully and deeply we breathe is determined by how we breathe, which typically is more habitual than conscious. In "normal" breathing there is relatively little volume, around five hundred milliliters (depending on physique, fitness, and health), while our respiratory capacity is four to seven times that much. The ability to breathe more deeply, steadily, and calmly—and to more consciously move energy throughout the body—can be developed through practices that make the skeletal and muscular components of breathing stronger and more limber. The movement of breathing itself maintains the suppleness and elasticity of the ribs, costal cartilage, and the muscles that support and mobilize the spine, although lifestyle, age, and genetics can diminish these qualities. The tendency is for the rib cage to expand either front-to-back or laterally, rather than mobilizing the ribs in both directions and thereby expanding breath capacity. Asana practice is an effective tool for developing the mobility of the rib cage in support of balanced breathing.

The movements of the rib cage are blended with the positioning and movement of the pelvis, legs, and shoulders. The pelvis and rib cage are linked through the lumbar spine, where several respiratory muscles attach. Movement of the pelvis affects movement in the rib cage—and vice versa—along with movement of the organs contained in the pelvis and thorax. Movement of the legs into extension stretches the iliopsoas muscles from their insertions on the lesser trochanter of the femoral heads up through the pelvis and to their origin on the lumbar vertebrae and twelfth thoracic vertebra. This is the same place where the diaphragm attaches at the central tendon. The shoulder girdle, consisting of the sternum, clavicles, and scapulae, is involved in breathing via its bony articulations and muscular attachments with the rib cage. The arms and shoulders will enhance or constrain inhalations and exhalations depending on their positioning.

The diaphragm and muscles acting on the rib cage do the primary work of respiration. The diaphragm is responsible for about seventy-five percent of inhalation. It is a double-dome-shaped muscular and fibrous wall located in the middle of the chest just below the lungs and heart, draping like a parachute over the stomach and liver (Netter 1997, plates 180–181). Its base is formed at the back by asymmetrical vertebral fibers that attach to the third lumbar vertebra. It has a fibrous central tendon out of which muscular fibers rise to attach to the entire circumference of the rib cage, sternum, and deep surface of the lower eight ribs. The diaphragm flattens and draws down as it contracts, varying in shape depending on pressure from the ribs, lungs, and the muscles and organs in the abdomen. Like the heart, it works incessantly. As it contracts and lowers, displacing the soft contents of the abdomen, lung volume increases, reducing air pressure in the lungs and drawing in air from outside. As the diaphragm relaxes, it moves up as the lung's natural elasticity pushes the air out, completing a cycle of breath.

Muscles acting on the rib cage, particularly the intercostal muscles between the ribs, assist the diaphragm. The pectoralis minor lifts the ribs forward, opening space in the upper chest and allowing breath more easily to fill the upper lungs. The sternocleidomastoid and scalene muscles also raise the upper rib cage, contributing to breathing into the upper regions of the lungs. Pectoralis major spreads the lower ribs and lifts the sternum, creating a more spacious inhalation that is lower in the lungs. Several muscles with attachments to the side and back ribs play additional roles: the serratus interior helps maintain the posture of the rib cage (and assists with exhalation); the transversospinal muscles extend the spine and thereby help lift the rib cage; serratus posterior spreads the back ribs and eases breath into the back of the lungs. Intercostal muscles also assist complete exhalation by drawing the ribs closer together and compressing the lungs. Lung volume is further reduced by contracting the abdominal muscles: transversus abdominis girdles the waist; the obliques lower the ribs and compress the abdomen; and rectus abdominus further closes the anterior abdomen by drawing the pubis and sternum toward each other. Pelvic floor muscles provide an adaptable foundation that withstands the pressure from above while initiating the active lifting of core abdominal muscles with complete exhalations (Calais-Germain 2005, 101), actions that are closely related to mula bandha and uddiyana bandha.

TEACHING BASIC BREATH AWARENESS

Breathing happens naturally, involuntarily, and unconsciously. This "natural breathing" varies considerably depending on the person's physical, emotional, mental, and spiritual condition. It is compromised by depression, anxiety, tight or weak respiratory muscles, distraction, lethargy, or flighty energy.[5] Under these conditions, the breath is typically shallow, inefficient, and overrelies on secondary respiratory muscles rather than the diaphragm. Instead of assuming that students share a common baseline quality of breath, it is better to guide pranayama practices starting with the natural conditions of each individual student and build from that initial foundation. This starts with guiding students in developing basic breath awareness. "Learning to breathe well is not an additive process in which you learn specific techniques for improving the breath you already have," says Donna Farhi (1996, 72–73). "It is a process of deconstruction where you learn to identify the things you are already doing that restrict the natural emergence of the breath." This observation process anticipates and develops insight into the possibilities of pranayama as well as deeper somatic awareness, helping students to consciously connect breath, body, and mind.

You can guide this initial awakening of breath awareness by asking students to lie on their backs, eyes closed, and to tune in to the natural flow of their breath. In this type of exercise, "We do nothing," suggests Richard Rosen (2002, 72), "but observe the what is." Guiding your students' awareness, emphasize perception of breath sensation through each phase of the breathing cycle:

- *Inhaling. Ask:* What does it feel like? What do you feel initiates the inhalation? What first happens in your body? How does the sensation of the breath change as it flows in? Where do you feel the breath? What parts of your body are moving? What is the succession of movement? Does the flow slow down, speed up, or seem to get stuck along the way? What does the breath sound like as it flows in? How fully do you inhale? What changes in sensation do you feel in your heart center, across your face, between your temples as the breath draws in? What fluctuations do you sense in your mind?

- *Filled with breath. Ask:* What do you feel at the crest of each inhale? What is the length of the natural pause? What sensations do you feel in your body? What fluctuations do you sense in your mind?

- *Exhaling. Ask:* Where do you first feel the movement into exhalation? Does the breath tend to rush out? How does the pace of the exhale change as the breath continues to flow out? What changes do you feel in your body and overall awareness as the breath leaves? How completely do you exhale? What fluctuations do you sense in your mind?

- *Empty of breath. Ask:* What do you feel when empty of breath? How long do you tend to hold the breath out? Do you feel any gripping or holding? What is the quality of your awareness when empty of breath? What fluctuations do you sense in your mind?

Repeat this process with students sitting in an upright position. Guide students through the same questions, cueing awareness of differences in sensation in this new relationship to gravity. Once past this initial awareness practice, students can gain deeper insight, making these observations in a variety of different positions, particularly amid the flow of an asana practice.

REFINING THE FLOW OF BREATH

With this baseline of breath awareness, you can teach students how to explore the development and refinement of their breathing more subtly, helping them to discover how to cultivate sthira sukham asanam more easily while breathing in a variety of different ways. This starts by guiding students into feeling the contraction and release of their respiratory muscles and the related movements in their body with two types of inhalation and exhalation, as follows:[6]

Puraka—The Inhalation

A single inhalation is termed *puraka*, referring to "the intake of cosmic energy by the individual for his growth and progress" (B. K. S. Iyengar 1985, 99). Depending on what other actions one is doing—certain asanas, pranayamas, or sitting in meditation—the breath can be received in ways that support those actions. The following exercises are designed to help students develop and refine their awareness and practice of puraka. In guiding these practices, encourage students to be receptive to the breath rather than grasping for it. With practice, the breath is received delicately yet fully, steadily yet easily, causing as little disturbance as possible to the body-mind.

Diaphragmatic Inhalation

- Lying on the back, flex the hips and knees as if preparing for Setu Bandha Sarvangasana, placing one palm on the belly, the other on the heart center. Feel how complete exhales cause the abdominal muscles to contract.

- With the following inhalation, feel how the belly expands outward. Continue to focus on this movement, which is caused by the contraction and descent of the diaphragm.

- Play with varying the extent of exhalation, feeling how this affects the subsequent movement of the belly. Try to allow the spine and ribs to remain relaxed and move only with the movement of breath caused by the diaphragm.

- Play with starting, stopping, and varying the rate and volume of each breath, concentrating this effort in the diaphragm while feeling the effects elsewhere in the body. Continue this exploration with the palms farther down the belly.

- Explore directing different volumes of diaphragmatic inhalations into different areas (one side and the other, front and back, lower and higher) in various body positions: lying on the back with the arms extended overhead, curled on the sides, lying on the belly.

- Finally, explore diaphragmatic inhalations while keeping the abdomen from expanding, using the hands on the ribs to feel the gradual spreading and lifting of the ribs. Try to allow this movement to arise from deep in the thorax rather than at the more superficial level of the ribs. Explore this in different positions.

Costal Inhalation

- Sitting comfortably tall in Vajrasana (Thunderbolt Pose, propped if necessary to establish pelvic neutrality and neutral spinal extension), place the palms high on the side ribs.
- Exhale completely, feeling the side and back ribs draw together and downward.
- With the inhalations, push the ribs into the hands while allowing the ribs to expand away from one another as the serratus anterior muscles contract, lifting and pulling the ribs back and out. Try to create the movement just in the ribs, keeping the shoulders and belly relaxed while feeling the full expansion of the rib cage and lungs.
- Next, activate inhalations with the pectoralis major muscles on the top of the chest: pulling the shoulder blades down gently against the back ribs, place your fingertips of one hand in front of the shoulders and the other fingertips on the front ribs in line with the xiphoid process (just below the line of the breast).
- Inhaling and exhaling, try to feel the contraction of the pectoralis major raising the sternum while spreading the lower and middle ribs apart.
- Drawing awareness into the higher regions of the chest and lungs, place the fingertips just under the clavicle and try to feel the ribs.
- Keeping the shoulder blades relaxed down against the back ribs, try to concentrate the inhalation as if breathing into the clavicles, activating the pectoralis minor muscles to open the heart center fully.
- Try to alternate inhalations using the pectoralis minor and major muscles, feeling how the difference in their resulting movements opens distinct areas of the rib cage.
- Now explore the highest breathing using the sternocleidomastoids (SCM) and scalenes.
- With your fingertips in and slightly above the hollow space between your collarbones, lean the head slightly back to feel the SCMs awaken. Create quick "sniffing" inhalations to feel the SCMs contracting. Explore doing this after

taking in and holding a full inhale, lifting the sternum, and noticing how this allows you to draw in more breath.

- Place the fingertips lightly onto the sides of your neck and feel into the texture of the scalenes muscles, which descend from the transverse process of upper cervical vertebrae down and outward to the first two ribs. These muscles assist high respiratory movements.

Rechaka—The Exhalation

The exhalation is termed *rechaka*, "the process by which the energy of the body gradually unites with that of the mind," says B. K. S. Iyengar (1985).

Abdominal Exhalation

- Sitting in Vajrasana, slowly and completely exhale out the breath while maintaining the neutral positioning of the lower ribs, feeling the natural contraction of upper belly just beneath the lower ribs. Notice the tendency of the spine to round forward into flexion.
- Placing your palms on your belly, repeat this exercise while the spine is extended.
- Now add mula bandha, lightly contracting and lifting the transverse perineal and deep pelvic muscles.
- Explore connecting the energetic and muscular lift of mula bandha with the gradual contraction of the abdomen, increasingly awakening the transversus abdominis muscles.
- Next, try to successively engage the abdominal muscles from below the navel up to the lower ribs as the breath is flowing out.

Costal Exhalation

- Placing one palm on your heart and one on your belly, slowly exhale while pulling your sternum back toward your spine and minimizing the abdominal muscles' contraction. This practice brings awareness to the transversus thoracis muscle, which closes the rib cage in the front. Try to feel the slight flexion of the upper spine as the breath flows out.
- With the palms on the side ribs, repeat this exercise, feeling how the side ribs lower as the obliques contract and the spine slightly flexes.
- Place the fingertips on the xiphoid process and repeat this exercise, feeling the lower front ribs draw lower and in.

Use these basic inhalation and exhalation practices in your regular classes to help students develop the balance and integrity of their breathing. Most students will initially find the inhalations and exhalations differing in pace, texture, sound, intensity, and duration. Later we will explore teaching variations in the pace of inhalation and exhalation, including equal and unequal ratios between them (*sama-vritti* and *vishama-vritti*). With practice, puraka and rechaka come into balance and form the foundation for all other pranayama practices, including ujjayi pranayama.

UJJAYI PRANAYAMA: BASIC YOGIC BREATHING

The basic breathing technique in Hatha yoga is ujjayi pranayama. Here we breathe through the nose with a very slight narrowing of the throat at the epiglottis (where you feel sensation when coughing or gargling). This increases the vibration of the larynx, creating a soft sound like wind breezing through the trees or the sound of the sea at the seashore. The effects of ujjayi are threefold: (1) the breath is warmed when breathing just through the nose, thus warming the lungs, which warms the blood, which warms the body and helps to awaken the body to natural movement in asanas; (2) the sound and sensation of ujjayi helps in maintaining awareness of the breath flowing with steadiness, ease, and balance; and (3) the rhythmic sound of ujjayi helps to calm the nerves and create a quieter internal practice.

Some teachings insist that the technique of ujjayi, like other aspects of the practice, is a "secret" that will (and should) reveal itself if the breath is left free in the asana practice.[7] Others directly guide students in ujjayi as part of both asana and pranayama practices. Whether one approach is better than the other is a question that is best resolved in practice, which creates a seeming conundrum: How would a person know if it is beneficial to learn it unless they learn it? While there does not seem to be any danger in doing ujjayi pranayama in asana practice, it can be taught and practiced in a way that overly restricts the breath, especially when it is taught through the application of jalandhara bandha (an essential part of many other pranayama techniques, but not of ujjayi). As with much of the practice, keeping it simple allows students to utilize an initial sensitizing technique while refining it through their own practice. Here is a simple way to guide students in discovering and cultivating ujjayi:

1. Sitting comfortably or standing in Tadasana, ask students to close their eyes, open their mouths, and breathe as if trying to fog up a mirror. This immediately creates the sound and sensation of ujjayi, bringing awareness to the epiglottis area.

2. Instruct your students to try to create the same sound and sensation while inhaling *and* exhaling. (The tendency is to do it only on the inhale.)

3 Ask them to close their mouth and breathe through their nose with the same sound and sensation.

4. Encourage them to play with it a little, creating more or less constriction in their throat and noticing how that affects the flow of breath, its sound, and the overall sensation.

5. Finally, ask them to begin treating their ujjayi with a sense of delicacy, exploring how they can breathe more deeply and strongly—yet just as delicately and softly.

Students can immediately apply ujjayi pranayama in their asana practice. Here are some tips on teaching the connection between ujjayi pranayama and asanas:

- Suggest making the steady, rhythmic, balanced, strong yet soft flow of ujjayi just as important as anything else in their asana practice, cultivating it in a way that changes as little as possible from the beginning to the end of the asana session.

- Ujjayi can be deliberately varied, using more intensity to fuel more difficult movements, and more ease to generate a deeper sense of calm.

- Encourage students to explore the deepening of their asana practice around the integrity of the breath rather than trying to force the breath in attempting asanas.

- Tune in to ujjayi as a barometer of the energetic effort and physical intensity of the practice, a source of immediate feedback that students can use in refining their practice.

DEEPENING THE PRANAYAMA PRACTICE

The following pranayama techniques are designed to further refine the awakening of subtle energy and awareness in connecting body, breath, and mind. Each of these techniques builds upon the natural breathing and disciplined puraka-rechaka practices discussed earlier. Invite students to explore these deeper methods only after finding stability and ease with puraka-rechaka and ujjayi. As with teaching other breathing practices, encourage students to find greater interest in relaxation than full performance of the breathing technique. Offer the concept of sthira sukham asanam as a tool for safely exploring pranayama. Instruct students to steadily maintain mula bandha through all of these practices and to variously engage jalandhara bandha and uddiyana bandha as explained here.

There are several contraindications for the following pranayama techniques. Pregnant students should stay with ujjayi. Students with high blood pressure, a heart condition, or pressure inside the head or specifically around the eyes should not do the retentions or kapalabhati. Students with high or low blood pressure should be counseled to explore these techniques more gently, doing the beginning level of each practice and evaluating how they feel before proceeding.

Vritti Pranayama: Fluctuating Breath

The breath fluctuates in a variety of ways, including in the relative length or duration of inhalations, exhalations, and the pauses in between. In vritti pranayama, the ratios of these durations are regulated. There are two practices: sama-vritti (equal fluctuation) and vishama-vritti (unequal fluctuation). We will first look at teaching these with the inhale and exhale; later, as part of introducing kumbhaka practices, we will apply these qualities to retention.

Sama-Vritti Pranayama

- Begin by guiding natural breath observation. Ask students to simply observe the breath without changing it in any way, noticing how it feels flowing in, out, and in the pauses in between. Guide them into making the breath flow smoothly.
- Then ask students to begin counting the duration of their inhalations and exhalations, noting the difference.
- Next, ask them to bring a uniform duration to the inhalations and exhalations, starting with a comfortable count (for most students this will be three to five).
- Gradually, practice by practice, expand the length of the inhalations and exhalations while keeping them in balance.
- Encourage students to make steadiness and ease more interesting than longer or deeper breaths, breathing only as deeply as they can while staying relaxed and comfortable.

Vishama-Vritti Pranayama

- Start teaching vishama-vritti pranayama with sama-vritti. At the end of a natural and balanced exhalation, instruct students to lengthen the inhalation by a one-count over the exhalation, staying with this for several rounds of breath.
- Encourage the class to watch and sense changes in the quality of the breath as well as subtle physical and mental reactions.

- Gradually increase the uneven ratio by further lengthening the inhalations, eventually inhaling for twice as long as exhaling.
- Stay with this several minutes before returning to the natural breathing and reversing the ratios, gradually lengthening the exhalations over the inhalations.

Kumbhaka: Breath Retention

Kumbhaka is the practice of staying with and expanding the natural pause between inhalations and exhalations.[8] In holding the breath in these pauses, the body-mind becomes more still and clear. There are two forms: *antara* kumbhaka is retention of the inhalation; *bahya* kumbhaka is retention of the exhalation.[9] It is important to develop these practices slowly, gradually refining the neuromuscular intelligence of the diaphragm, intercostals, and other secondary respiratory muscles. This practice should not cause any strain in the body or mind. Give students repeated encouragement to take it easy in expanding the duration of retention. Instruct as follows:

Antara Kumbhaka

- With students sitting in a comfortable upright position, guide the class into natural breathing with balanced puraka-rechaka (sama-vritti pranayama).
- Bring in ujjayi pranayama, guiding the gradual deepening of the breath. The spine should be naturally erect and relaxed, the heart center spacious and soft, the brain as light and quiet as possible in that moment.
- Using the basic breath awareness practices discussed earlier, ask students to focus their attention on the natural pause at the crest of the inhalations, noticing what happens in their body, mind, and larger sense of being in that space.
- Offer verbal cues that encourage a feeling of seamless movement into and out of the pause, staying with this simple practice for several rounds of breath.
- Introduce antara kumbhaka, asking students to retain the inhalations for a few seconds.
- Cue students to hold the breath with as little effort as possible while tuning in to the shifting sensations in their body and mental awareness.
- In transitioning into the exhalation, the tendency is for the breath to rush out; if that happens, instruct a shorter duration of retention.
- After one antara kumbhaka, guide several rounds of ujjayi pranayama, restoring the lungs to their natural condition. The rhythm of inhalation and exhalation should be smooth and steady before initiating further antara kumbhaka.

- Next, gradually lengthen the duration of retention, but only so far as there is no strain, imbalance in inhalations and exhalations, or gripping or collapsing in the lungs.
- Students should explore expanding the retention by one or two counts in each sitting, eventually holding the breath as long as they can with complete comfort.
- When students can easily retain the breath for fifteen seconds, they can fully develop the antara kumbhaka practice by engaging mula bandha, uddiyana bandha, and jalandhara bandha, thereby containing the pranic energy.

Bahya Kumbhaka

- Introduce bahya kumbhaka after students are at ease doing antara kumbhaka.
- Guide them into ujjayi, bringing attention to the natural pause when empty of breath. Do several rounds of ujjayi, refining awareness of the movement in and out of that pause.
- With the first few retentions of the exhalation, hold for just one count and then do several rounds of seamless ujjayi before repeating.
- Gradually expand the count, staying with simple retention. Encourage students to keep their eyes, face, throat, and heart center soft and not to grip in their belly.
- Unlike inhalations, exhalations naturally stimulate mula bandha and uddiyana bandha. Guide students into activating the bandhas along with bahya kumbhaka, starting with asking them to try to sustain mula bandha while breathing and retaining the breath.
- Introduce uddiyana bandha when students can comfortably hold the breath out for three counts. When pulling the belly back toward the spine and up toward to diaphragm, many students feel a gripping in the chest, throat, and head. If this happens, back off.
- To release bahya kumbhaka, it is important first to completely relax the belly and thereby allow the diaphragm to do its natural work; then consciously ease the breath in.
- If the breath rushes in, it was held in bahya kumbhaka for too long.
- Gradually develop this practice by lengthening the duration of retention and by adding antara kumbhaka in the same rounds of breath.

After students have refined their vritti pranayama and kumbhaka practices, begin guiding them in blending these practices, as follows:

- Applying vritti pranayama to kumbhaka practice, first instruct sama-vritti in each of the four phases of the breath cycle: cultivate an equal duration in puraka, rechaka, antara kumbhaka, and bahya kumbhaka, starting with a three-count and gradually lengthening.

- Remind students to pay close attention to the transitions between each phase while maintaining mental focus, emotional calm, and physical ease. When students can comfortably sustain this practice for a few minutes with at least a five-count in each phase, gradually introduce vishama-vritti, varying the duration of puraka, rechaka, antara kumbhaka, and bahya kumbhaka in a gradual manner.

- Working with breath ratios, start by increasing antara kumbhaka by 2:1 over puraka and rechaka, allowing the natural pause when empty of breath. Then gradually increase this ratio, working up to 4:1. When at 3:1, begin gradually extending the duration of rechaka eventually to a ratio of 2:1 over puraka.

- Add bahya kumbhaka, starting with a two-count retention and working up to the same duration as puraka.

- Continuing this practice, eventually puraka and bahya kumbhaka are the same duration, antara kumbhaka is 4:1 over puraka, and rechaka is 2:1 over puraka.

- The tendency in this practice is to gasp for air; extend durations only as much as the rhythm remains steady.

Viloma: Against the Grain

The term *viloma,* which in literal translation means "anti-hair," refers to going against the natural line or movement of the breath. In viloma pranayama, one repeatedly pauses during puraka and/or rechaka while changing as little as possible in the positioning and engagement of the diaphragm, rib cage, and lungs. With practice, one's awareness is steady throughout each cycle of breath, the nerves calm and quiet in support of both flow and pause. Begin by inviting students to sit up comfortably tall and do several rounds of ujjayi pranayama, focusing on the balance and ease in the breath, then guide as follows:

- After a complete exhalation, guide students to inhale to half their capacity and hold the breath there for a few seconds before completing the inhalation.

- Repeat several times before adding a second interruption to the inhalation, continuing in this way until reaching five pauses, and only so long as there is no strain or fatigue.

- Follow this with several rounds of ujjayi pranayama before resting in Savasana.

- Next, repeat this exercise with pauses in the exhalations only. With each interruption, bring slightly greater awareness and engagement to mula bandha and a light, gradual uddiyana bandha.
- When the lungs are empty, let the diaphragm relax and the belly draw farther back and up before easing into the inhalation.
- After resting in Savasana for a few minutes, guide students into viloma pranayama on both the inhalation and exhalation.

Experienced students whose basic viloma pranayama is free of strain can be introduced to the full practice of this technique in which kumbhaka is performed.

- Start with antara kumbhaka following a viloma pranayama inhalation in which there are one or more interruptions, keeping the diaphragm soft during the pauses.
- With the antara kumbhaka, retain the inhalation for two or three seconds before rechaka, gradually holding for longer with mula bandha and uddiyana bandha.
- After gradually developing this practice for up to ten minutes in each sitting, do viloma pranayama exhalations as described above, followed by bahya kumbhaka, gradually increasing the viloma interruptions and the length of bahya kumbhaka.
- For the full practice of viloma pranayama, invite students to explore viloma inhalations and exhalations along with antara and bahya kumbhaka, slowly lengthening the practice.

Kapalabhati: Cultivating Light

Kapalabhati (from *kapala,* "skull," and *bhati,* "luster") pranayama energizes the entire body by tremendously oxygenating the blood supply and creating a feeling of exhilaration.[10] In natural breathing, the inhalation is active, i.e., activated by muscles, while the exhalation is passive, resulting from contraction of the elastic lungs. This is reversed in kapalabhati pranayama: the exhalations are made active and inhalations passive. The technique described here is from the Hatha Yoga Pradipika (II.35). The Gheranda Samhita offers other forms of kapalabhati that blend this technique with nadi shodhana pranayama (see below).

- Start by guiding students into several rounds of ujjayi pranayama, warming and awakening the lungs while activating mula bandha.

- After completion of an ujjayi exhalation, the breath is drawn in halfway and then rapidly and repeatedly blasted out through the nose, with a slight pause when empty of breath. The sound is in the nostrils, not the throat.
- The inhalation happens naturally.
- In the early development of this practice, ask students to do twenty-five rapid exhalations, then fill their lungs and perform antara kumbhaka for a few counts before releasing the breath and relaxing.
- After this and each successive round, draw students' attention to the sensations they feel in their heads, suggesting the calming and clearing effects of this practice.
- Gradually increase to several minutes of sustained kapalabhati followed by kumbhakas.
- Complete the kapalabhati practice with Savasana or move into the asana practice.
- Explore kapalabhati sitting still, sitting while taking one to two minutes to reach the arms outward and up overhead, in Shishula Phalakasana (Dolphin Plank Pose) or in Ardha Navasana.

Bhastrika: Bellows Breath

Bhastrika ("bellows") pranayama is similar to kapalabhati, though more intense in fanning the flames of inner fire. Introduce students to this technique only after they are comfortable in the kapalabhati practice. Here both the inhalations and exhalations are done through the nostrils vigorously and in rapid succession. Unlike kapalabhati, there is no pause after the exhalation.

- Start students sitting and doing ujjayi pranayama.
- Initiate bhastrika by quickly blasting out the breath after a half inhalation.
- Make the following inhalation just as strong and quick as the exhalation, followed by a strong and quick exhalation, completing one round of bhastrika. The sound should come from the nose, not the throat.
- Do five to ten rounds, ending with an exhalation and several rounds of ujjayi pranayama, then repeat three or more times.
- Gradually increase the number of cycles in each round and the number of rounds in each sitting, eventually sustaining bhastrika for five or ten minutes.
- Rest in Savasana.

Sitali: Cooling Breath

The purpose of sitali ("cooling") pranayama is to cool and calm the physical body and mind. It can be done at any time, including during asana practice and after fiery pranayamas such as kapalabhati. Here the tongue is extended slightly out of the mouth and its sides curled up to form a channel. (The ability to create this channel is genetic; some people can do it, others can't. If a student can't curl his or her tongue, instruct that person to visualize the curling and continue with the practice.) Give cues as follows:

- Sitting comfortably, close the eyes and relax.
- Extend the tongue and curl its sides to create a channel for moisture.
- Slowly and deeply draw in the breath across the tongue, sensing the breath becoming moist and cool as it passes across the tongue.
- Then close the mouth and slowly exhale through the nose.
- Repeat this ten times, then relax.
- Gradually build up the sitali practice for up to fifteen minutes.
- Offer more advanced students variations that include antara kumbhaka (with mula bandha and jalandhara bandha) and viloma pranayama.

Anuloma and Pratiloma: Delicate Regulation of Breath

Anu, meaning "along with," and *prati,* meaning "against," give us pranayama practices in which one uses the fingers to delicately prolong the exhalations (in anuloma) and inhalations (in pratiloma). Done in stages, these practices help students to cultivate stronger breath control amid deepening ease. Guide as follows:

- Sit comfortably and do several rounds of ujjayi pranayama.
- Draw the fingers to the nostrils as described in the sidebar.
- Beginning with anuloma pranayama, exhale completely and then slowly and deeply inhale through the nose.
- At the crest of the inhalation, use the fingers to partially close the nostrils, being attentive to applying pressure evenly on each side of the nose.
- Slowly and completely exhale, feeling the natural pause when empty of breath.
- Release the fingers and take a deep inhalation, then reapply the fingers for a controlled exhalation. Make the exhalation about twice as long as the inhalation.
- Continue for five to twenty minutes, then rest in Savasana.

- For pratiloma pranayama, practice as described for anuloma, but switch to using the fingers and slowing the breath with the inhalations instead of the exhalations.
- Experienced students able to remain calm with basic anuloma pranayama and pratiloma pranayama can explore variations that include antara kumbhaka (with mula bandha and jalandhara bandha), bahya kumbhaka (with mula bandha, uddiyana bandha, and jalandhara bandha), viloma pranayama, and nadi shodhana (see below).

Suryabheda: Stimulating Vitality

Suryabheda (from *surya*, "sun," and *bheda*, "to pierce") pranayama is said to pierce the pingala nadi and activate pranic energy. The pingala nadi receives prana through the right nostril. In suryabheda pranayama, the fingers are applied to the nostrils to regulate the breath:

- Sit comfortably and do several rounds of ujjayi pranayama.
- Draw the fingers to the nostrils as described in the "Nadi Shodhana" section below, blocking the left nostril.
- Inhale slowly and deeply through the right nostril, close both nostrils, and perform antara kumbhaka for a few seconds with mula bandha and jalandhara bandha.
- Release jalandhara bandha, open the left nostril, and exhale slowly and completely.
- This completes one cycle of suryabheda pranayama. Repeat for up to thirty minutes, followed by Savasana.
- Introduce more experienced students to bahya kumbhaka, holding with uddiyana bhanda.
- Explore the permutations of viloma pranayama, as discussed earlier, with suryabheda.

Chandrabheda: Calming Energy

In Chandrabheda (from *chandra*, "moon," and *bheda*, "to pierce") pranayama, energy is directed in through the left nostril to the ida pingala, calming the body and mind. The practice is precisely the opposite of suryabheda pranayama. There is nothing written about chandrabheda pranayama in the traditional Hatha yoga literature, but it is described in the Yoga Chudamani Upanishad (Satyadharma 2003,

230–231).[11] Teach this practice with the same techniques applied in suryabheda, reversing sides and applying antara kumbhaka.

Nadi Shodhana: Alternate Nostril Breathing

We explored the subtle energy channels called nadis in Chapter Three. Here we look at teaching a pranayama technique that offers *shodana*, "purifying," of these channels. The Hatha Yoga Pradipika and other classical yoga texts describe nadi shodhana pranayama without giving it this name. This practice is said to activate and balance the ida and pingala nadis and harmonize the hemispheres of the brain

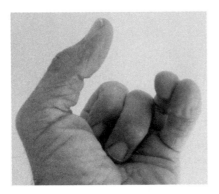

(Muktibodhananda 1993, 166). In its basic form, nadi shodhana combines puraka as performed in pratiloma and rechaka as in anuloma. More advanced variations add kumbhakas and bandhas.[12] This highly contemplative practice is, as B. K. S. Iyengar (1985, 210) puts it, "one of delicate adjustments. The brain and the fingers must learn to act together in channeling the in and out breaths while in constant communication with each other." It is, he continues, "the most difficult, complex, and refined of all pranayamas. It is the ultimate in sensitive self-observation and control. When refined to its subtlest level it takes one to the innermost self." Teach this technique as follows:

- Sit comfortably and practice ujjayi pranayama for a few minutes.
- Position the fingers as shown above. Place the fingertips on one side of the nose, the thumb on the other side, just below the slight notch about halfway down the side of the nose. Try to place the fingers with even pressure on the left and right sides of the nose, maintaining steady contact while keeping the nostrils fully open.
- While continuing ujjayi pranayama, play with slightly varying the pressure of the fingers, becoming more sensitive to the effects of the fine finger adjustments.

Technique 1: Basic nadi shodhana (with suryabheda and chandrabheda pranayama)

- After a complete exhalation, close the left nostril and slowly inhale through the right.
- At the crest of the inhalation, close the right nostril and slowly exhale through the left.

- Empty of breath, fully inhale through the left, close the left, and exhale through the right.
- Continue with this initial form of alternate nostril breathing for up to five minutes, cultivating the smooth and steady flow of the breath while remaining relaxed and calm.

Technique 2: Nadi shodhana with viloma pranayama

- Begin as described for Technique 1 and do two or three rounds of basic nadi shodhana.
- After a complete exhalation through the right nostril, inhale through the right to the halfway point of the inhalation, firmly close both nostrils and hold for a few seconds, then slowly complete the inhalation through the right nostril.
- Whenever cued to hold the breath, use the fingers to close both nostrils.
- Exhaling through the left nostril, stop halfway, hold the breath for a few seconds, then complete the exhalation through the left nostril.
- Inhaling through the left nostril, hold at the halfway point for a few seconds, then complete the inhalation through the left nostril.
- Exhaling through the right nostril, stop halfway, hold the breath for a few seconds, then complete the exhalation through the right nostril.
- This completes one round. Explore deepening this practice by adding pauses and extending their duration, eventually pausing five times on each side for ten seconds each.
- Most students find this practice very challenging. Remind them to make the steady, comfortable flow of the breath more important than the number or duration of pauses.

Technique 3: Nadi shodhana with kumbhakas

- Begin as described for Technique 1 and do two or three rounds of basic nadi shodhana.
- Start with antara kumbhaka. After a complete exhalation through the right nostril, slowly inhale through the right nostril and hold the breath in for a few seconds, closing both nostrils and engaging mula bandha and jalandhara bandha.
- Maintaining mula bandha, release jalandhara bandha and slowly ease the breath out through the left nostril.

- Ease the breath in through the left nostril and hold the breath in for a few seconds, closing both nostrils and engaging mula bandha and jalandhara bandha.
- Maintaining mula bandha, release jalandhara bandha and slowly ease the breath out through the right nostril. Continue for several cycles.
- Add bahya kumbhaka. Continuing as just described, at the end of the exhalation hold the breath out and engage uddiyana bandha as described in introducing bahya kumbhaka.
- Completely release uddiyana bandha before easing in the breath. Continue for several cycles, exploring longer retention with both antara and bahya (up to thirty seconds with antara and fifteen seconds with bahya).

Technique 4: Nadi shodhana with vilomas and kumbhakas

- Start with the practice described in Technique 1, adding viloma pauses.
- Start with one pause for a few seconds, then add more pauses, each held for a few seconds. When comfortable with three pauses held for three seconds each on both the inhalations and exhalations, add antara and bahya kumbhakas for a few seconds.
- Gradually lengthen the pauses and retentions, working up to five pauses of five seconds each, antara kumbhaka of thirty seconds, and bahya kumbhaka of fifteen seconds.

Technique 5: Nadi shodhana with kapalabhati pranayama

- This innovative pranayama technique should be practiced only when comfortable with the previous nadi shodhana practices. The effect is far more intense than the other techniques. Practice only as strongly as you can remain calm and quiet inside.
- Do five rounds of nadi shodhana as described in Technique 1. After a complete exhalation, inhale halfway through the right nostril, keep the left nostril closed, and engage mula bandha.
- Repeatedly and quickly blast the breath out through the right nostril for up to one minute (eventually several minutes), as described for kapalabhati pranayama.
- Inhale deeply through the right nostril and hold the breath, antara kumbhaka, for as long as can be comfortably maintained, then slowly exhale through the left nostril. Inhale through the left and exhale through the right.
- Do several rounds of soft ujjayi pranayama and switch sides.
- Rest in Savasana.

TABLE 8.1—**When and to Whom to Teach Pranayama**

PRANAYAMA	WHEN	WHOM
Natural breathing	Excellent way to initiate all classes.	All students.
Ujjayi	Teach at the beginning of every class.	All students.
Sama-vritti	Teach in conjunction with natural breathing and ujjayi.	All students.
Vishama-vritti	Teach in conjunction with natural breathing and ujjayi.	All students.
Antara kumbhaka	Teach in conjunction with ujjayi as a means of expanding and refining breath capacity.	Intermediate students at ease with ujjayi and experienced with bandhas; not when pregnant, experiencing eye or ear complaints, or with high blood pressure.
Bahya kumbhaka	After developing ease with antara kumbhaka.	Same as above.
Viloma	Teach in conjunction with ujjayi as a means of expanding and refining breath capacity.	All students, especially when experiencing fatigue or anxiety.
Kapalabhati	At beginning of class to stimulate energy, awaken the breath, and more quickly warm the body; during asana sequences, especially as part of core awakening. If during asanas, teach with students either sitting (ideally in Virasana) or in Shishula Phalakasana.	Intermediate students; not when pregnant, experiencing eye or ear complaints, or with high blood pressure.
Bhastrika	Pranayama class or as final energizing practice immediately before Savasana.	Same as above.
Sitali	For cooling down.	All students.
Anuloma	Pranayama classes.	Students familiar and comfortable with ujjayi.
Pratiloma	Pranayama classes.	Same as above.
Suryabheda	Teach in conjunction with ujjayi.	All students.
Chandrabheda	Traditionally practiced on alternate days from suryabheda.	All students.
Nadi shodhana 1	Beginning of class.	Intermediate students.
Nadi shodhana 2	When comfortable with Technique 1.	Intermediate students.

PRANAYAMA	WHEN	WHOM
Nadi shodhana 3	When comfortable, steady, and at ease with Technique 2.	Intermediate students at ease with ujjayi and experienced with bandhas; not when pregnant, experiencing eye or ear complaints, or with high blood pressure.
Nadi shodhana 4	When comfortable with Technique 3.	Same as above.
Nadi shodhana 5	When comfortable with Technique 4.	Same as above.

CONSCIOUSLY CULTIVATING ENERGY

The heart of yoga practice is the conscious awakening and movement of energy that creates a feeling of being fully alive and aware of the wholeness of one's being in the world. While asana practice is an essential part of this awakening, conscious pranayama most distinguishes yoga from physical exercise. If all you do as a yoga teacher is motivate and guide your students to breath consciously and feel themselves more subtly through the breath as they explore in the universe of their body, mind, and spirit, they will be well served. Blending pranayama practices with asana classes and meditation will take your students even farther along the path of living joyfully and consciously.

CHAPTER NINE

TEACHING MEDITATION

The pearl is in the oyster.
And the oyster is at the bottom of the sea.
Dive deep.
—*Kabir*

As part of the beauty of yoga, meditation is the seed that can always immediately blossom into the thousand-petal lotus flower of happiness, wellness, and fullness as an awakened human being. It is both the ultimate form of yoga practice and an integral part of the entire path of discovering, loving, healing, and transforming the totality of one's being. All the various paths of practice lead to meditation becoming a deeper yet easier method of feeling whole within one's self and connected as part of the whole of the universe. In meditating, we open the windows of the mind to clearer consciousness. To the extent that we refine the temple of the physical body through consistent asana practice, it gives us more unwavering support in allowing the windows to open smoothly. Similarly, consistent pranayama practices awaken subtle energy in a way that creates a stronger inner invitation to the currents of clear awareness, leading to a lighter and more balanced sense of being. Yet to meditate, we do not have to wait for some requisite level of asana or pranayama practice; rather, it can start the first time a student steps onto his or her mat, or even before, without ever having done a single asana.

Many yoga students say they can't meditate because their minds won't stop chattering. Frustrated, they often give up exploring meditation. This mind-set expresses the common misunderstanding that meditating means having no thoughts. While moving into inner stillness is one of the many fruits of meditation practice, it is not the goal of the practice itself. In fact, there doesn't have to be a goal. Much like the asana practice, when we go into meditation with a specific goal in mind, such as a perfectly quiet mind, it is frustrating because even the most practiced meditators have only rare moments of complete inner quiet and stillness. If, just like the asana practice, we practice meditation as a process of self-exploration, self-discovery, and self-transformation, we can experience the joy of it the first moment we try.

My first meditation teacher, Alan Watts, whose mid-1970s radio broadcasts offered mind-blowing kernels of insight into Eastern spiritual philosophy and practices, offered simple analogies to drive home the point that meditation is a process. "When we dance," he said, "the journey itself is the point. When we play music, the playing itself is the point, and the same is true of meditation. Meditation is the discovery that the point of life is always arrived at in the immediate moment" (Watts 1980, 5–6). He thought that meditation should be enjoyable, not a chore. "It is an appreciation of the present, a kind of 'grooving' with the eternal now, and it brings us into a state of peace where we can understand that the point of life, the place where it is at, is simply here and now." This take on meditation reflects a Buddhist influence; since thoughts will always come and go, much like clouds floating by overhead, they are something to play with. Interested without being attached, the playful practice of watching *is* the practice.

The Buddhist nun Pema Chödrön (2007, 29) comments that by meditating we come to four realizations: (1) thoughts have no birthplace, (2) they are unceasing, (3) they appear but are not solid, which, since there's nothing to react to, together lead to (4) awareness of "complete openness." But what about the Yoga Sutras, which define yoga practice as chitta vritti nirodaha, "to still the fluctuations of the mind"? The problem is that we do react to our thoughts, despite knowing they are just thoughts, and it is in these reactions that we find ourselves distracted, suffering, confused, unhappy, or hurting. The ancient yogis identified this problem as kleshas, a deep form of confused perception. Traditional yoga philosophy, much like Buddhism, holds out the hope that through its practices, from asana and mantra to pranayama and puja, we can come to a place of samadhi, a blissful state free of thoughts where we realize our true Self.[1]

While the various strands of yoga philosophy offer different maps to attaining samadhi, most offer a path through pratyahara, dharana, and dhyana. Here we will consider these as useful tools for helping students cultivate clearer self-awareness, self-understanding, and self-acceptance, which, taken together, tend to yield a steadier, easier, and ultimately happier and more meaningful life. But rather than looking on all this as leading to certain promised outcomes, it is more fruitful to explore these tools as sources for guiding students into deeper insight right here and now.[2] After looking at this classical yoga meditation process, we will explore

how to infuse asana classes with other practical meditation techniques, offering
a variety of ways to help your students discover the full joy of meditation.

PATANJALI'S PATH OF MEDITATION:
PRATYAHARA, DHARANA, DYANA

In Chapter One, we explored Patanjali's eight-limbed path of yoga, which begins
with essentially material practices: yamas to guide us in our social relations, niyamas for our intrapersonal life, asana and pranayama as tools of awakening that prepare us for a deeper journey into the Self. Yet with these practices we are still
scratching the surface, still working with *bahiranga,* the external life of the senses.
Moving into the mystical realm of samadhi first requires relieving our senses of
their external distractions, developing a single-pointed mental concentration, and
then a meditative state. This is the path from bahiranga to *antaranga,* or internal
meditative practice. In this traditional yogic view, before stepping into meditation
and blissful supraconsciousness, we must first cross a bridge departing the material realm of sense awareness. Patanjali describes this practice as pratyahara, "de-
taching at will from the senses." We are led to this bridge by following the path
of yama, niyama, asana, and pranayama. Nothing is forced as we abide in the self-
revealing truth of our being along this path. With asana we finally come to the
physical and mental health that allows us to work easily and steadily with the breath;
as we refine the breath and cultivate the life-force energy of prana, then "all that
veils clarity of perception is swept away . . . and thought becomes fit for concentration." But before we can completely concentrate, we must tame the mind's attachments to the wake of our senses. As Patanjali notes, "Withdrawal of the senses
occurs when the sensory organs, independent of their particular objects, conform to the nature of the mind" (Sutra II.54 as quoted in Bouanchaud 1999, 142).
In other words, we can bring our mind into its own inner space, freed from external stimulation. Only then can we can completely concentrate.

It is helpful to offer students a backdrop to pratyahara. Wherever we are, there
are always sounds, sights, aromas, and other vibrations entering our senses—or,
put differently, to which our senses are attaching. Sitting in class, it is likely that
sounds are reaching you from outside and from others in the room. If there is any
light, then there are visual impressions coming about through the eyes. The heart
is felt beating in the chest, clothing or a draft is felt on the skin, and perhaps there
is a sense of more subtle energy pulsating through one's entire being. There are all
these vibrations, what Alan Watts (1980, 8) termed "so many happenings." With
pratyahara, the idea is to just let them all be there. Sounds and other vibrations will

come and go. Meanwhile, there are the happenings of the mind, habitually taking all these vibrations and reacting to them with more thoughts. The thoughts are also reacting to other thoughts, the mind typically chattering away, reactively and imaginatively adding more vibrations. Without focusing on the breath or anything else, just following the breath as another source of vibration, you will notice that when empty of breath there is a natural quieting, an opening to the bridge from the world of the senses to the world of the true self. Staying in that awareness, without thinking about it, you are on the other side, the inside, in pratyahara, even as vibrations intrude.

So how do we guide students to stay inside without thinking about it and reintroducing intrusions? This is the practice of dharana, single-pointed focus of concentration. By intently focusing the mind on one thing, there's no space for anything else. It doesn't matter what you focus on. Commenting on Patanjali's advice that we "concentrate wherever the mind finds satisfaction," Sally Kempton (2002, 61) suggests that we can recognize satisfaction when the experience is one of natural joy, peace, and relaxation. "If you have to work too hard at it," she writes, "that may be a sign that it is the wrong practice for you." In concentrating, a person is aware that he or she is concentrating, aware of being in the practice of single-pointed awareness, conscious of being a meditator who is meditating.

In traditional dharana practice, the focus is a mantra, "a tool for the mind" (Kempton 2002, 67), but it could be the breath or, as we'll explore shortly, even

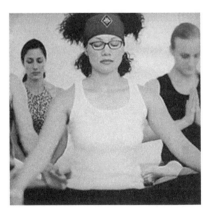

an activity such as gardening or surfing in which our attention is wholly connected with what we're doing. For many years, I found my mind quite satisfied—in a state of natural joy, peace, and relaxation—when fully concentrating on carefully placing my foot on a tiny lip of granite on the face of a cliff hundreds of feet off the ground, my life literally in the balance. In this intense circumstance, I was definitely "in the moment." What about complete concentration in less intense circumstances? Around this period I also had the privilege of sharing time with a group of visiting Tibetan Buddhist monks I was working with in the juvenile facilities of the County of Los Angeles. When we were together one weekend I suggested hiking to a tranquil meditation spot on top of a mountain overlooking the Pacific Ocean. They openly laughed at this idea, gently admonishing me that one could just as easily meditate while washing the dishes.[3] While appreciating their experience and wisdom, it also occurred to me that I hadn't grown up meditating in Dharamsala, India, and wasn't at their level of easy concentration. I was still with the yogis of old who had discovered that when we repeat a word or phrase over and over, it not only occupies our mental space, but opens up an inner rhythm of quieting awareness. In some meditation traditions, the mantra is said to contain "the throb of shakti," the "original pulsation of divine energy that creates the universe and remains embedded within every particle of it" (Kempton 2002, 72). Whether or not that is what is happening with mantra practice, one thing is clear: focusing the mind on a single thing, whether it's repetition of a word or phrase, following the breath or some other recurrent energy, the effect is a steadier mind in which thought slows down.

At the heart of Patanjali's approach to meditation is the idea that a steadier mind is a clearer mind. Clarity arises when "the senses are perfectly mastered" through pratyahara and dharana (Sutra II.55 as quoted in Bouanchaud 1999, 144), bringing us farther along the path to the pure meditative state of dhyana, "a current of unified thought."[4] In this state of consciousness, the truth of one's being as an expression of pure love is made manifest, as "perfect concentration on the heart reveals the contents of the mind" (Sutra III.34 as quoted in Bouanchaud 1999, 187). Mantra now disappears as the person's awareness is completely at one with the divine (spirit, nature, the universe, the Self). "When purity of the peaceful mind is identical with that of the spiritual entity," Patanjali relates, "that is liberation" (Sutra III.55 as quoted in Bouanchaud 1999, 216). Free of external stimulation, present in the moment, there is only the truth of one's being as love and light. There is a sense of directly knowing the essence of whatever one is meditating on, of being part of the whole of existence.

Where does this effort lead? Samadhi (Kempton 2002, 114). The alternative origins of the term are insightful: sam ("together"), a ("towards"), and dha ("to get"); sama ("equal") and dhi ("intellect"). In either case, samadhi means moving into a sense of wholeness and balanced awareness. Pure bliss. The eight-limbed path of Patanjali's raja yoga is the classical formulation of moving into this state of blissful being. There are many other schools of yogic thought with different approaches to samadhi, ranging from laya samadhi's trance dance into joy to the vaishnava bhakti yogis' pathway through purely devotional love of God.[5] But as exemplified by the Tibetan Buddhists visiting Los Angeles several years ago, it's entirely possible to find that state of bliss doing practically anything. What Patanjali and others have bequeathed to us are some practical tools that we are free to adapt and apply in our lives here and now in ways that make blissful being that much more abundant and accessible.

TAKING ONE SEAT

When Patanjali summarized the received wisdom of earlier yoga traditions in the Yoga Sutras, he was succinct on asana: sthira sukham asanam. In earlier chapters we have focused on steadiness and ease. Asanam, "to take one seat," is a foundation for chitta vritti nirodaha, "to still the fluctuations of the mind." Regular asana practice creates a foundation for the physical steadiness and ease we want when sitting in meditation. Similarly, refining the breath and cultivating life-force energy through pranayama yields more naturally awakened awareness in meditation. Through these practices we can sit more comfortably tall with the spine in its natural form, the heart center spacious, and the breath flowing effortlessly; pratyahara comes more naturally, it is easier to stay with dharana, and dhyana appears more frequently and stays longer.

In helping students set up for seated meditation, ask them to choose a comfortable sitting position. The most important quality in sitting is comfort; over time, alignment of the spine will lead to greater comfort in sitting for longer periods. With practice, most students will eventually be able to sit on top of their sitting bones with a neutral pelvis that allows their spine to be more easily held naturally erect. For some students, this requires a chair, high cushion, or wall for back support. Over time and with practice (along with a supportive lifestyle and favorable genetics), students may find they are able to sit comfortably in Padmasana, the ultimate asana for sitting (although in reality, few Westerners, including those with lifelong meditation practices, can sit in this position for extended periods, perhaps because of having grown up sitting in chairs, and as a consequence can injure their hips when sitting in Padmasana). Guide students into sitting with whatever props it takes to establish and maintain a neutral pelvis, then ask them to consciously root down into their sitting bones, feeling how that grounding action leads to a taller spine, more open heart center, more natural flow of breath, and a sense of their head floating on top of their spine. Exploring this stable and eventually more sustainable position, ask students to feel their spine and the crown of their head extending taller as they feel more grounded through their sitting bones, from there allowing the shoulder blades to release down their back and their chin to release slightly down. The palms can rest together in the lap or in a mudra on the knees.[6]

SIX GUIDED MEDITATION TECHNIQUES

All the basic meditation techniques involve focusing the mind on a single thing. Here we look at five different guided meditations using various objects of attention. Each approach tends to evoke different qualities of meditative awareness. Play around with how these feel in your own meditation practice before offering them in class. Explore doing each technique at different times of the day, in different moods, before and after practicing asanas, and after experimenting with some of the pranayama techniques described in Chapter Eight. As with the asana practice, there is no one correct or best path, only infinite paths that you and your students will find different and change resonance with during the course of your lives.

One: Breath[7]

1. Sit comfortably tall, drawing your attention to the breath.

2. Allow the breath to flow softly and quietly, simply watching it without trying to change it in any way.

3. Feel and visualize the breath flowing in through your nostrils, down through your throat, and into your lungs, receiving the breath as a pure form of beauty or a gift from the universe of the divine.

4. As easily and naturally as the breath flows into your body, let it flow back out just as effortlessly, a sense of giving back the gift we all share.

5. Allow your mind to become completely absorbed in the flow of the breath, noticing how and where it arises and what it feels like along the way.

6. When your mind wanders away from the breath, gently bring it back to the steadiness, the rhythmic flow of your inhales and exhales.

7. Staying fully absorbed in the breath and allowing it to continue flowing freely, notice the natural pauses between each inhale and exhale.

8. Notice the natural quieting and stilling of the mind that happens when you are empty of breath, allowing that sense of quiet to ride along with the following inhale.

9. At the crest of your inhale, feel a sense of the rising quiet expand into a feeling of openness and spaciousness in you mind, and just as simply let the breath flow out.

10. Stay with it, continuously coming back to the feeling of your thoughts as though enveloped in the breath, at one with the breath as it flows in and out of your body.

Two: Mantra[8]

1. Choose a mantra that works for you. If this is your first mantra meditation, consider using the words *inhale-exhale* or *so-hum: so* meaning "that," *hum* meaning "I am." Although you can use any word, keep it simple and consider using words that you want to embed more deeply in your consciousness, such as *calm, clear, peace,* or *love.* If you feel a deeper resonance using ancient Sanskrit words, try *aum* or *shanti* ("peace").

2. Do the breath-focused meditation for a few minutes, letting your awareness settle into the natural flow of the breath.

3. After completing an exhale, with your inhale slowly say the word *inhale* (or *so*) while absorbing your awareness in the word, not the breath.

4. As easily as the breath draws in, allow it to flow out while saying the word *exhale* (or *hum*).

5. As with the breath meditation, notice and allow the natural stillness that happens in the pauses between the breaths, then just as the breath moves, begin repeating the mantra.

6. As with all meditation techniques, your mind will wander—it will think. This is what it is good at and likes to do! Without thinking about the thoughts or judging yourself for thinking (or for judging), come right back to the mantra.

7. Rather than jumping from one mantra to another, stay with one for at least ten sessions to see what happens. One of the benefits of repetition is that the words themselves become less and less significant, the sound of the mantra in your mind gradually becoming like a neutral vibration, the "grooving" awareness described by Alan Watts (1980, 6).

Three: Counting[9]

1. Do the breath-focused meditation for a few minutes, letting your awareness settle into the natural flow of the breath.

2. With an inhale, say "one hundred" to yourself as the breath draws in, then say "ninety-nine" to yourself as it flows out.

3. With the next cycle of breath say "ninety-eight" with your inhale and "ninety-seven" with your exhale, continuing in this way until exhaling on "fifty-one."

4. As other words and thoughts intrude, just come back to breathing and counting down.

5. Now inhale *and* exhale saying a single number to yourself, starting with stretching "fifty" across one complete cycle of inhale-exhale, continuing in this way until exhaling on "twenty-one."

6. After exhaling on "twenty-one," stop counting and simply follow the breath. As words and thoughts arise, just watch and come back to the breath.

7. Continue sitting and watching for longer than it would have taken to count down to zero, noticing how the mind slows and quiets along the way.

Four: Chakras

1. Do the breath-focused meditation for a few minutes, letting your awareness settle into the natural flow of the breath.

2. More consciously grounding down through the sitting bones, bring more awareness to the floor of the pelvis, feeling with each breath a deepening sense of stability and rootedness. Watching the breath, with each exhale say to yourself *lam*, visualizing the vibrations of that silent sound stirring the upward release of energy, drawing in the energy of the earth. Repeat the mantra five times, bringing consciousness to the muladhara chakra.

3. Staying with the breath, bring your awareness up into the center of your pelvis, opening your imagination to the deep reservoir of creativity resting in the svadhisthana chakra. With each of five exhales, say the word *vam* to yourself while visualizing that silent sound stimulating your creative juices. Feel the richness of that creativity deepen with each sound of *vam*.

4. Drawing your awareness to the center of your belly, sense the latent determination resting in the manipura chakra. With each of five exhales, say the word *ram* to yourself, visualizing the vibrations of that silent sound sparking the fire of willful consciousness that opens you to easier laughter and joy.

5. Breathing as though you are doing it through your spiritual heart center, tap into feeling the love that you are in your essence. Connected with the breath, with each of five exhales, say the word *ham* to yourself, visualizing the vibrations of that silent sound opening your heart to the light and wisdom pulsating there along with each beat of your heart, each breath a sense of the love that you are radiating from your anahata chakra all through and around you.

6. With your awareness resting in the light of love and innate wisdom, draw your awareness to your throat, imagining your every word arising from the love and wisdom in your heart. Following the breath, with each of five exhales, say the word *vam* to yourself, visualizing the vibrations of that silent sound emanating from the vishuddha chakra creating a peaceful resonance with all the other sounds in the universe.

7. Feeling energy drawing up from the base of your spine, through your heart, and to your third eye, imagine light drawing into your third eye, opening your

inner visual landscape to the purity of light. With each of five exhales, say the word *ke-sham* to yourself, visualizing the vibrations of that silent sound opening your ajna chakra to clearer awareness of yourself and your connection with the universe.

8. Now let your awareness rest more gently in the breath, feeling a sense of blissful being as energy rises effortlessly from the base of your pelvis out through the crown of your head. Visualize a feeling of the crown of your head opening like a thousand-petal lotus flower, the sahasrara chakra expanding the light of your being. Stay with it, with a sense of being whole and complete in this moment of blissful being.

Five: Light

1. Either following the chakra meditation or breath meditation, draw your palms together at your heart in a prayer position, anjali mudra, the reverence seal.

2. Bring your awareness to the sense of energy rising from the base of your spine and out through the crown of your head. Imagine this energy like warm white light beaming out toward the sky.

3. With your awareness resting in the effortless breath and keeping your palms together, with an inhale raise your palms up past your face and slowly overhead through that beam of light, grounding down while reaching toward the sky, spaciousness all through you.

4. As you exhale, slowly extend your arms out and down, a sense of drawing that light out and around you as you bring the backs of your hands to rest softly on your knees, feeling a sense of being warmly enveloped as though in a cocoon of nourishing light.

5. Staying with the breath, spread your fingers and palms wide open, a sense of radiating energetically from your heart center out through your fingertips and the crown of your head.

6. Bringing the tips of your thumbs and index fingers together into jnana mudra, let your thumbs symbolize all that you consider divine or beautiful in the universe, your index fingers all that is divine or beautiful in yourself, the touching of your thumb and fingertips representing that yoking, the union, the whole of these qualities.

7. Breathing and following the natural flow of the breath, allow the three extended fingers on each hand to represent your release of the illusions in your life that keep you from feeling more whole, happy, and complete—the ego, fear, anger, and greed giving way to contentment and clarity of being.

8. Staying in the light of this awareness, keep following the breath, breath by effortless breath creating a sense of deepening self-awareness and self-acceptance in this perfect moment.

Six: Mala

1. Holding a string of *mala* beads (108 beads) across the middle finger of your left hand, palms resting in your lap or on your knees, do the breath meditation for a few minutes.

2. Placing your thumb against the *semuru* (head bead), as the breath draws in, circle your thumb around the next bead.

3. As the breath flows out, use your thumb to move the mala to the next bead, circling it with your thumb as the breath flows in, rotating the mala to the next bead as the breath flows out.

4. Continue in this fashion until completing one mala, eventually going around 108 times.

5. In using your thumb to move the beads, become completely absorbed in doing just that, opening your awareness to each gentle push from your thumb drawing the energy of the divine, or the essence of nature, deeper into your consciousness.

WHEN TO MEDITATE

One can meditate at any time and place. When teaching classes, we can offer brief or extended periods of seated meditation at the beginning or end of class. Amid the flow of the class, you can always bring the students to samasthihi or to sitting for a few moments of self-reflective meditation. Going beyond asana classes, you may want to offer classes devoted entirely to meditation or a combination of pranayama and meditation. In giving students more meditation tools, they can also explore the time and settings they find the most conducive to deeper meditation. Most people find the most natural inner peace and quiet in the early morning hours, before the day fills their mind with new thoughts. Others find the asana-pranayama practice lends to the most favorable inner conditions for meditation. Here we will look at one approach to bringing meditation into the asana-pranayama practice itself.

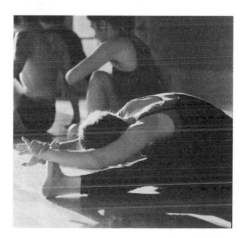

MEDITATING AMID THE FLOW OF BODY AND BREATH

In guiding Hatha yoga classes, we want to help students explore at a place of intensity in their physical, mental, and emotional experience because pure consciousness is especially close to us in moments of intensity, moments that might seem the opposite of peace. The entire yogic paradigm is based on the idea that there is something vast, loving, and spacious in the heart of reality; the practice is to live from that vast spacious source, going to the very core of ourselves to include the totality of our experience and dissolve it to its essence. Anything in our experience can provide a doorway to this quality of consciousness; developing the fortitude to hold steady with this intensity can bring us a to place of synchronicity, so we are not "doing" yoga but just being in that state of grace, in that awareness that it is all just happening.[10] This is where tantric awareness utilizing micropractices can gain practical traction, and where tantra brings deeper meditative awareness to the flow of asanas.

A good example of this: standing asana sequences. In most classes, we usually do standing asanas after warming up the entire body with Sun Salutations or other dynamic movements. The standing asanas continue to heat the body while opening and strengthening the hips and legs. But if you teach an inappropriately long, sustained sequence of standing poses requiring strength mostly from one leg, then muscle fatigue will eventually set in, compromising neuromuscular functioning and leading to the wrong muscles being recruited to do the required work. If you are coaching your students to "go for it" or to "push harder to find your true self," strain or even serious injury is probably not an "if" but a "when."

Surely our own thoughts can misguide us in various ways, leading us either to push too hard or to shy away from challenges, usually reflecting to some degree the behavioral patterns in our larger lives. One of the purposes of doing yoga is to cultivate a clearer mind and more balanced life. This clarity arises in the practice of yoga asana with the interplay of body-mind-breath, especially as we "play the edge" of the intensity of experience with increasingly subtle awareness of what we are feeling. Ignore the feeling and there you are, back in the world of aerobics, or maybe yoga-robics.

There is a far deeper level in guiding a yoga practice as one of conscious awakening to spirit, bliss, or inner peace. The key is in guiding students in:

- Working with what they are feeling in the totality of their experience.
- Exploring going with that feeling to a place of sensible intensity.
- Opening themselves through refined breath and nuanced movement to a greater sense of spaciousness around that intensity.

- Tapping more deeply into the source(s) of their feeling/experience.
- Moving along with their shifting edge as their body-mind-breath invites them into a place of expanded awareness, openness, inner strength, and harmony.

In applying this approach to the flow of asana practice, students can embrace the fullness of energy in a way that makes the asana practice itself a form of meditation. When fully absorbed in the flowing connection of breath-body-mind, students come to experience the present moment in a nonthinking state of awareness, so direct that it leads to spontaneity and gives way to a joy that is no longer dependent on external circumstances of freedom or attainment. This is the essence of tantra as expressed in Hatha yoga. Guiding students into creating the inner space to really feel takes them to the core of being by including everything in their experience—the feeling of their feet grounding into the earth, the rhythmic pulsation of their breath and heart, the vibration of energy in their legs and through their spine, the emotions and thoughts swirling all through and around them—bringing them ever closer to a sense of essence. This practice fruitfully and ultimately extends well off the mat. In the simplest of experiences—tasting an apple, riding a bicycle, weeding the garden, standing in Tadasana, flowing from Up Dog to Down Dog—it is the same: to be conscious, to give yourself the space to breathe completely, to feel completely, to move with intuitive spontaneity in each moment of freedom and find there more bliss for an expanding moment.

CHAPTER TEN

SEQUENCING AND PLANNING CLASSES

Acomplete and effective yoga class is one that allows students to progress steadily and simply from one place to another in their personal practice. Here we are blending two essential concepts: (1) *parinamavada*, the understanding that constant change is an inherent part of life; and (2) *vinyasa krama,* from *vinyasa,* "to place in a special way," and *krama,* "stage," referring to the sequencing of asanas, pranayamas, and other yoga techniques to accommodate different intentions and abilities.[1] These concepts apply equally to planned group classes, individual instruction, and personal practice in which one is listening inside for intuitive guidance. The art of teaching yoga is creatively expressed in how you craft asana, pranayama, and meditation sequences that honor the needs and intentions of the students in your classes. Your creativity is given form by yoga philosophy, the style of yoga you are teaching, the biomechanics and energetic requirements and effects of asanas, and by your personal sense of purpose in meaningfully sharing yoga. Here we look to our full palette of knowledge and skills to create classes that resonate with the needs and expressed intentions of our students, offering them a clear pathway to more radiant well-being. The teacher's role in this process is threefold: (1) intelligently plan the route based on the realities of the terrain and students in class; (2) observe and communicate with students to ascertain when they have integrated the experience with stability and ease; and (3) provide informed guidance and inspiration along the path.

Sequences are designed based on the style of yoga, the level and condition of students in the class, special themes, and your choice of peak asanas. Generally speaking, every class should offer a balanced practice that includes dynamic warming of the body, standing asanas that build further stamina and strength, a well-thought-out pathway to the peak asanas, time to fully explore the peak, and from there a calming pathway to Savasana. Within each week and month of classes, variations in sequences should be offered that allow students to gradually move more

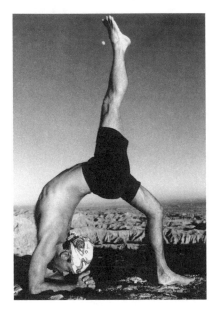

deeply into their practice while still giving an overall balanced practice in each class. Part of the challenge to you as a teacher is that student attendance is typically uneven and inconsistent, with new students appearing each day and others disappearing. This makes it largely impractical to offer a highly structured curriculum in which you plan classes across a period of weeks or months around certain practice objectives. Still, you can bring more coherence to the parinamavada process and the overall vinyasa krama of your classes by regularly alternating between different asana focus areas. This requires thinking about what you have recently taught, addressing tension that might have set in after previous classes, and introducing new asanas that encourage students to deepen and expand their practice. By applying basic principles of sequencing in planning your classes, you can offer students a rich variety of practices that are sustainable and self-transforming.

PRINCIPLES OF SEQUENCING

There are infinite possibilities for structuring and sequencing yoga classes. By following these five sequencing principles, you can ensure that each class is safe, effective, and integrated:

1. Applied Parinamavada:
Know and Teach Appropriately for Your Audience

The Tao of Pooh begins with Piglet asking Pooh, "Where will you begin the story, Pooh?" Pooh replies, "Well, Piglet, we'll begin at the beginning" (Hoff 1982). The idea is to begin from where you are, for a student to begin his or her practice based upon his or her present physical, emotional, and mental condition. The power of this insight is in its simplicity: Acknowledge where you are and progress from there, as opposed to jumping ahead at the expense of sthira and sukham. For a teacher, this means letting go of preconceptions about students and classes, instead observing where they are and, guided by the concepts of parinamavada and vinyasa krama, moving from there. Based on your assessment of your students, plan a class that includes asanas and pranayama techniques that are safe and accessible for that group. Apply the observation and assessment tools discussed in Chapter Six. Carefully consider the physical requirements of each asana and the class as a whole:

physical strength, stamina, flexibility, risks, and contraindications. Most yoga studios distinguish classes by levels, most often on a scale of 1, 2, and 3 with level 1 being easiest and level 3 most difficult. While this usually helps to separate students by their ability, almost invariably you will find many students in a class above their safe and effective ability level. In crafting specific classes, consider your students' age range, level of experience, physical condition, emotional condition, lifestyle, and overall health as well as your own experience. It is important to have substantial personal experience practicing and studying an asana or asana sequence prior to teaching it to others. Ideally, you will explore what you want to teach under a variety of conditions—different settings, seasons, moods, etc.—as a means of deepening the insight required for safely and effectively guiding others in that practice.

2. Move from Simple to Complex Asanas

This principle applies to asanas within a common family and to the movement across families when building toward a peak asana. Simpler asanas are those in which the body feels a relatively deeper sense of natural familiarity, steadiness, and ease. If Salamba Sirsasana I is in your sequence, start the class standing on their feet in Tadasana, teaching students about grounding and the principle of roots and extension discussed in Chapter Six, which will directly apply later in the Headstand. Progressing farther toward Salamba Sirsasana I, offer students Uttanasana, which stretches the back and gives students a sense of what it is like breathing while inverted. In classifying asanas as more or less simple, explore which ones feel more demanding. This will vary with different students, but there are still common patterns. Sustained standing poses that strongly stretch the hamstrings, such as Utthita Trikonasana, and require considerable strength to support the lateral positioning of the torso and spine are sensibly sequenced after Virabhadrasana II because it more gently opens the hips while warming and awakening the legs and the core muscles that give support to the spine. We will further explore and apply the principle of moving from simple to complex when looking at creating anticipatory sets below.

3. Move from Dynamic to Static Exploration

In dynamic exploration, we move in and out of asanas with the rhythmic flow of the breath. Dynamic movement allows the body to open more slowly, gently, and deeply so that the positioning that students are moving toward becomes more assimilated into the body. This method of practice more fully awakens the sense of connection of breath to movement, strength, and release within and between the asanas, making the breath more of the focal point of the overall practice. This both prepares the body for safer and deeper exploration of statically held asanas and deepens the ultimate effects of the asana. Surya Namaskara is the classic example of dynamic movement in the practice. In Ashtanga Vinyasa–style yoga, dynamic movement spices up the entire practice as students perform the vinyasa of Tolasana, Lolasana, Chaturanga, Up Dog, Down Dog, Dandasana between most of the statically held asanas. You can play with offering a variety of other dynamic movements. In reality, the entire practice is dynamic because we are always breathing and moving, even when moving into a sense of deepening inner stillness. We are inherently dynamic beings, and the asana practice should express, never suppress, this natural quality of our being. The heart is always beating, blood is always circulating, and in the asana practice hopefully the breath is always flowing. Rather than thinking of long-held asanas as static, it is important to encourage very small refining movements that bring stronger stability and lighter ease to the breath, body, and mind. Opening to our natural dynamism is a surer path to deeper inner peace and clarity than the determined effort to be perfectly still.

4. Sattvic Effect: Cultivating Energetic Balance

Hatha yoga is a practice of moving into energetic balance. The *ha* part of *hatha* is more energizing, the *tha* part more relaxing. Generally, classes should cultivate a sustainable balance of energy, a sattvic effect in which students feel fully awakened yet calm and clear. Sometimes you may want to offer a more stimulating or calming class. When students display low energy or depression, a stimulating practice can help bring them into energetic balance. If students have high anxiety or stress, a more calming class will help them find that balance. What asanas you put in a sequence as well as their order will make a class more or less energizing or calming. Dynamic movements, backbends, and standing asanas with spinal extension are more energizing. Forward bends, seated hip openers, and static holding in asanas are more calming.

5. Pratikriyasana: Integrating the Effects of Asana

As part of parinamavada, each asana works and stretches the body in particular ways that create new needs and possibilities for further exploration and change. For instance, after practicing Urdhva Dhanurasana, your body will feel like neutralizing the spine with twists and forward bends in order to come into a new balance. This neutralizing practice is pratikriyasana (*prati,* meaning "against," and *kr,* meaning "action"). The objective of pratikriyasana is to integrate prior actions in a way that prepares students to move forward into the next asana, sequence, class, or later activity free of tension and as balanced and blissful as possible. This principle is often applied with its literal meaning of "opposite pose," or "counterpose." This can be problematic, especially when applied asana by asana. In this narrow conception of pratikriyasana, one would counterpose Salamba Sirsasana I with

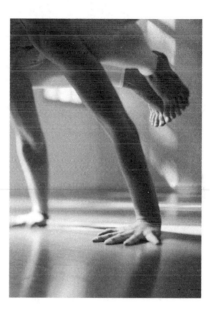

its opposite, Tadasana, likely causing many students to become dizzy and possibly fall. Similarly, this approach of pose-counterpose would place deep forward bends immediately after deep backbends, possibly straining the muscles and ligaments along the spine. What we want to do instead is to neutralize, integrate, refine, and deepen. There are many ways to sequence asanas for effective pratikriyasana. Generally, first offer students the simplest form of a neutralizing asana, and then offer variations or successively more complex asanas to reduce accumulated tension and restore overall stability and ease. Rather than approaching pratikriyasana asana by asana, it is better to take a broader view of entire practices, considering where in the small sequences that make up an entire class neutralizing and opposing asanas can help students to integrate their practice.

THE BASIC ARC STRUCTURE OF CLASSES

Most yoga classes should follow an arc-like structure. There are five elements of this structure:

1. Initiating the Yogic Process

In Chapters 5 and 6, we looked at several aspects of starting classes. Bringing the qualities discussed there together initiates the process of unification that is Hatha yoga: relieving the senses of their external distractions by focusing the mind on the breath and energetic awakening. Always create space for this initiation of the practice, setting the tone, intention, theme, and other overarching aspects of the class. The most fundamental part of this process is breath awareness, which extends as the unifying thread—sutra—throughout the entire class. By guiding students into a more focused inner awareness connecting body, breath, and mind, you help students to establish the fundamental foundation of their practice.

How students sit—usually in a cross-legged position or Virasana—or lie during this opening of the class should be determined by the larger class plan and your assessment of student ability. Regardless of students' body position, suggest props as described in Chapter Seven. Sitting in a cross-legged position is most stable and accessible for most students. In intermediate to advanced classes, Virasana is an excellent starting asana. In restorative, prenatal and postnatal, children's, and therapeutic classes, lying on the back offers a more calming introduction to the practice. Observe and try to get a feeling for the mood, energy level, and mental focus of the class. Let this observation and intuitive assessment inform how long to sit and what to include in this initial sitting part of the practice. This is an excellent time to go into further depth with pranayama techniques that move the class more immediately toward a sattvic state of being. Stimulating pranayamas like kapalabhati will help raise the energy level of a tamasic group of students; nadi shodhana will help calm a more rajasic group. Also consider a longer meditation practice at the beginning of class; if students seem to be focused in the initial sitting, consider staying with it for several more minutes, whether as silent or guided practice.

2. Warming the Body

Gradually warming the body increases flexibility, reduces the risk of injury, and generates tapas, inner fire, to burn away toxicity. In the traditional science of flexibility, warm-up is divided into two broad categories: passive, which uses an outside force such as a heated room or hot bath; and active, which is self-initiated (Alter 1996, 149–150). Studies show that passive warming, as found in Bikram and other "hot" yoga styles, is significantly more effective than active warming in increasing hip flexion (for example, releasing into Balasana).[2] However, increased temperature reduces the tensile strength of connective tissue, potentially leading to ruptures (Troels 1973, 1–126), due in part to the less conscious awareness of what is happening in the body with passive versus active sources of warming. While passive warming is helpful in preparing the body for intense activity, active warming has several added benefits in yoga: increased heart rate, which prepares the cardiovascular system for more intense activity; increased blood flow through active muscles; increased metabolic rate; increased speed of nerve impulses, which facilitates more subtle awareness of body movements; and increased reciprocal innervation in which opposing muscles work more efficiently.

There are two types of active warming: general and targeted. General warming consists of activities that bring overall warmth to the body. These warming activities should be done at the beginning of the practice, either immediately following or incorporated into the earlier initiation of the yogic process discussed above.

- The most basic warming activity is ujjayi pranayama, which can be safely practiced by all students (with caution to pregnant students not to overheat their body).

- Kapalabhati pranayama is a far more intensely warming activity that stimulates the cardiovascular system and generates warmth throughout the body. Doing this after a few minutes of ujjayi pranayama is excellent preparation for bringing more extensive movement into the body.

- The classic physical warm-up in Hatha yoga is through Surya Namaskara, the Sun Salutations discussed in detail in Chapter Seven. While warming the entire body, Surya Namaskara also offers targeted warming and awakening as it involves every asana family except twists: forward bends, backbends, standing poses, arm support, and inversion. The number, form, and duration of Sun Salutations should be varied depending on the level and overall plan of the class.

- Level 1 and level 1–2 classes can effectively warm up with undulating movement through the pelvis, spine, and shoulder girdles into alternating forms called Cat and Dog tilts.[3]

- Adho Mukha Svanasana is a great initial warming asana that gently opens the shoulders, chest, upper back, hips, and the backs of the legs, as well as the hands and feet. Introduce this asana with dynamic movements, including moving forward into Plank Pose and back to Down Dog several times, bicycling the legs, and extending one leg back and up.

Targeted warming mimics the more intense actions to come later in the practice. These activities can be incorporated into the general warming practice and/or the more in-depth anticipatory sets as described below. For example, if the class will focus on backbends, you can integrate deeper warming (and opening) of the pelvic girdle, spine, and shoulder girdle in Surya Namaskara by holding the related asanas longer, doing more of them, and offering variations within them (Anjaneyasana and Virabhadrasana I with Gomukhasana or Viparita Dandasana arms, Urdhva Mukha Svanasana, Adho Mukha Svanasana).

Sustained standing sequences, deep core work such as Navasana, Tolasana, and Lolasana, and core movements such as yogic bicycles and Jathara Parivartanasana are excellent ways to further warm the body. You can also effectively weave a variety of shoulder and pelvic girdle stretches into the standing asanas to further prepare for specific actions in arm balances, backbends, deeper hip opening, and forward bending, thereby offering students a clearer path to the peak pose while continuing to build general and targeted warmth. The dynamic sequence of Plank, Chaturanga, Up Dog, Down Dog is an excellent way to build further warmth, stoking the inner fire while integrating pratikriyasana amid standing asana sequences.

3. Pathway to the Peak

Each asana requires certain muscular actions, contracting or releasing in a way that supports stability, ease, and balanced integration within the asana. Rather than creating a random sequence of asanas, it is important to place asanas in relationship to each other in a way that makes each one more accessible. The basic principle is to move progressively from simple to complex actions that lead to the deepest and easiest possible exploration along the entire path to the peak asana, and eventually to Savasana. Like a child learning to crawl before walking and to walk before running, yoga students benefit from first learning basic asanas before attempting complex ones, playing the edge with each breath along the way. Similarly, within a single class, students benefit from moving from simple to complex poses, each pose and breath cultivating a deeper awareness of how the body can open and stabilize in

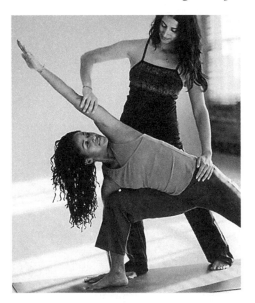

certain forms. This gradual learning process ideally involves anticipatory experiences along the path, giving students the opportunity to successively explore—with clear guidance from you—the various alignment forms, energetic actions, and other qualities of engagement they will be asked to apply at the peak. By introducing the constituent elements of the peak in simpler form, you will help students to grasp intellectually and to embody consciously the more complex combination of elements found in the peak asana. For example, when introducing Adho Mukha Svanasana in a level 1 class, start on all fours with the arms extended forward in the Puppy Dog variation; here you can guide students into the hand, arm, shoulder girdle, and spine elements of the full asana without the added challenge of opening through the legs and pelvis. Cat and Dog tilts can then be explored as a way to experience pelvic neutrality in relationship to the spine, while Uttanasana can be tapped for teaching about pada bandha, internal rotation of the thighs, and activation of the quadriceps. Now students will find it easier to integrate these elements in the complete asana.

Consider the following questions in breaking down the peak asana into its constituent elements, then apply that analysis to crafting a specific sequence leading to the peak asana (basic preparatory and integrative asanas are given in Appendix D):

- What needs to be open? What needs to be cooperative in allowing that specific opening?
- What needs to be stable? What are the sources of that stability?
- What are the alignment principles of the peak asana?
- What other asanas have the same or similar alignment principles?
- What are the energetic actions of the peak asana?
- What other asanas have the same or similar energetic actions?

Your ability as a teacher to accurately analyze all the asanas in a complete class sequence requires studying the functional anatomy and biomechanics of the asanas. The complexity of the human body, particularly when teaching a diverse student body, makes this a lifelong process of learning and professional development. Yet from the beginning you will express your own creativity in the particular ways you structure and guide each class.

4. Exploring the Peak

The peak asana or asanas are simultaneously the easiest and most challenging part of the class. They are the easiest if the pathway to the peak offers a clear and simple view of the peak, so there are few surprises and much joy in the feeling of exhilaration in exploring what might have otherwise been unattainable. They are the most challenging because they require the greatest strength, openness, or balance. Most arc classes place backbends at the peak. This is perfectly sensible but certainly not the only option. The peak asana can be from any asana family and chosen based on the type of class, students, theme, and other considerations. Once at the final approach to the peak, it is important to create space for students to completely relax, balance the breath, and tune in to their personal intention in the practice. This is a good time to remind students, as noted in Chapter Six, that the practice is not one of attainment of idealized physical postures, but a process of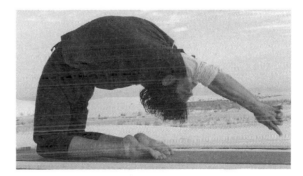

self-exploration, self-acceptance, and self-transformation. Reinforce the concept of playing the edge, encouraging students to abide by the core principle of sthira sukham asanam. Since there are invariably students with different abilities and interests in all classes, offer appropriate modifications and variations. As you develop your skill and comfort as a teacher, you will increasingly be at ease in offering multiple options to the class while remaining responsive to what is happening with each student in the class.

5. Integration

As noted earlier, pratikriyasana applies to individual asanas, sets of asanas, and to entire class sequences. With experience, students will learn to sustain a balance of effort and relaxation from the beginning of each practice until completely letting go in Savasana. Still, in an arc-structured class, it is important to offer more deeply integrating and restorative asanas following the peak of the practice. There are three stages in this integrative process:

1. Specific pratikriyasana for the peak asana: Teach simple asanas to neutralize any tension arising from the practice of peak asanas.

2. Deep and relatively more static relaxing asanas: After neutralizing tension, teach a series of asanas that calm the body and allow students to move into deeper release. Focus on seated forward bends and hip openers, calming inversions such as Salamba Sarvangasana, Halasana, or Viparita Karani, and calming pranayama and meditation.

3. Savasana: Conclude all classes with at least five minutes in Savasana, the ultimate restorative asana. Remind students that Savasana allows them fully to assimilate the effects of the practice while offering a feeling of completeness, openness, and wholeness.

SEQUENCING WITHIN AND ACROSS ASANA FAMILIES

This section identifies when certain families of asanas and individual asanas are best placed in an ordered sequence of asanas making up a class. Please refer to the asana descriptions provided in Chapter Seven for more detailed discussion about these families and asanas.

Surya Namaskara and Fluid Flow Sequences

- Excellent for initiating the conscious connection of breath to movement in the body.

- Excellent for warming the entire body and preparing for all other asanas.
- Classical Surya Namaskara offers a gentler sequence of asanas appropriate for beginning level and early-morning classes. Excellent dynamic awakening of the spiral erector muscles, hip flexors, and shoulder girdle.
- In beginning classes, consider preparing for Surya Namaskara with Cat/Dog, supine hamstring stretches, and basic shoulder openers.
- Surya Namaskara A more deeply warms and awakens the entire body.
- Surya Namaskara B is a strong sequence appropriate for more experienced students (levels 2 and 3) and offers a deeper exploration of the hip flexors.
- Dynamic movement of the arms and shoulders in the flowing phases plus shoulder flexion in Urdhva Hastasana, Utkatasana, Anjaneyasana, and Virabhadrasana I are excellent preparation for backbends and inversions.
- Stretching the hamstrings prepares the body for deeper forward bends and standing asanas.
- Creative flow sequences such as Dancing Warrior can be designed to focus on specific areas of opening in preparation for a specific peak asana.

Standing Asanas

- Following the warming effects of Surya Namaskara, standing asanas are the safest asana family for warming and opening the entire body in preparation for more complex asanas.
- Use Tadasana, Adho Mukha Svanasana, and the preparatory position of Prasarita Padottanasana as a starting stance for other standing asanas.
- Separately sequence externally rotated standing asanas (e.g., Utthita Trikonasana, Virabhadrasana II, Parsvakonasana) and internally rotated standing asanas (Utthita Parsvottanasana, Parivrtta Trikonasana, Virabhadrasana I, Virabhadrasana III).
- In creatively sequenced classes (i.e., not set classes such as Ashtanga Vinyasa), refrain from moving back and forth between internally and externally rotated-hip standing asanas.
- Aside from Anjaneyasana in Classical Surya Namaskara and Virabhadrasana I in Surya Namaskara B, generally teach externally rotated-hip standing asanas prior to internally rotated-hip standing asanas.
- When transitioning from Virabhadrasana I to Virabhadrasana II, carefully guide students to keep the knee of their front leg aligned directly above or

behind the heel (never beyond it toward the toes) and aligned toward the little-toe side of their foot. This is a difficult transition for students with tight hips, the typical result being the inward splaying of the front knee (and risk to the knee ligaments).

- Introduce twisting standing asanas in a sequence that allows the gradual rotational opening of the spine (e.g., Parivrtta Utkatasana, Parivrtta Ashta Chandrasana, and Parivrtta Trikonasana before Parivrtta Parsvakonasana).

- Twisting standing asanas are excellent preparation for backbends, especially those that open the hip flexors (Anjaneyasana, Ashta Chandrasana, Virabhadrasana I and II).

- Prepare for twisting standing asanas by first practicing twist-free standing asanas that open the hamstrings, hips, spine, and shoulder girdle.

- In classes with an arm balance focus, creatively integrate shoulder openers (e.g., Gomukhasana arms, Garudasana arms, Prasarita Padottanasana C arms, and reverse namaste) into the standing asana sequence.

- In intermediate and advanced classes, offer arm balances as transitions out of related standing asanas (e.g., Parsvakonasana to Eka Pada Koundinyasana to Chaturanga).

- In classes with a backbending focus, explore the standing asanas that open the iliopsoas (Virabhadrasana I, Anjaneyasana) and shoulder girdle as well as twisting standing asanas.

- In beginning-level classes, sequence standing balance asanas toward the early part of the standing pose sequence, when students' legs are less likely to be fatigued.

- Never transition from internal to external or external to internal rotation in standing balance asanas (such as Ardha Chandrasana to Parivrtta Ardha Chandrasana) because the extreme downward pressure of the femoral head can injure that bone or the hip joint.

- Except with very experienced and physically adept students, do not do more than two or three sustained asanas in a linked sequence on one side.

- Standing asanas relate mostly to the manipura, svadhisthana, and muladhara chakras. They are also energetically stimulating, helping to focus the mind in the early part of the practice.

The Abdominal Core

- Excellent preparation for arm balances.
- Warm the body.
- Never sequence deep backbends immediately following deep abdominal core strengthening practices. If core work is done prior to backbends, first neutralize the core.
- Effective for restabilizing support for the lumbar spine following backbends.
- See guidelines in Chapter Eleven on abdominal pressure during pregnancy.

Arm Balances

- Sequence following the warming effect of Surya Namaskara and standing asanas.
- Following core work to better feel the abdominal lift and stability that lends to levity.
- Interweave with standing asanas, applying the intelligence and opening developed in successive standing asanas to the foundation of each arm balance, as follows:
- Utthita Trikonasana, Prasarita Padottanasana, Utkatasana, and Malasana in preparation for Bakasana and Tittibhasana.
- Uttanasana, Malasana, and Prasarita Padottanasana in preparation for Bhujapidasana.
- Parivrtta Trikonasana and Parivrtta Utkatasana in preparation for Parsva Bakasana.
- Parivrtta Parsvakonasana and Ardha Chandrasana in preparation for Eka Pada Koundinyasana.
- With Sirsasana II vinyasa: Bakasana, Parsva Bakasana, Dwi Pada Koundinyasana, Eka Pada Koundinyasana, Urdhva Kukkutasana in either a broken or continuous series. This is a strong series that should be practiced with sensitivity to the neck and wrists.
- Adho Mukha Vrksasana and Pincha Mayurasana are excellent preparation for shoulder flexion backbends such as Urdhva Dhanurasana and Natarajasana.
- Always offer a variety of wrist therapy stretches following sustained arm balance sequences.

Backbends

- Backbends are naturally integrated into Surya Namaskara as part of the warming and initiating practice.
- Deep and sustained backbends should be sequenced at the peak of a practice when the body is warmest and most prepared for these relatively complex asanas.
- Allow time for neutralizing and calming asanas after backbends, especially in the evening.
- "Active" backbends that require the use of spinal erector muscles (i.e., contraction backbends such as Salabhasana) should be sequenced before backbends in which the arms, legs, or a wall leverage the asana.
- Specific sequences of standing asanas can open the quadriceps, hips, and groin, which contribute to greater hip extension.
- Use shoulder flexion openers (opening the latissimi dorsi, pec majors, and rhomboids) to prepare the shoulders for safe flexion in backbends: Adho Mukha Svanasana, Gomukhasana arms, Garudasana arms.
- Supta Baddha Konasana and Anjaneyasana, both of which have mild backbend elements, offer excellent opening of the hips and thighs in preparation for backbends. Both asanas can incorporate shoulder flexion stretches for greater ease in shoulder flexion backbends.
- Use asanas like Prasarita Padottanasana C to open the shoulders for shoulder extension in Setu Bandha Sarvangasana.
- Amid a backbending sequence, do not draw the knees into the chest or do other forward bending positioning of the spine until the sequence is complete —stay in a backbending or neutral spinal position until it is finished.
- Create the space to lie still in a neutral spine position before beginning counterasanas: Savasana, Ananda Balasana, and Supta Baddha Konasana.
- Use gentle twists for initial counterposing, then move into successively deeper forward bends, hip openers, and deeper twists. Give time for students to drop slowly and deeply into these counterposes, encouraging them to continue following their breath while enjoying the awakened consciousness that backbends naturally stimulate.
- Core integration movements following backbends will help to stabilize the lower back.

Twists

- Releasing the large outer layers of the trunk muscles with forward bends, backbends, and side bends allows easier and fuller rotation at the deep level of the small spinal muscles.

- As neutralizing asanas, twists are excellent for calming anxiety and relieving lethargy.

- Excellent preparation for backbends and excellent initial neutralizing (including calming) asanas following backbends.

- Twists will mildly simulate the nervous system and reawaken energy following deeply relaxing sequences of forward bends and hip openers.

- After an intensive twisting sequence, a slight passive backbend such as Setu Bandha Sarvangasana feels good and helps integrate the effects of the twists.

- Practice twists evenly on each side, promoting balance.

Forward Bends

- All forward bends should be approached with conscious attention to a deep sense of sukham, beginning with the warming movements of Surya Namaskara when folding into Uttanasana.

- Although forward bends can be practiced at any time, they are most safely approached when the body is warm and awakened through other asanas.

- As deeply calming asanas, forward bends are ideally sequenced as part of the *tha* practice following the practice's peak asana, especially backbends and arm balances.

- Following backbends or arm balances, lying in Supta Baddha Konasana will give an abdominal and pelvic release, and Supta Padangusthasana will give a hip opening and hamstring stretch that physically prepares your students for greater openness and ease in seated forward bends.

- Seated forward bends are well initiated through the intelligence of Dandasana.

- Hip openers like Balasana, Baddha Konasana, and Kurmasana are excellent preparation for seated forward bends.

- Following a deep forward bending practice, offer gentle backbends such as Setu Bandha Sarvangasana as a counterpose to reintegrate the hamstrings.

Hip Openers

- Surya Namaskara initiates the journey into the hips.
- Most standing asanas are hip openers that warm and open the lower body in effective preparation for deeper hip opening requirements in many arm balances, backbends, and deep seated hip openers and forward bends.
- In Adho Mukha Svanasana, offer the option of extending one leg up and passively stretching the hip in a "scorpion tail" positioning.
- Specific hip openers can be intelligently sequenced in preparation for many arm balances that require open, awakened, activated hip flexors or adductors.
- Hip openers can be creatively adapted to include shoulder openers in preparation for arm balances and backbends.
- In the *tha* part of the practice, sustained hip openers are deeply calming and allow deeper integration of strong sequences of standing asanas, arm balances, backbends, and inversions.
- Easily combined energetically with forward bends, side bends, and twists.

Inversions

- Generally sequenced as part of the finishing practice.
- Sirsasana I is an excellent warming asana when held for more than two minutes and as such can be done early in class. In doing so, Adho Mukha Svanasana and Uttanasana are excellent preparation.
- In a finishing sequence, do Salamba Sarvangasana after Sirsasana (not vice versa) to calm the body more deeply.
- Variations in Salamba Sarvangasana include alternately releasing one leg toward or to the floor overhead, Baddha Konasana legs, Upavista Konasana legs (including revolving through the torso and hips), and releasing the legs forward into Setu Bandha Sarvangasana.
- From Salamba Sarvangasana, offer the option of Urdhva Padmasana and Pindasana to students who are stable and can safely fold their legs into Padmasana. Otherwise offer Halasana and Karnapidasana. Explore the same variations in Urdhva Dandasana in Sirsasana.
- Counterpose Sirsasana with Balasana.
- Counterpose Salamba Sarvangasana with Matsyasana and Uttana Padasana.
- Inversions are excellent preparation for meditation.

PLANNING SPECIFIC CLASSES

Every yoga practice should flow like a good story, with a beginning, middle, and end that takes the class to a new and different awareness, experience, or ability (Ezraty 2006). As teachers, how we structure each class gives it a basic story line. The plot could be a theme or overarching intention, the principle characters the specific asanas, while the setting derives from the mood or vibe of the class. How we put this together to form a coherent class is "the art form of yoga practice" (Gannon and Life, 2002), which is inherently creative yet ideally based on an applied understanding of how asanas work in relationship to one another in the flow of the class.[4] Each class should be planned and taught with a storyline that takes students on a journey into themselves. The basic idea is to start from where students are and guide them to move consciously—"in a special way"—as they progress from simpler to more complex practices, gradually refining the body-mind and awakening to a clearer self-awareness, sense of balance, and harmony in life—a more sattvic state of being. This is the heart of vinyasa krama and parinamavada. This step-by-step process helps students to deepen their practice gradually, developing greater capacity for steadiness and ease amid the ever-increasing complexity and challenge of whatever they are doing, on or off the mat.

TABLE 10.1—**Basic Template for a Complete Arc Class**

1. Seated meditation, ujjayi pranayama	7. Arm balances (can be omitted)
2. Initial warming	8. Backbends (contraction then leveraged)
3. Surya Namaskara (Classical, A and B)	9. Twists
4. Standing asanas: externally rotated hips	10. Forward bends and hip openers
5. Standing asanas: internally rotated hips	11. Inversions
6. Abdominals (can be omitted)	12. Savasana

TABLE 10.2—**Basic Template Applied to Different Level Flow Classes**

	LEVEL 1: 75 MINUTES	LEVEL 2: 90 MINUTES	LEVEL 3: 108 MINUTES
Seated meditation and ujjayi pranayama	2–3 minutes; Introduce ujjayi	3–5 minutes; Refine ujjayi	3–5 minutes; Expand ujjayi
Initial warming	No kapalabhati; Cat/Dog tilts; Extended Cat/Dog; Puppy Dog; Balasana	Introduce kapalabhati, 1–3 rounds of 45 seconds; Cat/Dog tilts; Adho Mukha Svanasana 1–2 minutes	Kapalabhati, 1–3 rounds of 1–2 minutes; Adho Mukha Svanasana 2–3 minutes
Surya Namaskara	3 Classical; 1–3 A's 1–3 B's	1–3 Classical; 2–3 A's 2–3 B's	3–5 A's 3–5 B's
Standing-external	From Prasarita stance: Virabhadrasana II; Utthita Parsvakonasana; Utthita Trikonasana; From Tadasana: Vrksasana Hold each asana 5–8 breaths before changing sides.	From Prasarita stance or in fluid transition from Virabhadrasana I: Virabhadrasana II to Utthita Parsvakonasana on each side, then transition to: Tadasana to Vrksasana or Utthita Hasta Padangusthasana Utthita Trikonasana to Ardha Chandrasana.	From Virabhadrasana I: Virabhadrasana II to Utthita Parsvakonasana; optional transition to Chaturanga through Eka Pada Koundinyasana I; Utthita Trikonasana; Ardha Chandrasana. Hold each 1–2 minutes; offer variations.
Standing-internal	Prasarita Padottanasana A; Parsvottanasana; Ashta Chandrasana Hold each 5–8 breaths.	Prasarita Padottanasana A and C; Parsvottanasana; Parivrtta Trikonasana. From Down Dog: Ashta Chandrasana to Parivrtta Parsvakonasana Prep Pose Hold each 5–8 breaths.	Prasarita Padottanasana A (with Bakasana option), then variation C; Parsvottanasana; Parivrtta Trikonasana to Parivrtta Ardha Chandrasana on each side. From Down Dog: Ashta Chandrasana to Virabhadrasana III to Parivrtta Hasta Padangusthasana to Virabhadrasana III to Adho Mukha Vrksasana to Chaturanga.

	LEVEL 1: 75 MINUTES	LEVEL 2: 90 MINUTES	LEVEL 3: 108 MINUTES
Standing-internal *continued*			From Down Dog: Virabhadrasana I to Parivrtta Parsvakonasana; Optional transition to Chaturanga through Eka Pada Koundinyasana II.
Abdominals	Paripurna Navasana Prep 3 times; Yogic bicycles 1 minute	Paripurna Navasana to Ardha Navasana 2–3 times; Yogic bicycles 1–2 minutes; Jathara Parivartanasana 3–5 times; leg lifts.	Paripurna Navasana to Ardha Navasana to Tolasana 3–5 times; Tolasana to Lolasana 3–5 times, holding 5–10 breaths; Yogic bicycles 2–3 minutes; Jathara Parivartanasana 5–10 times; kapalabhati pranayama concluding with bahya kumbhaka and uddiyana bandha.
Arm balances	Handstand Prep 1 at wall; Forearm Balance Prep 2 at wall. Wrist/shoulder stretches.	Bakasana; Bhujapidasana; Handstand Prep 1 and 2 at wall; optional Handstand at wall. Forearm Balance Prep 1 and 2 at wall; optional Forearm Balance at wall. Wrist/shoulder stretches.	Handstand, Forearm Balance; Sirsasana II Arm Balance Vinyasa (options: Bakasana, Tittibhasana; Parsva Bakasana, Eka Pada Koundinyasana, Urdhva Kukkutasana). Astavakrasana, Galavasana, Uttana Prasithasana.
Backbends	Salabhasana A 3 times; Setu Bandha Sarvangasana 1–3 times.	Prep: Anjaneyasana with shoulder stretches. Salabhasana A 1–3 times; Salabhasana C Prep 1–3 times; Setu Bandha Sarvangasana 1–3 times;	Prep: Anjaneyasana, Virasana, and shoulder stretches. Salabhasana A 5 breaths to Chaturanga vinyasa to Salabhasana B 5 breaths to Chaturanga vinyasa

	LEVEL 1: 75 MINUTES	LEVEL 2: 90 MINUTES	LEVEL 3: 108 MINUTES
Backbends *continued*		or Dhanurasana 1–3 times Optional Urdhva Dhanurasana 1–3 times.	to Salabhasana C 5 breaths to Chaturanga vinyasa to Dhanurasana 1–3 times to Chaturanga vinyasa to Urdhva Dhanurasana 1–3 times to Viparita Dandasana 1–3 times. Optional Eka Pada in Urdhva Dhanurasana and Viparita Dandasana; optional drop–backs.
Twists	Jathara Parivartanasana with both knees bent; Bharadvajrasana I; Marichyasana C Prep. Hold each 1–2 minutes.	Jathara Parivartanasana; Ardha Matsyendrasana Prep; Marichyasana C; Swastikasana. Hold each 1–2 minutes.	Jathara Parivartanasana; Ardha Matsyendrasana; Marichyasana C; Bharadvajrasana II; Marichyasana D; Swastikasana. Hold each 1–2 minutes.
Forward bends and hip openers	Dandasana; Paschimottanasana; Baddha Konasana; Upavista Konasana.	Dandasana; Paschimottanasana; Janu Sirsasana A; Parivrtta Janu Sirsasana; Baddha Konasana; Upavista Konasana.	Dandasana; Paschimottanasana; Janu Sirsasana A; Baddha Konasana; Tiriang Mukha Eka Pada Paschimottanasana; Krounchasana; Parighasana; Upavista Konasana; Kurmasana.
Inversions	Viparita Karani; Salamba Sarvangasana Prep	Viparita Karani, or Sirsasana I; Balasana; Halasana; Salamba Sarvangasana; Karnapidasana; Uttana Padasana.	Sirsasana I (or I–6); Halasana, Salamba Sarvangasana; Urdhva Padmasana; Matsyasana; Uttana Padasana. Add optional Tolasana with kapalabhati for 1 minute, then vinyasa.
Savasana	5 minutes or longer.	5 minutes or longer.	5 minutes or longer.
Meditation	Up to a few minutes.	Several minutes.	As long as possible.

TABLE 10.3—**Level 1—Theme: Basic Class**

1. Meditation, set intention, aum	14. Utthita Trikonasana (5–8 breaths)
2. Sukhasana, ujjayi pranayama	15. Prasarita Padottanasana C (5–8 breaths)
3. Cat/Dog tilts (5 times)	
4. Balasana—Salabhasana B—Balasana (5 times)	16. Parivrtta Prasarita Padottanasana (5 breaths)
5. Puppy Dog (10 breaths)	17. Setu Bandha Sarvangasana (3 times, 5–8 breaths)
6. Adho Mukha Svanasana (10 breaths)	
7. Tadasana (1 minute; teach pada bandha)	18. Supta Parivartanasana (1 minute each side)
	19. Supta Padangusthasana (1 minute each side)
8. Classical Surya Namaskara (3 times)	20. Baddha Konasana (2 minutes)
9. Surya Namaskara A (1–3 times)	21. Upavista Konasana (2 minutes)
10. Surya Namaskara (1–3 times)	22. Paschimottanasana (1 minute)
11. Vrksasana (1 minute each side)	23. Viparita Karani (2 minutes)
12. Virabhadrasana II (5–8 breaths)	24. Savasana (5–8 minutes)
13. Utthita Parsvakonasana Prep (5–8 breaths)	

TABLE 10.4—**Level 2—Theme: Heart Opening (Backbend Peak)**

1. Meditation (in Virasana), set intention, *om*	19. Anahatasana (1 minute)
2. Kapalabhati pranayama (2 minutes)	20. Ardha Matsyendrasana (1 minute each side)
3. Adho Mukha Svanasana (2 minutes)	21. Setu Bandha Sarvangasana (1–3 times, 5 breaths each)
4. Classical Surya Namaskara (Anjaneyasana 5 breaths)	22. Urdhva Dhanurasana (1–3 times, 5 breaths each)
5. Surya Namaskara A (3 times)	23. (Offer Dhanurasana as an alternative to Urdhva Dhanurasana)
6. Surya Namaskara B (3 times, Virabhadrasana I 10 breaths on last round)	24. Supta Baddha Konasana (1 minute)
7. Virabhadrasana II (5–10 breaths)	25. Supta Parivartanasana (1 minute each side)
8. Utthita Parsvakonasana (5–10 breaths)	26. Paschimottanasana (2 minutes)
9. Utthita Trikonasana (5–10 breaths)	27. Upavista Konasana (2 minutes)
10. Prasarita Padottanasana A and C (5 breaths each)	28. Parivrtta Janu Sirsasana (1 minute each side)
11. Parsvottanasana (5 breaths)	29. Baddha Konasana (2 minutes)
12. Parivrtta Trikonasana (5 breaths)	30. Gomukhasana (1 minute each side)
13. Garudasana (1 minute each side)	31. Halasana (1 minute)
14. Surya Namaskara A	32. Salamba Sarvangasana (2–3 minutes)
15. Parivrtta Parsvakonasana Prep (5–10 breaths)	33. Karnapidasana (1 minute)
16. Adho Mukha Svanasana (1 minute)	34. Uttana Padasana (5 breaths)
17. Virasana (1 minute)	35. Savasana (5–8 minutes)
18. Supta Virasana (2 minutes)	36. Meditation

TABLE 10.5—Level 3—Theme: Grounded Levity through Integrated Standing Asanas and Arm Balances

1. Meditation, set intention, om	26. Tadasana—wrist therapy, samasthihi, revisit intention
2. Kapalabhati pranayama (2–3 minutes)	27. Utkatasana in transition to:
3. Adho Mukha Svanasana (2–3 minutes)	28. Galavasana (5 breaths, vinyasa)
4. Surya Namaskara A (3–5 times)	29. Tadasana in transition to:
5. Surya Namaskara B (3–5 times)	30. Parivrtta Garudasana Prep in transition to:
6. Virabhadrasana I with Garudasana Arms (vinyasa)	31. Uttana Prasithasana (5 breaths) vinyasa
7. Tolasana/Lolasana (10 breaths each)	32. Dandasana (10 breaths)
8. Malasana (5 breaths) to:	33. Eka Pada Salamba Sirsasana (5 breaths) transition to:
9. Bakasana (5 breaths, float to Chaturanga, vinyasa)	34. Astavakrasana (5 breaths) transition to:
10. Adho Mukha Svanasana (1 minute)	35. Eka Pada Koundinyasana A, (5 breaths), vinyasa
11. Parsva Utkatasana (5 breaths)	36. Shishulasana
12. Parsva Bakasana (5 breaths, float to vinyasa)	37. Pincha Mayurasana (1 minute)
13. Utthita Trikonasana (1 minute) to:	38. Balasana
14. Ardha Chandrasana (1 minute)	39. Wrist Therapy
15. Virabhadrasana II (1 minute)	40. Prone Shoulder Cross Pose
16. Utthita Parsvakonasana (1 minute)	41. Salabhasana C Prep (hands clasped, shoulder stretch)
17. Eka Pada Koundinyasana A (5 breaths, vinyasa)	42. Dhanurasana (3 times, 5–10 breaths)
18. Prasarita Padottanasana A	43. Balasana (1 minute) (5 breaths) to:
19. Bhujapidasana (5–10 breaths) to:	44. Bharadvajrasana II (1 minute)
20. Tittibhasana (5–10 breaths) to Bakasana to vinyasa	45. Paschimottanasana (2 minutes)
21. Parsvottanasana (5 breaths)	46. Halasana (1 minute)
22. Parivrtta Trikonasana (5 breaths), vinyasa	47. Salamba Sarvangasana Cycle (5 minutes)
23. Ashta Chandrasana with Gomukhasana Arms (1 minute)	48. Matsyasana (10 breaths)
24. Parivrtta Parsvakonasana (5 breaths) transition to:	49. Uttana Padasana (5 breaths)
25. Eka Pada Koundinyasana B	50. Savasana (5–8 minutes) (5 breaths, vinyasa)

SEQUENCING FOR THE MENSTRUAL CYCLE

Just as each student comes to the practice in a unique way, women experience their menstrual cycle in different ways. For some women, menstruation is simple and easy, while for others it can be painful and distressing. Most of the literature on yoga for women advises a highly modified practice emphasizing basic restorative poses and no inversions.[5] Yet many active yoga students maintain their regular practice while menstruating—including inversions—with no signs of ill effects. (The question of whether or not to invert when menstruating is a topic of considerable debate. There is no medical evidence supporting the widely held assumption that inversions cause retrograde menstruation. Even B. K. S. Iyengar recommends inversions for some menstrual conditions.) The best guide to practice when menstruating is each student's personal intuition. The following sequence is a relaxing practice to reduce pressure in the uterus and abdomen:

TABLE 10.6—**Sequence to Help Relieve Menstrual Discomfort**

1. Balasana (2–3 minutes, knees wide apart)	8. Paschimottanasana (3–5 minutes)
2. Virasana (2–3 minutes)	9. Supta Parivartanasana (2–3 minutes each side)
3. Supta Virasana (5–7 minutes, bolstered)	10. Setu Bandha Sarvangasana (3–5 minutes, bolstered)
4. Supta Baddha Konasana (5–7 minutes, bolstered)	11. Balasana (2–3 minutes, knees wide apart)
5. Janu Sirsasana A (2–3 minutes each side)	12. Viparita Karani (5 minutes, bolstered)
6. Parivrtta Janu Sirsasana (2 minutes each side)	13. Savasana (5–10 minutes)
7. Tiriang Mukha Eka Pada Paschimottanasana (2 minutes each side)	14. Meditation

THE CHAKRA MODEL OF SEQUENCING

In Chapter Three we looked at the chakra model of subtle energy. Taken as a whole, the chakra model offers an approach to integration in the entire being, unifying the physical, emotional, and spiritual. This model provides a useful approach to sequencing asanas while exploring deeper qualities of self-awareness that embody a more multidimensional self-understanding. Whether applied as the model for a complete class or to stimulate specific areas of energetic balance or self-awareness, a chakra model class has a variety of creative possibilities.[6] Use this table to design specific chakra sequences.

TABLE 10.7—**Sequencing around Chakras**

CHAKRA	EXPLORATION	ACTIONS
Muladhara	Physical security, grounding, basic self-identity, personal stability	Pada bandha, Tadasana, strong standing asanas, balancing asanas
Svadhisthana	Desire, impulse, creativity, pelvic balance	Surya Namaskara, Dancing Warrior, mula bandha
Manipura	Clarity of purpose, self-manifestation	Core strength and suppleness, uddiyana bandha
Anahata	Harmony, love, spiritual clarity	Heart opening backbends, heart-centered breathing
Vishuddha	Personal truth, spiritual wisdom, communication	Jalandhara bandha, Pursvottanasana, Matsyasana
Ajna	Levity, inner peace, clear mind	Meditation, mindfulness in flow, nadi shodhana pranayama
Sahasrara	Pure consciousness	Meditation, Savasana

POPULAR HATHA YOGA SEQUENCES

As a learning exercise, try applying the basic sequencing principles to the following standard sequences found in the major styles of Hatha yoga. What is the vinyasa krama? Do the asanas seem to be ordered in a way that eases students from asana to asana? What do you think are the contrasting energetic effects of each sequence? What risks do you think are heightened or reduced by the order of asanas? What is the appropriate audience?

Anusara—General Template

This arc-structured template is applied by starting at the top of the list and moving down sequentially, with specific asanas chosen to support the class theme, level, and intention (Friend 2006, 69). The Anusara system offers teachers an extensive list of asanas categorized by class level of asana family from which to choose in designing classes.

TABLE 10.8 — **Anusara Sequence**

1. Sitting and centering: meditation and/or breathing	9. Abdominals
2. Warm-up exercises	10. Supta Virasana
3. Adho Mukha Svanasana	11. Inversions/Salamba Sirsasana and variations
4. Surya Namaskara	12. Backbends
5. Adho Mukha Vrksasana and/or Pincha Mayurasana	13. Sarvangasana
6. Standing asanas	14. Twists and forward bends
7. Basic hip openers	15. Meditation
8. Hand-balancing	16. Savasana

Ashtanga Vinyasa—Primary Series

The Ashtanga Vinyasa sequences are sometimes described as a "sandwich" (Swenson 1999), referring to the three phases found in each series: (1) the standing sequence, (2) the unique sequence of each of the six series, and (3) the finishing sequence. The first and third phases are generally practiced in all six series, with the specific series distinguished by the middle sequence. Most of the asanas are held for five breaths. There are specific transitions prescribed between each asana, most often involving Tolasana–Lolasana–Chaturanga–Up Dog–Down Dog–Dandasana as a fluid movement.

TABLE 10.9—**Ashtanga Vinyasa Sequence**

1. Tadasana/Samasthiti	25. Kurmasana
2. Surya Namaskara A (5 times)	26. Supta Kurmasana
3. Surya Namaskara B (5 times)	27. Garbha Pindasana
4. Padangusthasana	28. Kukkutasana
5. Padahasthasana	29. Baddha Konasana A, B
6. Utthita Trikonasana (from Prasarita stance)	30. Upavista Konasana A, B
7. Parivrtta Trikonasana	31. Supta Konasana
8. Utthita Parsvakonasana	32. Supta Padangusthasana A, B, C
9. Parivrtta Parsvakonasana	33. Ubhaya Padangusthasana
10. Prasarita Padottanasana A, B, C, D	34. Urdhva Mukha Paschimottanasana
11. Parsvottanasana	35. Setu Bandhasana
12. Utthita Hasta Padangusthasana A, B, C, D	36. Urdhva Dhanurasana
13. Ardha Baddha Padmottanasana	37. Paschimottanasana
14. Utkatasana (from vinyasa)	38. Salamba Sarvangasana
15. Virabhadrasana I	39. Halasana
16. Virabhadrasana II	40. Karnapidasana
17. Dandasana	41. Urdhva Padmasana
18. Paschimottanasana A/B	42. Pindasana
19. Pursvottanasana	43. Matsyasana
20. Ardha Baddha Padma Paschimottanasana	44. Uttana Padasana
21. Tiriang Mukha Eka Pada Paschimottanasana	45. Salamba Sirsasana I
22. Janu Sirsasana A, B, C	46. Baddha Padmasana
23. Marichyasana A, B, C, D	47. Padmasana
24. Paripurna Navasana	48. Tolasana
25. Bhujapidasana	49. Savasana

Bikram Sequence

The Bikram forms of asanas differ from the forms bearing the same name in other styles of Hatha yoga. For clarification, see Choudhury (2000). Each asana is done twice.

TABLE 10.10—**Bikram Sequence**

1. Pranayama series	14. Pavanamuktasana
2. Ardha Chandrasana with Padahasthasana	15. Sit up
3. Utkatasana	16. Bhujangasana
4. Garudasana	17. Salabhasana
5. Dandayamana—Janu Sirsasana	18. Poorna—Salabhasana
6. Dandayamana—Dhanurasana	19. Dhanurasana
7. Tuladandasana (Balancing Stick Pose)	20. Supta—Vajrasana
8. Dandayamana—Bibhaktapada—Paschimottanasana	21. Ardha—Kurmasana
9. Trikonasana (Triangle Pose)	22. Ustrasana
10. Dandayamana—Bibhaktapada—Janu Sirsasana	23. Sasangasana
11. Tadasana	24. Janu Sirsasana with Paschimottanasana
12. Padangusthasana	25. Ardha—Matsyendrasana
13. Savasana	26. Kapalabhati pranayama

Iyengar Sequence

This sequence is drawn from the first third of Iyengar's basic twenty-week course (B. K. S. Iyengar 2001, 390), offering a representative sample of how asanas might be ordered in a level 1 or 2 Iyengar class. Most of the asanas are held for one to two minutes, with the final form of some asanas held as long as possible. Props are utilized in most of these asanas.

TABLE 10.11—**Iyengar Sequence**

1. Tadasana (with various arm positions)	14. Upavista Konasana
2. Utthita Trikonasana	15. Adho Mukha Virasana
3. Utthita Parsvakonasana	16. Adho Mukha Swastikasana
4. Virabhadrasana I	17. Paschimottanasana
5. Virabhadrasana II	18. Janu Sirsasana
6. Adho Mukha Svanasana	19. Paschimottanasana
7. Prasarita Padottanasana	20. Bharadvajrasana
8. Uttanasana	21. Marichyasana C
9. Dandasana	22. Parsva Virasana
10. Virasana	23. Supta Baddha Konasana
11. Janu Sirsasana (upward facing— i.e., without folding forward)	24. Supta Padangusthasana
12. Swastikasana	25. Setu Bandha Sarvangasana
13. Baddha Konasana	26. Savasana

Power Yoga Sequence

Like Vinyasa Flow–style yoga, there are as many variations of Power yoga sequences as there are Power yoga teachers. The following sequence is from Baron Baptiste (2000, 73–159).

TABLE 10.12—**Power Yoga Sequence**

1. Balasana	24. Ustrasana
2. Adho Mukha Svanasana	25. Setu Bandha Sarvangasana
3. Uttanasana	26. Urdhva Dhanurasana
4. Sun Salutation A (3–5 repetitions)	27. Supta Baddha Konasana
5. Sun Salutation B	28. Leg lifts
6. Anjaneyasana	29. Supta Baddha Konasana
7. Parivrtta Ashta Chandrasana	30. Yogic bicycles
8. Utthita Parsvakonasana	31. Supta Baddha Konasana
9. Vasisthasana	32. Navasana
10. Parivrtta Utkatasana	33. Supta Baddha Konasana
11. Padahasthasana	34. Salamba Sarvangasana
12. Bakasana	35. Halasana
13. Garudasana	36. Karnapidasana
14. Utthita Hasta Padangusthasana A, B	37. Adho Mukha Eka Pada Raj Kapotasana
15. Virabhadrasana III	38. Dwi Pada Raj Kapotasana
16. Natarajasana	39. Bhekasana
17. Vrksasana	40. Janu Sirsasana A
18. Trikonasana	41. Paschimottanasana
19. Parivrtta Trikonasana	42. Pursvottanasana
20. Prasarita Padottanasana A	43. Matsyasana
21. Parsvottanasana	44. Ananda Balasana
22. Salabhasana	45. Supta Parivartanasana
23. Dhanurasana	46. Savasana

Restorative Yoga

In restorative and deeply relaxing classes, asanas are usually held for five to ten minutes. The following classic restorative sequence is from Judith Lasater (1995, 33–53).

TABLE 10.13—**Restorative Yoga Sequence**

1. Simple Supported Backbends (bolster under heart center, neck supported, knees bent)

2. Supported Supta Baddha Konasana

3. Mountain Brook Pose (same as the first pose, except legs are extended and knees bolstered)

4. Supported Bridge (legs extended, entire body elevated on level bolster, with shoulders and head draped off and neck supported)

5. Reclining Twist (laying on side with ample bolsters to hug and give support)

6. Supported Upavista Konasana (high stack of pillows to fold forward onto)

7. Supported Cross-Legs Pose (sitting bones elevated on bolster, arm crossed onto a chair seat)

8. Savasana (lower legs elevated on bolsters, neck and head supported)

Sivananda—the Basic Sequence

The basic Sivananda sequence offers a comprehensive routine in which each asana is said to augment or counterbalance the one before. Each series (read: family) of asanas "is followed by one that provides the opposite stretch" (Sivananda Yoga Center 1983, 30–31).

TABLE 10.14—**Sivananda Sequence**

1. Savasana (2–3 minutes)	10. Matsyasana
2. Seated position—pranayama	11. Paschimottanasana
3. Neck, shoulder, and eye exercises	12. Bhujangasana
4. Classical Surya Namaskara (using Cobra in place of Locust)	13. Salabhasana
5. Leg raises	14. Dhanurasana
6. Salamba Sirsasana I	15. Ardha Matsyendrasana
7. Salamba Sarvangasana	16. Bakasana
8. Halasana	17. Utthita Trikonasana
9. Setu Bandha Sarvangasana	18. Savasana

CREATING YOUR CLASSES

While there are effective and ineffective ways to sequence asanas, there is not a singularly correct way to sequence asanas in creating complete classes. Rather, sequencing can tap into all the aspects of yoga along with your intention and creativity as a teacher to offer students a variety of experiences in the practice. Using the resources provided throughout this book, play around with designing sequences for different class levels, physical benefits, energetic effects, seasons, and other qualities that you find interesting and inspiring. Practice them on your own, share them with your fellow teachers, and refine them as you teach them in classes and observe how students respond. Continuously coming back to your own creative sensibilities, have fun with this while working to offer students the best classes you can for their needs and interests.

CHAPTER ELEVEN

SPECIALIZED TEACHING

It's not about how far you go,
but how you go.

Students come to yoga classes with a variety of physical, mental, and emotional conditions that should be given special attention and support by teachers. While making clear the distinction between yoga teacher and licensed medical or mental health professional, as teachers we are responsible for creating a safe and supportive environment for all students, including those with injuries, depression, age-related needs, and conditions such as pregnancy and menopause. Here we will look at practical approaches to working with students whose bodies, hearts, and minds (which are not really separate) indicate the need for special accommodation in classes or in one-on-one sessions. Bringing a specifically yogic perspective to this aspect of teaching starts with looking at and appreciating every student as the whole person he or she is, offering tools and techniques for using various challenging conditions to heal, feel better, and move into a deeper quality of integration.

NEW TO YOGA

People first come to yoga with a variety of conditions and motivations. Most new yoga students have previously participated in group exercise classes and may have high body intelligence. But very few have experienced a physical practice in which they are invited to move and explore in the specific ways asked of them in yoga: consciously connecting breath-body-mind amid increasingly complex and challenging positioning of the body. With most new students starting off in regularly scheduled classes rather than introductory workshops, they find themselves diving into a flowing stream surrounded by unfamiliar words, techniques, and challenges.

Yoga teacher Max Strom (1995) recalls being "completely confused" and feeling "anger and despair" when taking his first yoga class in 1991. Add a spiritual dimension—even chanting *aum*—and many new students put up such defenses that complicate their experience.

Teaching new students is an opportunity to deepen our own practice of "beginner's mind" and to encourage it among others in class. In this mind-set, we open ourselves to whatever we are doing as if it is the first time. Although the body-mind knows from prior experience where it is going and what to expect, the idea is to soften that preconditioned mind-set in order to feel what is happening more freshly and free of preconceptions. When we do this as teachers, it allows us to have a more

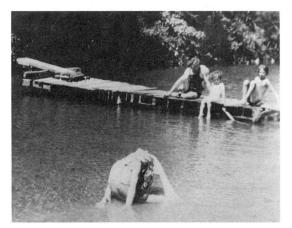

The author's mother, Royal Sarah Stephens, age 8, 1931

empathetic understanding of new students' experiences, thereby making it easier to give them the guidance and support it takes for them to do the most they can. This is actually far more challenging than teaching highly complex asanas to advanced students, so, inevitably, teaching new students deepens your skill as a teacher.

All new students deserve an individualized welcome from their teacher. Along with asking about prior experience, injuries, and intentions, this initial contact is essential in helping new students feel more comfortable in class. It is important to tell them explicitly that in yoga we are interested in *how* we go, not how *far* we go; that it is a process of consciously connecting breath-body-mind while exploring the development of strength, flexibility, and balance as part of a long-term sustainable practice of integration. In yoga, perhaps more than in any other physical activity or discipline, change comes slowly, often over years, as sustained practice undoes habits cultivated over a lifetime. This change, moreover, is rarely linear. Emphasize the importance of steadiness and ease, show them Balasana, and encourage them to rest in that or any other asana whenever they feel the need. Whether or not they think they need props, ask them to have a block, strap, two blankets, or a bolster next to their mat since is it likely they will benefit from using some or all of them during class. If possible, group new students close to one another so you can more easily give demonstrations and more specific guidance to them while remaining attentive to the larger class. Also try to position them behind more experienced students whom you can count on to stay with the basic asanas (rather than behind a show-off student whose fancy variations will be confusing and possibly lead the new student beyond a safe practice).

Use the presence of new students in class to review the basics of ujjayi pranayama and the foundational elements of each asana; all experienced students will benefit from the review, including those students whose patience this might test. During Surya Namaskara, position yourself immediately next to new students to demonstrate more closely and explain each asana and transition. While the rest of the class is holding Adho Mukha 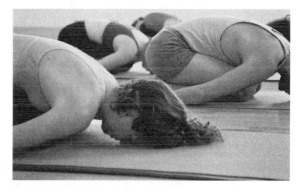 Svanasana, bring new students back into Surya Namaskara asanas in which they seemed confused or especially challenged, giving them more elaborate guidance and modification options.

Try to talk with new students after class to find out how they felt during class. This is a good time to give them information about resources that are helpful to new students, including basic etiquette guidelines that should be shared with all students (discussed in Chapter Five).

WORKING WITH INJURIES[1]

Many students come to yoga to heal injuries or chronic pain sustained off the mat. Many others are injured or experience pain while doing yoga, often as a result of nonyoga activities but just as often due to inappropriate sequencing of asanas, forceful adjustments, or pushing too hard in their practice. Knowing the source of the injury or painful sensation, including patterns of activity that may have created the underlying conditions, can provide insights about working with students in their healing process. Is the problem the result of imbalances in strength, flexibility, and alignment in an otherwise healthy body and brought on by excessive use, disuse, or abuse? Or is it a pathological condition such as arthritis or scoliosis? Are the student's age, weight, or lifestyle likely factors? How severe is the condition? When is it experienced? Are there other possibly complicating conditions such as pregnancy, heart problems, asthma, or hypertension?

In discussing the origin, nature, and manifestations of injuries with students, it is important to remind them that you are a yoga teacher, not a doctor or physical therapist (again, unless you are, in which case you need to adhere to that profession's ethics). You can then proceed to offer three forms of support: (1) a safe setting in which they can explore within their own bodies how to move and hold in ways that facilitate the natural healing process; (2) modifications of asanas and use of props in those asanas that help reduce further injury; and (3) asanas that enhance healing. The primary focus here is on how to support students with asanas that are aligned with the physical therapy protocols for certain injuries. We will address the most common injuries seen in yoga classes: ankle sprains, knee strains (and repairs), hamstring strains, lower-back pain, scoliosis (a disease, not an injury), wrist tendinitis and carpal tunnel syndrome, shoulder impingement, and rotator cuff problems. All the suggestions here should be offered to students with the clearly stated reminder that they are provided by a yoga teacher, not a licensed medical professional.

In Chapter Six we discussed how painful sensation can be tapped as a friend and teacher, its unique language announcing and guarding the edge of our safe limits in the asana practice. Rather than fighting this expression of the body's intelligence, it is important for students to learn to cooperate with it, exploring pain's messages for direction on where and how to create safe space and movement. Focused on cultivating healing, wholeness, balance, and radiant well-being, your role as a teacher working with injured students and those with chronic pain is to help them create a healing resonance, doing only what feels good in the practice, consciously moving energy in the sensitive areas, going slowly enough to listen, feel, adapt, and enjoy the process.

Ankle Sprains

Ankle sprains occur when the foot twists, turns, or rolls beyond its normal range of motion, causing the ankle ligaments to stretch beyond their normal length and, in extreme cases, tear. Because the ligaments are overstretched, reinjury is often a chronic problem. More than ninety percent are inversion sprains in which the ankle turns excessively out. A small percentage are "high" sprains in which the syndesmosis ligaments that join the tibia and fibula are strained, requiring screws and a cast for healing. The vast preponderance of ankle sprains can be successfully treated using the RICE method: rest, ice, compression, and elevation. Depending on the severity of the sprain, healing should proceed in five phases:

1. Using the RICE method, first decrease pain and swelling while protecting the ankle ligaments from further strain. Rest is essential. A healing ligament also requires a light amount of stress to heal properly, although overdoing it early in the rehabilitation process can inhibit healing. Isometric exercises can be performed early on as long as they are not painful. It is important to avoid

both inversion and eversion of the ankle. Several asanas are contraindicated: Virabhadrasana and Utthita Trikonasana positioning of the back foot, and Baddha Konasana (unless the knees reach the floor and there is no inversion of the ankle joint).

2. When the swelling stops and pain diminishes, the ligaments are at minimal risk of being re-strained from mild stress. Still use caution in asanas where the feet are bearing weight and the injured ankle is in inversion. This is the time to begin improving mobility and flexibility, using manual joint manipulation for plantar flexion/dorsiflexion only in Dandasana, Sirsasana, and other non-weight-bearing asanas. Use the dorsiflexion to bring more stretching to the Achilles tendon, and ice afterward.

3. After doing the initial mobility/flexibility movements for however long it takes to move the ankle without pain, begin initial strengthening, using a strap around the feet in Dandasana to create isometric resistance. Focus on strengthening the peroneus muscles by mild eversion resistance exercises using the strap as described with Dandasana. Standing on both feet, do toe raises to awaken pada bandha, stimulating the awakening and strengthening of the peroneus longus and tibialis posterior muscles. Do low heel raises to stimulate the slow-twitch fibers in the gastrocnemius and soleus muscles. Continue icing after exercising.

4. Only with comfort and ease, begin to reestablish proprioception (neuromuscular control and coordination) using Vrksasana and other standing balance asanas; consider using a wall to support balance and help prevent reinjury. Also do daily "ankle ABCs," sitting on a chair and writing the entire alphabet on the floor with the big toe.

5. Several asanas will effectively develop further strength and flexibility: Ashta Chandrasana to stretch the gastrocnemius, toes on a block in Tadasana to stretch the soleus, Balasana to stretch the top of the leg, Anjaneyasana to stretch the Achilles tendon, tiptoe movements in Tadasana to strengthen the gastrocnemius and soleus, Virasana to stretch the top of the ankle and thighs, Baddha Konasana to gently work into inversion (or eversion if the opposite side sprained). Gradually apply more weight to the foot when placed in back when doing Utthita Trikonasana and Virabhadrasana I and II.

Knee Strains and Repairs

Knee pain is a common complaint both in and out of yoga classes. There are widely varied causes, including arthritis, ligament strains, cartilage injuries (including meniscus tears), patellar tendinitis, and bursitis. The specific condition indicates what to do and not to do in healing the knee. Where asanas present the risks to the knees, it is primarily to the ACL, MCL, and medial meniscus, typically through the cumulative effects of repetitive stress or incorrect alignment, or due to excessive force (by the student or teacher). Here we will focus on a healthy knees program and healing ACL, MCL, and medial meniscus repairs.

Healthy Knees Program

Healthy knees start with not abusing them. Unfortunately, accidents happen, and repetitive use can rise to the level of abuse without a person realizing it. Several exercises done regularly can help ensure the stability and integrity of the knee joint and help alleviate minor strains. As a casual practice, students with slight knee pain should do regular ankle ABCs and massage the patella daily to maintain mobility. The muscles acting on the knee from above—the abductors (primarily the glutei and tensor fasciae latae, acting through their attachment to the iliotibial band), adductors (primarily the gracilis), the quadriceps (for extension), the hamstrings (for flexion), and the sartorius (synergist in flexion and lateral rotation)—help the ligaments to stabilize the knee when contracting from their various origins on the front, back, and bottom of the pelvis. The following asanas and non-asana exercises offer balanced strengthening and stretching of these muscles and ligaments supporting the knees; all should be done with progressively greater repetition and resistance:

1. Strongly contract the quadriceps in Dandasana, Paschimottanasana, Adho Mukha Svanasana, Navasana, and Utthita Hasta Padangusthasana to maintain a healthy relationship between the quadriceps and the patella tendon while stretching the hamstrings. Strongly contract the quadriceps in Tadasana for further quadriceps and patella stability.

2. Virasana—sitting high on a prop if necessary—and Dhanurasana stretch the quadriceps and stimulate circulation around the avascular areas of the knee joint.

3. Lying as though in Savasana and slowly sliding the feet in as if to prepare for Setu Bandha Sarvangasana while resisting with the heels (bridge slides) strengthens the hamstrings and helps to maintain the healthy attachment of their ligaments behind and below the knee.

4. Sitting on a chair or table with the lower legs and feet dangling free, (1) cross the ankles and pull the heels back to flex the knees, and (2) extend the knees to engage the quadriceps.

5. Move back and forth from Tadasana to Utkatasana and from Utkatasana to Malasana, strengthening the quadriceps while moving the knee joint through its full range of motion while progressively weighted.

6. In Setu Bandha Sarvangasana, squeeze a block between the knees to strengthen the muscles wrapping across the knee from above and attaching to the medial tibia (gracilis, sartorius, semitendinosus).

7. Standing in Tadasana, slowly lift the heels as high as possible, holding for several breaths before slowly releasing the heels to the floor.

8. Starting with straight legs in a long stance and the hips squared toward the front of the mat, slowly bend and then straighten the front knee into and out of Ashta Chandrasana, focusing on the steady tracking of the knee toward the center of the foot and the gradual release into a deeper lunge; try to keep the back knee extended by pressing the heel back.

Anterior Cruciate Ligament (ACL) Rehabilitation

Damage to the ACL is common among athletes and one of the greatest risks in yoga classes where there is little or no detailed guidance in alignment of the knees in high lunge asanas such as Virabhadrasana I and II. Students returning to class following an ACL repair should closely follow the rehabilitation exercises from their physical therapist and, if free of pain, incorporate the following asanas and non-asana exercises:

1. During the first month after surgery, do healthy knees program exercises that focus on strengthening and stretching the hamstrings, quadriceps, gastrocnemius, and patellar mobilization without bearing significant weight. Never force full knee extension or flexion. Use Apanasana (not Balasana or Virasana unless highly propped, which may be contraindicated for up to a year) to explore gently increasing knee flexion.

2. Gradually progress to weight-bearing gastrocnemius stretches in Ashta Chandrasana and Parsvottanasana prep (hands on a wall), begin toe raises in Tadasana, balancing in Vrksasana, ankle flexion resistance using a strap in Dandasana, and hamstring curls lying in Salabhasana Prep.

3. Once knee swelling decreases and the student can stand evenly and easily on both legs, work gently toward full knee extension in Dandasana. Do heel raises in Tadasana. Hold Dandasana for two or more minutes several times a day to stretch the hamstrings, and begin moving dynamically in and out of Utkatasana with the feet at hip-distance apart.

4. Gradually start to maintain full knee extension, starting in Dandasana, Supta Padangusthasana, and Utthita Hasta Padangusthasana, and further increase flexion in Apanasana, Utkatasana, Balasana, and finally Virasana.

5. Use standing balance asanas such as Vrksasana and Utthita Hasta Padangusthasana to enhance proprioception, the full restoration of which typically takes longer than restoration of full extension and flexion.

6. To develop full flexion and strength, begin exploring lunging gradually more deeply in Ashta Chandrasana, Anjaneyasana, Utkatasana, and Malasana while continuing the overall healthy knees program.

Medial Collateral Ligament Sprain

The medial collateral ligament (MCL) joins the inner surfaces of the femur and tibia, preventing the inner knee from widening under stress. Force against the outside of the knee can strain or tear its fibers, with symptoms ranging from mild tenderness (grade 1) to significant tenderness with some swelling (grade 2) to a complete tear and significant joint laxity (grade 3, which often hurts less than a grade 2 strain). The rehabilitation process starts with RICE; grade 2 and 3 strains may indicate the need for a brace. With all MCL strains, the initial focus is on decreasing swelling, maintaining range of motion (particularly flexion), and strengthening the musculature around the knee; strengthening exercises should not be initiated until swelling has decreased significantly and range of motion is restored. Be careful not to adduct the leg while under stress until all pain is relieved. Explore as follows:

1. To initially maintain range of motion: use ankle ABCs, bridge slides, and isometric quadriceps strengthening (such as in Dandasana as described above).

2. To strengthen: from standing, raise the leg using hip flexion (as moving into Utthita Hasta Padangusthasana) with no adduction, first working dynamically and then holding for five to ten breaths; in Setu Bandha Sarvangasana, squeeze a block between the knees; from Tadasana do heel raises (using a wall for balance to ensure against accidental adduction); move back and forth from Tadasana toward Utkatasana with the feet at hip-distance apart.

3. When the above movements can be done with little discomfort and no increase in swelling or point tenderness, begin to explore standing in Prasarita Padottanasana Prep, move more deeply into Utkatasana, and begin exploring dynamic movement into and out of Ashta Chandrasana while being vigilant in steadily tracking the knee toward the center of the foot.

4. When step 3 can be done free of pain, swelling, and point tenderness, begin exploring lateral movement as well as weighted adduction as in Garudasana.

Medial Meniscus Tears

The menisci are crescent-shaped cartilage resting on top of the tibia and provide shock absorption and even movement of the femur above the tibia. The medial meniscus is more prone to injury than the lateral meniscus because its attachment to the MCL and joint capsule reduces its mobility; it is also commonly torn along with ACL injuries. Excessive twisting of the knee in asanas such as Padmasana or Ardha Matsyendrasana as well as twisting the knee when it is bearing weight in standing balance asanas are common causes of medial meniscus tears in Hatha yoga. The injury is usually experienced as pain on the inner surface of the knee and may involve swelling, pain in flexion, and inability to bear weight without sensitivity. The tears are also caused by degenerative changes such as arthritis and repetitive stress.

1. Begin treatment with RICE and an anti-inflammatory diet rich in turmeric and ginger.

2. Gently massage the area around the knee several times daily. If the tear is mild, once pain has subsided begin exercises as described for healthy knees to increase range of motion, balance, and to maintain the strength of the quadriceps and hamstrings.

3. With more severe tears ("bucket handle") or deterioration that requires surgery, begin the rehabilitation process immediately with RICE, gentle massage, ankle ABCs, bridge slides, and mild strengthening of the quadriceps (such as isometric contraction in Dandasana), then proceed with the next step when free of pain, swelling, and point tenderness.

4. Do the strengthening exercises as described in step 2 with MCL rehabilitation, focusing primarily on the quadriceps and hamstrings. Gradually add weight-bearing lunges and heel raises to further develop strength.

5. Gradually do the entire healthy knees program as described above.

Hamstring Strains

Hamstring strains are very common in Hatha yoga classes. They typically result from forcing forward bends, unknowingly overstretching when warm (more likely when hot), stretch reflex when eccentrically contracting muscles are fatigued, and from overexposing the hamstring attachments at the ischial tuberosities (sitting bones) by pulling the flesh of the buttocks away before doing seated forward bends. Most hamstring tears sustained in yoga are at the sitting bones, usually felt as a slight pinching sensation, not in the bodies of the muscles. Due in part to unavoidable use of the hamstrings in daily activities such as walking, tears are easily re-strained and require considerable patience to heal. Follow these steps to assist healing:

1. Try to rest the leg as much as possible, and ice the painful area for fifteen to twenty minutes every two hours.

2. With mild strains: begin static stretching by holding Dandasana for one to two minutes five times daily (there should be no sharp sensation in the muscle or its attachments); in Setu Bandha Sarvangasana, press the sitting bones firmly up to feel the hamstring attachments deepening; do prone hamstrings curls to gradually strengthen the muscles; get progressively deeper massage of the hamstrings; gradually explore deeper stretching with a yoga strap wrapped tautly around the leg as high up into the groin as possible (to focus the stretch away from the vulnerable attachment and more into the body of the muscles).

3. With more severe strains (not complete tears): proceed as above until there is no pain when doing isometric contractions in Dandasana and Setu Bandha Sarvangasana. Stay with static stretching until free of pain, then proceed with step 4.

4. Slowly introduce dynamic stretching and strengthening by moving back and forth between Tadasana and Utkatasana, and between Dandasana and Paschimottanasana (do not bounce!). If free of pain, introduce proprioceptive neuromuscular facilitation (i.e., reconnecting the brain, nerves, and muscles) by lying on your back and pressing down through the heel with increasing effort (start easy, patiently explore doing it more strongly), then gradually repeat this exercise with the heel placed on an increasingly high stack of blocks (or gradually up a wall, eventually into Viparita Dandasana).

5. Gradually introduce deeper stretching and strengthening, ideally combined with deep tissue massage of the hamstrings every other day. Practice Baddha Konasana to explore stretching the neighboring adductors and internal rotators, being sensitive to pain when pulling near the sitting bones. Be especially conscious in the initiating actions of all movements in which the stretching or contraction of the hamstrings changes (for example, in the Sun Salutations).

6. When completely free of pain, begin static stretching in Upavista Konasana, Paschimottanasana, Halasana, and Parsvottanasana (place the hands on a wall and gradually explore folding forward). Many students tend to reinjure the hamstrings in standing asanas such as Parsvottanasana and Utthita Trikonasana.

7. Along with pain-free static stretching, begin additional strengthening through prone hip extension: lifting the legs off the floor in Salabhasana, holding Setu

Bandha Sarvangasana, Virabhadrasana III with hands on a wall). As a final strengthening practice, it is important to do eccentric strengthening: being sensitive to overworking the hamstrings, take five breaths to fold forward from Tadasana to Uttanasana (bend the knees if necessary and consider using a wall for support).

Lower-Back Pain

Most lower-back pain results from degeneration of intervertebral disks and the consequent pressure on nerves. While this is part of the normal aging process, injuries, cigarette smoking, and poor posture speed up degeneration. Depending on the severity of degeneration, additional problems can develop, including annular tears, disk herniation, arthritis, segmental instability, and stenosis. Some lower-back pain is referred from areas away from the spine itself, including from spasms in the quadratus lumborum. Overstretching in forward bends is a common cause of lower-back strain in Hatha yoga, especially when not firmly grounding down through the sitting bones in seated forward bending or not firming the quadriceps in standing forward bends. The lower back is also frequently strained doing quick movements from forward-bending to backbending asanas (such as snapping, rather than gradually transitioning, from Urdhva Mukha Svanasana to Adho Mukha Svanasana), when forcing any forward or backbend, and in complex asanas and transitions involving simultaneous hip flexion, axial rotation, and spinal extension as when floating from Astavakrasana to Chaturanga Dandasana.

The surest way to prevent or minimize lower-back pain is through regular exercise that supports balanced posture, which depends on the balance of strength and flexibility throughout the body, especially in the muscles acting on the pelvis, spine, and shoulders. With the pelvis, it is important to have balanced strength and flexibility in the hip flexors and extensors to create a stable foundation for pelvic neutrality and neutral extension of the spine. Tight hip flexors combined with weak or hyper-flexible hamstrings, which can occur through an unbalanced yoga practice, is a recipe for excessive lordosis in the lower back, which over time contributes to disc compression and arthritis. With the spine, it is important to balance strength and flexibility of the spinal erector muscles, multifidi, and quadratus lumborum with strength and flexibility in the core abdominal muscles.

With students experiencing lower-back pain, emphasize doing a "seventy-percent practice" in which they back off from where they might otherwise go in all stretching and strengthening related to the lower back, even if free of pain in those asanas. Then proceed with the following sequence, moving progressively to each successive asana only when comfortable:

TABLE 11.1—**Healthy Lower-Back Sequence**

1. Supine pelvic tilts	14. Standing side bends
2. Supine bent knee to chest	15. Wall slides
3. Double knees to chest	16. Fire hydrant
4. Partial sit-ups	17. Supta Padangusthasana
5. Partial yogic bicycles	18. Upavista Konasana
6. Bent knee rolls—Jathara Parivartanasana	19. Utthita Hasta Padangusthasana with ledge
7. Setu Bandha Sarvangasana	20. Anjaneyasana
8. Naraviralasana	21. Eka Pada Raj Kapotasana Prep
9. Salabhasana A, B, C	22. Marichyasana C
10. Prone leg lift	23. Parsvottanasana Prep
11. Prone opposite arm/leg lifts	24. Jathara Parivartanasana with straight legs
12. All fours with opposite arm/leg lifts	25. Virasana
13. Cat/Dog	26. Full practice

Scoliosis

Scoliosis is a condition in which the spine is curved from side to side and possibly rotated. While a small percentage of scoliosis cases are congenital or a symptom of another condition such as cerebral palsy, most cases do not have a known cause. Most cases show a right thoracic curve: when viewed from the back, the thoracic segment of the spine curves outward (to the right) from the normal plumb line of the spine. In left lumbar scoliosis the lumbar spine curves out to left. Left lumbar and right thoracic are often found together, creating an S-curve, while right lumbar and right thoracic create a long C-curve. Scoliosis can be painful because muscles try to conform to the curvature, often creating muscle spasms. Scoliosis is typically detected by noticing uneven musculature across the back, uneven hips, ribs, and shoulders, and other asymmetries that suggest a structural anomaly. Women are about five times more likely than men to have scoliosis.

In teaching yoga to students with scoliosis, emphasize the importance of establishing a balanced foundation for the spine through the actions of the feet, legs, and pelvis. As with all students, focus on standing equally on the feet, cultivating pada bandha, awakening the muscles of the legs, and developing awareness of pelvic neutrality. Many students with scoliosis are likely to have muscular imbalances in the connection of the pelvis and spine, primarily due to compensation in the iliopsoas, quadratus lumborum, and piriformis muscles. All students with scoliosis will benefit from more extensive opening and balancing of these muscles on the right and left sides of the body through Anjaneyasana, Virabhadrasana I, Gomukhasana, and Ardha Matsyendrasana. They should also develop more balanced support for the spine by stretching and strengthening the muscles that support the spine, particularly the abdominal core muscles and the spinal erectors, multifidi, and quadratus lumborum (through contraction backbends).

Farther up the spine, it is important to compensate for the rounding of the spine by developing the muscular basis for keeping the shoulder blades rotating down against the back ribs while lifting the sternum. This involves strengthening and stretching the rhomboids and mid-trapezius muscles using Gomukhasana arms; stretching and strengthening the serratus anterior muscles in Phalakasana and Cat/Dog practices; and maintaining a general healthy shoulders practice using the asanas listed in the section below on shoulder issues. An essential part of this work involves using the breath to create more space in compressed areas of the ribs and chest, stretching and strengthening the intercostals and other respiratory muscles. As always, the breath should be drawn into areas of tightness and into the lengthening of the spine.

There are several ways to modify asanas to reduce or slow the further progression of the condition while helping to decrease pain.[a] If these modifications are not done, the normal alignment and energetic action principles might exacerbate the scoliosis. Asanas involving lateral flexion and spinal rotation are among the most important ones to significantly modify. For example, in Utthita Trikonasana, with the right foot turned out, students with a right thoracic curve should not try to lengthen the right side of their rib cage, focusing instead on lengthening on the left side from a stable and even foundation in the feet, legs, and hips. In Parivrtta Trikonasana with the right foot out, that same student should work to draw in the right-side ribs while lengthening the left side while twisting to the right; with the left foot out that student should not twist at all. There are similar important modifications in Utthita Parsvakonasana, Parsvottanasana, Janu Sirsasana, and all other asanas involving asymmetrical legs and positioning of the spine.

Wrist Tendinitis and Carpal Tunnel Syndrome

With the recent advent of flow-oriented Hatha yoga classes with repetitive movements through Chaturanga Dandasana, Urdhva Mukha Svanasana, and Adho Mukha Svanasana, along with numerous asanas in which the entire weight of the body is supported on the hands, students' wrists are increasingly at risk of injury. Meanwhile, many students' lifestyles potentially strain their wrists, whether from mountain biking, typing, or doing massage work. Problems include overstretching or tearing wrist ligaments, wrist tendinitis, and carpal tunnel syndrome (CTS). Students with severe wrist pain should undergo diagnostic tests (such as Phalen's and reverse Phalen's to identify CTS, and Finkelstein's test to identify De Quervain's tenosynovitis, common in new mothers). Note that many cases of CTS are misdiagnosed; rather than inflammation of the flexor tendons passing through the carpal tunnel causing pressure on the medial nerve, the pressure is often from compression of the nerve elsewhere, particularly in the neck and shoulder area. Regardless of the specific condition, treatment, including modification of asanas, should be based on the cause and diagnosis. In all cases, sharp pain contraindicates hand balances and other asanas in which the wrists are significantly weight-bearing.

Students experiencing mild wrist pain can benefit from warming up their fingers, hands, arms, and shoulders before beginning their practice. Wrist and forearm massage are also effective in helping reduce pain. So long as the pain is mild, the following exercises can be healing:

1. *Tadasana wrist therapy:* Gently rotate the wrists through their full range of circular motion, repeatedly changing direction, then gently shake out the wrists for around thirty seconds. This can be incorporated in brief form into every Sun Salutation.

2. *Uttanasana wrist pratikriyasana:* Whenever folding into Uttanasana amid Sun Salutations, place the backs of the wrists toward or onto the floor and make an easy fist. This is less intense on the wrists than Pada Hastasana (also, more students can do it and it can be easily done with the exhale into Uttanasana).

3. *Wrist pumps:* Holding the fingers of one hand with the fingers of the other hand, move the wrist forward and back while resisting the movement with the opposing hand. Repeat for one to two minutes if pain-free.

4. *Anjali mudra:* Press the palms and fingers (from the knuckles to the fingertips) firmly together at the chest in a prayer position for one to two minutes. This is also known as reverse Phalen's test; if there is a burning sensation inside the wrist joint within thirty seconds, this could indicate CTS. Reverse the position of the hands, placing the backs of the wrists and hands together, and press firmly for up to a minute (Phalen's test).

5. *Hand dance:* Kneeling comfortably, place the hands down on the floor with the fingers pointed forward, then turn the palms up, then down with the fingers out, up with the fingers in, down with the fingers back, up with the fingers back, continuing in this fashion with every permutation of palms up and down with the fingers forward, back, in, and out.

Persistent wrist tenderness or strain usually benefits from ice, splints worn during sleep, anti-inflammatory agents (including turmeric and ginger), acupuncture, and other alternative treatments. Encourage students to explore all possible measures and to consult a doctor for additional guidance.

Shoulder Instability and Impingement

Instability and impingement in the shoulder joint both arise from problems in the rotator cuff, the four muscles covering the head of the humerus that work together to lift and rotate the arm (see Chapter Four for shoulder details). When one or more of these muscles is weak, or when the supporting ligaments are overstretched, the humerus is at risk of subluxation (commonly called a dislocated shoulder). When one or more of these muscles is tight, in spasm, inflamed, or otherwise out of healthy balance, the deltoid is unopposed in abduction, jamming the humeral head up against the acromion process of the scapula when lifting the arm. Other causes of impingement include acromioclavicular arthritis, structural abnormalities, and calcified ligaments. Other sources of pain in the shoulder include inflamed tendons, bursitis, and tears in the labrum.

The key to healthy shoulders is balanced strength and flexibility. If imbalance is creating instability or impingement, first avoid painful activities and refrain from unstable movements in which the elbow is lifted above the shoulder, especially with any whipping motion such as throwing a ball. Treat persistent pain with ice and anti-inflammatory agents. To develop healthy range of motion and strength, explore the following asanas and exercises:

1. Lying prone on a table with the arm dangling down, simply swing it forward and back in Codman's pendulum swings and around in circles.

2. Stretch the rhomboids with Garudasana arms; use one arm to pull the other gently across the chest in horizontal adduction if unable to get into the Garudasana position.

3. Use Gomukhasana arms to stretch the triceps, latissimus dorsi, infraspinatus, teres minor, and pectoralis major of the upper arm and the pectoralis major, biceps, serratus anterior, and trapezius of the lower arm.

4. Use Parsvottanasana arms to stretch the infraspinatus, teres minor, serratus anterior, anterior deltoids, and pectorals.

5. Use Prasarita Padottanasana C arms to stretch the pectorals and anterior deltoids.

6. Stabilize the scapula by strengthening and stretching the serratus anterior and rhomboid muscles. on all fours and keeping the arms straight, slowly alternate

between lowering the chest toward and away from the floor; when easy, do this in Phalakasana and progress to moving slowly back and forth between Phalakasana and Chaturanga.

7. To strengthen the rotator cuff muscles: supraspinatus through abduction of the arms into Virabhadrasana II; infraspinatus and teres minor through external rotation of the arms in Adho Mukha Svanasana; subscapularis through isometric contraction in Parsvottanasana.

8. If free of pain, explore further strengthening of the shoulders by keeping the arms overhead in flexion in Salabhasana C and Virabhadrasana III. If still pain-free after these asanas, explore holding Adho Mukha Svanasana for up to one minute, eventually working up to five minutes. If still pain-free, explore Adho Mukha Vrksasana, eventually holding for up to two minutes.

WORKING WITH DEPRESSION

Students come to yoga classes with a wide array of emotional conditions. For those experiencing depression, whether mild or clinical, yoga can be helpful.[3] In Chapter Five, we discussed creating space for healing emotional traumas and moving into a steadier sense of santosa, contentment. It is important to note that feeling sad or "down," usually thought of as negative, can be subtly beneficial in helping a person cope with certain circumstances. The perceived sadness attracts social support, can help calm a person suffering from other ailments, and can have a "sadder but wiser" effect as a person comes to see the world more realistically.[4] However, in the traditional yogic perspective, depression is seen as reflecting either a rajasic state, with symptoms of anxiety and restlessness, or a tamasic state, characterized by inertia and hopelessness.[5] Looking at depression through this prism, one of the goals of yoga is to move into a sattvic state of clarity and ease using the tools of asana, pranayama, and meditation as follows:[6]

- If tamasic: Offer students a more vigorous, flowing style of asanas that includes a sustained series of stimulating backbends and twists and invigorating forms of pranayama such as kapalabhati along with meditation practices in which the eyes remain open with clear dristi and the quality of mindfulness is oriented toward being fully awake.

- If rajasic: Offer students a slower asana practice that includes long holds in forward bends, a long Savasana, calming forms of pranayama such as nadi shodhana, and meditation practices in which the eyes are closed and students explore the slowing rhythms of thought.

WORKING WITH PREGNANT STUDENTS

Which yoga asanas are beneficial or possibly risky during pregnancy and in the early postpartum period (and during extended periods of lactation)? Which asanas are indicated and contraindicated during each trimester? How do these prescriptions vary depending on the unique woman and specific conditions such as age, number of previous pregnancies, and other factors? These and other questions pertaining to working with pregnant students did not appear in the yoga literature until the late twentieth century. Looking more broadly to the general question of exercise and pregnancy, we find very different views in the modern historical literature, starting with Alexander Hamilton's 1781 "Treatise on Midwifery," which encouraged moderate exercise avoiding "agitation of the body from violent or improper exercise, as jolting in a carriage riding on horseback, dancing and whatever disturbs the body or mind" (Mittelmark et al. 1991). Nineteenth-century scientific examination of exercise and birth outcomes all have similar findings showing an association between robust activity and lower birth weight, leading to legislation in several countries (but not the United States) prohibiting employment of women in the weeks preceding and following delivery. By the early twentieth century we find a growing list of arbitrary restrictions on activity, derived more from cultural and social biases than scientific study. A 1935 issue of *Modern Motherhood* says to "bathe, swim, golf and dance, but no excessive walking, horseback riding or tennis," while noting that some expectant mothers experience no ill effects from such activities. Yet also in the 1930s, British writer and maternal advocate Kathleen Vaughan advocated improving joint flexibility through squats to widen the pelvic outlet as well as Baddha Konasana–like positions, and pelvic floor exercises to prevent tears of the perineum. Still, during the 1940s and 1950s, most of the literature suggested very moderate activity and no sports, giving way in the 1950s to Vaughan's criticism of the sedentary life of English women in *Exercises before Childbirth,* which presents both physical and psychological benefits of regular group exercise during pregnancy.

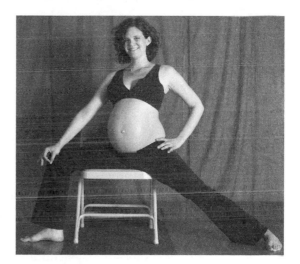

In the 1970s and early 1980s, we find the emphasis shifting to control over the body and a sense of well-being, but the advice typically ignores basic physiological changes such as aortal compression syndrome, laxity of joints and ligaments, exaggerated lumbar lordosis, and abdominal compression issues. We also start to find the unexamined assumption that some minor dietary error or failure to engage in some specific regimen of prenatal exercises could damage the unborn child or mother, motivating many pregnant women to quickly immerse themselves in exercise programs, often predisposing them (and their babies) to injury. In the past twenty years we have come to much greater insight into the relationship between exercise and pregnancy, including clear evidence that normal daily activities in no way compromise the mother or baby unless there's some significant pathological condition. The emergent conventional wisdom offers several suggestions regarding exercise during pregnancy: it should be regular, not intermittent, and not competitive; if vigorous, it should not be in intense heat or humidity or with high fever; ballistic and jarring movements as well as deep flexion and extension of joints should be avoided; and if starting from a sedentary lifestyle, begin with very simple exercises.

These insights come largely through the lens of a Western medical and scientific model, which still mostly assumes the separation of body and mind. Taken to the extreme, this perspective considers thoughts and feeling largely irrelevant to physical welfare, addressing physical anomalies and problems with purely physical therapy, drugs, or surgery. Yet we find considerable evidence that emotion is a highly significant factor in pregnancy and delivery; holding onto a secret fear, having commitment issues, and other emotional feelings can have a direct effect on the physiology of the body.[7] An increasing number of hospitals and birthing centers recognize that discharging emotions eases the way in labor, and so offer a more peaceful environment and even encourage conscious breathing and meditation practices to ease labor and delivery.

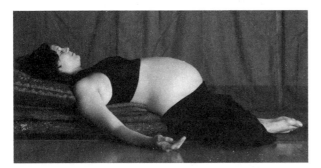

We can usefully divide pregnant students into two general categories: (1) those with sedentary lifestyles, poor physical health, or high-risk pregnancy, and (2) those with active lifestyles, good overall health, and minimal pregnancy risks. Women in the first category should be encouraged to attend yoga classes designed specifically for pregnant students, typically referred to as pre/postnatal yoga. Women in the second category should be encouraged to explore practicing in regular yoga classes with teachers who are prepared to give them informed guidance on when and how to modify their practices. Women in the second category and already regularly practicing yoga should be encouraged to do a maintenance practice along with the modifications discussed below; pregnancy is not the time to begin a vigorous yoga practice, nor the time to attempt new or more complex asanas.[8]

Pelvic Awareness and Health

All pregnant students can benefit from bringing greater awareness and support to the structure, muscles, and organs of their pelvis. This can usefully begin well before pregnancy with a more focused practice of mula bandha as a tool for toning and refining one's awareness of the lower pelvic muscles and organs. Mula bandha helps to develop a stronger and more flexible set of perineal muscles, more awareness of the lower pelvic organs and their surrounding support structure, greater ease in the delivery process, and a reduction in several physical risks that often naturally occur during pregnancy, labor, and delivery, including perineal tears (or reduced indication of episiotomy), urinary incontinence, and vaginal prolapse. Building on the basic mula bandha practice, women can develop more subtle awareness and control of all of the superficial muscles of the perineal floor and higher up into the layers of deep pelvic muscles that surround and give support to the bladder, vagina, and rectum.[9] With this awareness, women can participate in the birthing process in a more conscious fashion.

Practices by Stage of Pregnancy

Early Pregnancy—First Trimester

During the early period of pregnancy up to around the thirteenth week, students should take it easy as they adjust to changing hormones and energy during an often intense and delicate period of transformation. This is a time for getting more grounded, slowing down a bit, focusing more inside, and creating a favorable environment for the ovum to grow into a healthy fetus. Follow these guidelines:

- Stay with ujjayi pranayama. Do not do kapalabhati pranayama or other breathing techniques that involve pumping action in the belly.
- Do not jolt the body by jumping into asanas (if the student has a well-developed floating practice, she might feel comfortable staying with it).
- Minimize twisting (to minimize pulling on the broad ligament that attaches to the uterus); when twisting, focus the movement in the upper thoracic spine.
- Do basic pelvic awareness exercises.
- The fetus is very small and the uterus well protected inside the pelvis, so students can lie on their belly (until they are "showing").

- Develop more pelvic awareness by doing Bridge Rolls (undulating the pelvis and spine slowly in and out of Setu Bandha Sarvangasana), Supta Baddha Konasana, Swastikasana, Vajrasana, Virasana, Upavista Konasana, Gomukhasana, Ananda Balasana, and Eka Pada Raj Kapotasana Prep. Become very familiar with Malasana.

- Do a variety of shoulder strengtheners and openers (see the discussion on shoulders above).

- Explore Utthita Trikonasana, Virabhadrasana II, and Utthita Parsvakonasana as hip openers that stimulate circulation in the legs and contribute to strong feet and legs, creating a more stable foundation for the off-kilter weight distribution soon to come.

- While still in the first trimester, begin to explore asanas and props that are used in the second and third trimesters.

Second Trimester

With the placenta fully functional, hormone levels balance out and the pregnancy is generally well established. This is the perfect time to focus on cultivating strength and stamina, to refine awareness of the pelvis and spine, and to build more internal support for the inevitable challenge to balance and ease that will happen as the baby grows. The size of the belly varies greatly in the second trimester; different women show at different points in time. As a woman's pregnancy start to show, the pelvis no longer protects the uterus, so it is time to start adapting poses accordingly. Toward the middle of the second trimester, students should tune in more to any sense of numbness while lying on their back as the increasing weight of the baby may place pressure on the vena cava, restricting the flow of blood back to the mother's heart. Guide the practice as follows:

- Avoid jarring movements, intense abdominal work such as yogic bicycles and Navasana, and kapalabhati pranayama. It is important to avoid pressure on the abdomen and to develop a supple belly; female athletes with tight abdominal muscles are at highest risk of perineal tears and urinary incontinence arising from downward pressure.

- Use pelvic neutrality exercises in Tadasana and Urdhva Hastasana to cultivate alignment of the spine, and stay with the Bridge Roll practice.

- Practice Surya Namaskara with the feet apart in Tadasana, step back to Plank, and use folded blankets to support the ribs and hips when lying prone in preparation for either Salabhasana or Urdhva Mukha Svanasana. Integrate squats into the salutations.

- Practice standing asanas to develop or maintain leg strength and open the hips and pelvis (modify and use a wall or chair for support as needed): Vrksasana, Garudasana, Anjaneyasana, Ashta Chandrasana, Virabhadrasana I and II, Utthita Trikonasana, Parsvottanasana, Utthita Parsvakonasana.
- Explore a variety of seated hip openers and forward folds: Baddha Konasana, Upavista Konasana, Parivrtta Janu Sirsasana, Bharadvajrasana, Eka Pada Raj Kapotasana Prep, Gomukhasana, Dandasana, Paschimottanasana (with legs apart), Marichyasana A, and Janu Sirsasana. Release pressure in the sacroiliac joint with the knees wide apart in Balasana.
- For relaxation, explore Viparita Karani with legs straight up the wall, apart, and with the feet together and knees apart; elevate the feet in Baddha Konasana; raise the hips and legs onto a long bolster in Savasana.

Third Trimester

This is the time to refocus on cultivating energy, especially by resting amid the flow of asanas to allow the body to integrate the practice more fully. It is increasingly important to limit time lying supine as the weight of the baby puts greater pressure on the vena cava. Relaxin hormone levels are now sufficiently high to cause the softening of ligaments throughout the body (not just in the pelvis), potentially causing fallen arches (as the calcaneonavicular ligaments stretch), weakness in the knees, and instability in the sacroiliac and other joints throughout the body.

- Continue working on postural alignment to give support to the spine.
- Become increasingly familiar with using a chair to support a variety of standing and sitting asanas (including Virabhadrasana and Malasana).
- After the thirty-sixth week, be aware that Adho Mukha Svanasana and other inversions can cause (or reverse!) breech presentation.
- Begin doing birthing visualizations in squatting and other abducted hip opening positions.
- Explore using a high bolster for long holds in Supta Baddha Konasana.
- Increasingly rest in Savasana lying on the side of the body with props between the knees, under the head, and under the upper arm for easy comfort and relaxation.

After Delivery

It is important for new mothers to slowly increase energy, redevelop muscle strength, and cultivate more endurance after giving birth. There should be no abdominal pressure from core work or kapalabhati pranayama for at least six weeks (longer if there was an episiotomy or perineal tear, allowing complete healing before starting pelvic floor exercises); gradually move back into toning the abdominal core. There are heightened levels of relaxin hormone until around two months postpartum or postlactation if breastfeeding, so encourage students to stay with an eighty-percent practice when doing deep stretches (especially forward folds and backbends).

TEACHING IN ALTERNATIVE SETTINGS

Before teaching yoga, I spent more than twenty years working as a community organizer, academic teacher, and in various social service and policy roles related to public schools, juvenile institutions, prisons, drug rehabilitation, and mental health treatment centers. Soon after starting to teach yoga, I worked with others in the Los Angeles yoga community to create the Yoga Inside Foundation, developing sustainable yoga programs in a variety of alternative settings, eventually setting up more than three hundred programs in the United States and Canada. Similar initiatives in recent years by organizations such as Off the Mat, Art of Yoga, the Lineage Project, and others have expanded this work far beyond our early efforts, extending the gift of yoga to people and institutions otherwise off the yoga map. The unique challenges and opportunities in this *seva* (service) go far beyond what we ordinarily experience when teaching yoga in traditional settings:

- There is a greater diversity of students in any given class: different backgrounds, ages, conditions, and motivations.
- Many students will have deep emotional wounds, suffer from post-traumatic stress disorder, be on mood-modifying drugs, or are extremely vulnerable.
- The host agency may be less than wholly supportive of the yoga program, with some staff creating resistance while adamantly enforcing institutional rules.
- The practice room is not likely to have a finished hardwood floor, sound system for music, stage, candles, wall straps, or some of the other accoutrements you may have grown accustomed to while teaching at your local neighborhood yoga shala.
- There are likely to be time limits that vary from one class to the next, and you may have frequent and surprise interruptions.

The experience of teaching in alternative settings is shaped in part by whether the classes are voluntary or compulsory. Some yoga teachers choose not to teach in a setting where there is any constraint on a student's volition; it feels antithetical to yoga that someone would step onto a yoga mat without freely deciding to do so. While compulsory attendance is often associated with classroom behavioral management challenges, the larger emotional and behavioral issues will typically overshadow initial motivation to attend or not. It is therefore up to the teacher to manifest an energy and presence in the class that fosters a spirit of openness about doing the practice while managing the room in a way that encourages the most yogic feelings amid whatever else is going on. Many yoga students in public schools, prisons, treatment centers, and other places have only the vaguest notion of yoga before their yoga teacher arrives on the scene; here is your opportunity to introduce yoga by demonstrating yogic equanimity amid these challenges.

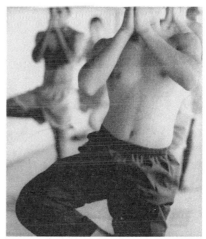

L.A. County Juvenile Facility, 1997

In a population that is struggling with emotional and psychological issues, yoga addresses several important matters. Most people in treatment centers have a pattern of obsessive-compulsive behavior and are typically depressed. It is very important to recognize and respect your own specific role as a yoga teacher in these settings. You are not a therapist, even if yoga can be therapeutic. Indeed, one of the goals in providing yoga in alternative settings is to help replace unhealthy behaviors or routines with healthy ones. Drawing on your knowledge and skills as a yoga teacher, you can contribute to your students' healing process. This includes connecting with the breath, creating a safe and contained environment where yoga students are not judged, regaining a sense of self, self-acceptance, self-confidence, a sense of balance, connecting to emotional pain, developing awareness of body-mind reconnection, being present, resting, bringing renewed meaning to life, and breaking out of patterns. With patient effort, you can help your students to gain self-acceptance, to detach from old unhealthy thoughts, to put the mind in one place—and to discover their authentic selves.

More practically, when teaching in alternative settings, give more attention to these elements:

- Introduce yoga and share personal yoga experiences, disclosing to connect with and give support to your students.
- Find a balance for all of the students in the room conveying safety, support, and acceptance. Give them tools for life by embodying the experience of healing and reflecting transformation and growth.

- Focus on the self-reflective aspects of the practice rather than "the perfect pose."
- Create strong, clear boundaries, and help your students recognize the gift of the class by insisting on mutual respect.
- Provide consistent encouragement to help build self-confidence, reinforcing and acknowledging self-transformation.
- Emphasize the body as a vehicle and container for self-transformation that can help students feel what they may be avoiding.
- In asanas, stay in the nonpainful discomfort—breathe and transform. Relate the discomfort in asanas to discomfort in life, encouraging students to stay with difficult feelings as a way to explore breakthroughs, cultivating balance and strength in the asanas and applying this to the healing process.
- Pranayama and meditation are important tools in alternative settings; explore using them to go more deeply and safely into hidden feelings and to stop cycles of obsessive thinking.

CHAPTER TWELVE

THE YOGA PROFESSION

Teach what is in you,
not as it applies to you, to yourself,
but as it applies to the other.
—*T. Krishnamacharya*

Yoga is a $5.7 billion industry, up eighty-seven percent since 2004 and showing no signs of slowing. More than sixteen million people are regularly practicing yoga in the United States alone (another eighteen million have dabbled). There are currently seventy thousand–plus yoga teachers at various levels of experience and competence in the United States, an increase of about fifty-five percent in the past five years. While the United States leads the way, this trend is worldwide and particularly strong in other English-speaking countries and Europe (there are more than eleven thousand yoga teachers in Great Britain). The growth is found in all styles of yoga, with the largest growth in eclectic styles such as Vinyasa Flow and Power yoga that blend the teachings of several different approaches. Yoga businesses and associations are quickly ramping up yoga teacher-training programs to meet the growing demand for qualified teachers, while thousands of new students are venturing into teaching with minimal or no training (less than twenty-five percent of teachers have completed a training program). Indeed, anyone can instruct yoga. There is no required background, experience, training, certification, or licensing. But whether you are interested in teaching informal classes to friends and family, teaching part-time or full-time, to be an effective teacher requires continuous personal practice, training, study, and a commitment to learning something new from every student and class. With an attitude toward teaching as a profession, you will do all you can to hone your skills and knowledge, enjoying the path of teaching as a learning journey unto itself.

YOGA TEACHER TRAINING AND CERTIFICATION

Teacher training begins with practicing yoga on a consistent basis and exploring every available opportunity to learn about yoga. If you have not yet explored the teaching path, begin by taking specialized workshops on specific yoga topics to help determine if you have the depth of interest and fortitude for the hard work involved in in-depth yoga studies. Deepen your studies through independent read-

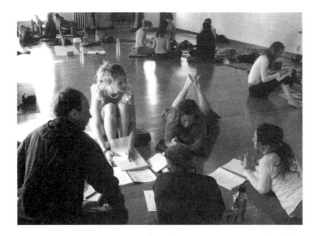

ing of classical and contemporary yoga literature. Look into teacher-training workshops that can give you a feel for the larger process of teacher certification. There are presently more than 1,400 yoga teacher-training programs worldwide, ranging from online distance learning and one-weekend certification to residential schools with rigorous curriculum standards requiring two years or longer to complete. In some styles, there are several levels of certification; some are strictly peer-reviewed and highly selective in conferring recognition as a teacher. At the very minimum, a credible yoga teacher-training program offers the following:

1. The opportunity to study, refine, and deepen your own practice, including asana, pranayama, and meditation.

2. A thorough exploration of asanas, including their alignment principles, energetic actions, modifications, use of props, variations, verbal and hands-on cues, risks, contraindications, and benefits.

3. Study of yoga philosophy, history, ethics, and lifestyle practices, the specific content reflecting the values of the school and its instructors.

4. Training and practical experience in planning classes and sequencing asana, pranayama, and meditation practices.

5. Opportunities to learn how to work with students who have injuries and other limiting conditions.

6. Opportunities to learn how to work with pregnant students.

7. Extensive opportunities for progressively more challenging practical experience teaching asanas and entire classes.

8. Opportunities for apprenticing with experienced teachers.

9. Guidance in finding your niche as a teacher and getting started in the profession.

10. Ongoing connection with other participants.

   In choosing a yoga teacher-training program, consider these questions:

1. What are the school's professional standards? How are these standards reflected in the school's curriculum and core faculty?

2. What are the school's philosophical values? Is the school part of a specific lineage, style, or tradition? Is there a guru or spiritual head of the school? If so, what do you know about him or her? Do you share the same or similar values?

3. What is the school's track record in training, certifying, and offering continuing guidance to graduates? What do recent graduates have to say about the program and its instructors?

4. What prior experience do the program's lead instructors have in training yoga teachers at the level of training you are pursuing (two-hundred-hour or five-hundred-hour certification)?

5. Is the school registered with the Yoga Alliance? If not, why not?

6. If the program offers a quick-immersion approach to training, how will you fully integrate the material into your developing repertoire of skills and knowledge?

7. How does the program provide hands-on practical experience in learning how to see, read, comprehend, and meaningfully relate with verbal and hands-on cues to a diverse array of students in each of the fifty or more basic asanas?

8. How does the program prepare you to work with students who are pregnant, new to yoga, injured, or limited in some other significant way?

9. How do the program's fees compare with those of other programs?

10. What is the time frame for completion and the requirements for certification?

APPRENTICING

Apprenticing is a timeless tradition in yoga. Here knowledge and skill are passed directly from teacher to student, with one intention being that the student is also on the teaching path. In this relationship the more experienced teacher has the opportunity to share wisdom, knowledge, and skill in the spirit or karma yoga, or seva (service), while the more amateur teacher has the opportunity to learn in closer interaction with the teacher willing to share his or her experience (Briggs 2001).

After completing a teacher-training program (or as part of it), apprenticing is among the most valuable ways to further develop your teaching skills.

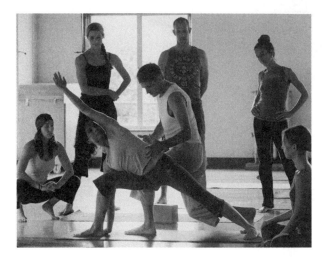

The purpose of an apprenticeship is to more closely observe regular classes, get hands-on experience in the classroom working closely with a qualified teacher, and to develop further the skills and confidence for conducting well-balanced, safe, and effective classes on your own. In the ideal apprenticeship, your mentor teacher will patiently explain the nuances of his or her craft, explaining sequences, exploring with you the various ways of giving hands-on adjustments in live classes, and addressing the multitude of questions that arise in every good teacher's mind in any given class. There are many ways to structure the apprenticeship. Here is one model:

- Assist once per week for six weeks in one type of class, then for another six weeks in a different type (or level) of class with the same mentor teacher or two different teachers.

- After each class, identify a topic that arose in the class as a question, issue, curiosity, etc., and focus on it that week. It can be something that either the apprentice or mentor thinks is an area where additional learning will benefit the apprentice.

- The mentor teacher gives the apprentice some initial thoughts on the question plus guidance on how to explore looking into it, including where the apprentice might read or research specific information, exploring something on one's own mat, or in some other way doing something that is thought to be the best way to approach the area where additional learning is being sought.

- After the apprentice has researched the question, he or she writes one page (no more than that) on the topic and gives this write-up to the mentor, thus providing the mentor the opportunity to further engage in a meaningful way with the apprentice in guiding him or her further along the teaching path. This is done each week.

In the class itself, the role and activities of the apprentice can vary considerably based on the needs and expectations of both parties and the students in the class.

- Often in the first session the apprentice actively observes and/or shadows the teacher as he or she moves about the room offering verbal and hands-on cues.
- With mutual confidence, this can evolve into the apprentice giving cues to individual students, giving isolated instruction to a new student to help that student more easily integrate into the class, or perhaps teaching part or all of a class. This is a judgment call primarily on the part of the mentor teacher, ideally made in kind and respectful consultation with the apprentice.

Most yoga teacher trainers offer apprenticeships as part of seva, taking on apprentices they have observed as being committed to excellence in the profession. Regularly taking a mentor teacher's classes or teacher-training workshops is one of the best ways to develop a relationship that might lead to an apprenticeship. When you are ready to apprentice, ask your teacher to be your mentor.

TEACHING OPPORTUNITIES AND REMUNERATION

Despite the seeming abundance of yoga teachers in many communities, there are equally abundant opportunities to teach. Those opportunities will manifest as soon as you decide that you want to teach and put your mind to it, asking yourself several questions to hone in on the best situations for you: What style of yoga do you want to teach? Who do you want to teach—whoever shows up in a public class, or a specific group such as children, athletes, actors, healers, or firefighters? How often do you want to teach? Is monetary compensation a consideration? At this phase in your development as a teacher, what teaching experiences do you think will most help you to further develop your skills? How do you want to share the gift of yoga? With clarity in each of these areas, consider these opportunities:

- *Informal classes:* Whether at home, in your workplace, or in another setting, this is among the best ways to get started with teaching. Here you can work out your sequencing, pacing, voice, music, adjustment, and most of the other skills you will need when teaching public classes. When the feeling is right, put out a donation box or set a price for classes. You might decide a home studio is right for you.
- *Substitute teaching:* Teachers on the regular schedule of yoga studios invariably miss classes, creating a steady demand for substitute teachers. As with apprenticeships, substitute teaching opportunities usually come from existing relationships with studios and teachers. Still, ask the studio director or other teachers about the studio's teacher-substitution policy. Many studios leave it up to individual teachers to find their own substitutes, while others

have an established substitute teacher list, some in order of preference in accordance with the regular teacher's style or requests. Compensation is usually set at some minimum for all substitutes.

- *Yoga studios:* Considered the plum of the teaching profession, teaching in a yoga studio offers you the opportunity to work with motivated students in a supportive setting. It ties you into the studio's culture, opening up new relationships with other teachers. As one of the most sought-after settings, there is often strong (even if unspoken) competition over time slots on the schedule at a yoga studio. Most studios give the best time slots to their most popular teachers (or to the studio owners). More than any other setting, teaching at a yoga studio depends on relationships and recognition of your potential as a teacher. Patience, perseverance, and popularity are usually the keys to moving from a challenging to a favorable time slot. Compensation varies considerably, usually with a base (the amount you are paid regardless of how many students attend), plus a bonus (starting at some threshold such as ten or twenty students).

- *Health clubs:* Heath clubs, fitness centers, and spas are among the fastest growing employers of yoga teachers. As these businesses have increasingly recognized the yoga market, many have created dedicated spaces that are just as supportive as full-fledged yoga studios, although many offer yoga classes in the same space where others are working out with machines. In hiring teachers, health clubs tend to rely on proof of training and experience, including Yoga Alliance registration, more than existing relationships. Classes are often scheduled for less than one hour, and teacher compensation is usually set at a specific amount per class (with no bonus).

- *Professional settings:* Large companies and organizations such as hospitals and schools often provide yoga classes to their employees before or after work and even at lunchtime. Some even have dedicated yoga spaces and a full schedule of classes. If they don't offer classes, you might be able to propose a yoga program through their human resources department. In some professional settings, the yoga program is subsidized by the organization; in others, the teacher sets a price.

- *Recreation and wellness programs:* Most cities and towns have recreation centers offering a schedule of activities in multipurpose rooms that are available for rent. Contact the recreation department to find out about renting space and getting your classes on their calendar.

- *Alternative settings:* Schools, prisons, drug rehabilitation centers, mental health treatment facilities, halfway houses, juvenile institutions, hospitals, hospices, senior citizen centers, veterans facilities, and many other settings are often open to yoga and other recreational, healing, and meditative arts programs. See Chapter Eleven for more on what is involved in teaching in these alternative settings. If you are not aware of an existing program in your area, take the initiative by contacting the facility to explore offering classes. Although usually done on a voluntary basis, many facilities come to so appreciate the effects of the yoga classes that they find a way to provide funding for both props and teacher compensation.

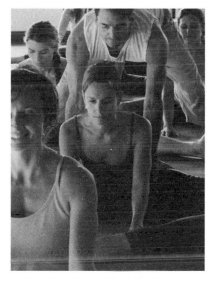

- *Private clients:* Many teachers prefer working one-on-one with students, and many students are either unable to attend public classes or prefer private instruction. In setting up private classes, use your intuition (and ask around) to ensure that the prospective private client has positive motives. If you are unsure of the student's motives, explain that you will bring an assistant; this usually dissuades those with ill motives. Set a standard rate (hourly or per class) and consider a surcharge to cover your travel costs, then agree to the rate before setting up a schedule. Have a clear cancellation policy (usually twenty-four hours in advance). Depending on your market area and your reputation as a teacher, you can charge from $50 per hour to more than $200 per class.

CULTIVATING ABUNDANCE: GETTING YOURSELF OUT THERE

Many yoga teachers have other sources of livelihood and teach yoga as an honored hobby. But many others are open to gaining a financial livelihood in exchange for their work as a teacher. The purpose of marketing is to let others know what you have to offer and to encourage them to try it out. The idea is to get the word out in places where you are most likely to communicate with prospective students. With time, your most effective marketing will be your reputation, which will spread wider than you can imagine through the oldest marketing tool in history: word of mouth. Meanwhile, here are several ways to publicize your classes:[1]

- *Flyers:* If you are new to teaching in the area, place flyers around town in spots where you think your potential students frequent, including health food stores, alternative healing centers, and community centers. Make sure the design of the flyer reflects your intention as a teacher.

- *Free class cards:* This can be your professional business card, with the words *first class free* appearing prominently. Go to every business in your neighborhood and ask if you can leave a stack of cards near their cash register, and while you are at it, invite the store staff to take a class for free.

- *Calendar listings:* Most local newspapers (daily and weekly) offer free calendar listings of upcoming events. Keep your listings simple and clear.

- *Web site:* Web sites are increasingly easy and inexpensive to set up and maintain. They are a great way to provide more detailed information about your classes, background, and other topics that you feel will attract students to your classes.

- *Social media:* Online social networking sites such as Facebook, Twitter, and Daily Om offer effective and essentially free resources for promoting yourself as a teacher.

- *Professional résumé:* Include all of your relevant training, including workshops, classes, conference attendance, CPR, and anything you've done that has involved teaching (even if it's topics such as physics or drawing). Be honest while highlighting your strengths. Include a list of your most influential teachers and note which ones are your references.

PRESERVING ABUNDANCE: LIABILITY INSURANCE

Accidents happen. So do unintended consequences of completely responsible actions. In either case, there can be liability. If you are teaching exclusively in a studio or health club, you might be covered by the company's liability policy. Even if you are, you still might want to have your own policy to cover private instruction and help to ease your way into other teaching opportunities, including workshops and retreats.

Here are the three major providers of insurance for yoga teachers:

Fitness and Wellness Insurance
380 Stevens Avenue, Suite 206
Solana Beach, CA 92075
Phone: 800-395-8075
Web site: www.fitnessandwellness.com

Sports & Fitness Insurance Corporation
214 Key Drive, Suite A
Madison, MS 39110
Phone: 800-844-0536
Web site: www.sportsfitness.com

Venbrook Insurance
22801 Ventura Boulevard, Third Floor
Woodland Hills, CA 91364
Phone: 800-991-3080
E-mail: sports@venbrook.com
Web site: www.myfitnessinsurance.com

REGULATION OF THE PROFESSION

In the mid-1990s, the rapidly expanding yoga profession caught the attention of several state legislatures and regulators, whose hearings and investigations raised the potential for state licensing and oversight. The ostensible motive, fueled in part by media reports of student injuries and abuse, was concern over student safety. With professions such as cosmetology, dental hygiene, and therapeutic massage under regulation, many considered yoga fair game for regulatory oversight. But one central question and obstacle revolved around the definition of yoga and just what was to be regulated: was it just physical yoga or all forms, including bhakti and meditation? This scrutiny of the yoga profession soon dissipated, in part because of demonstrable initiatives from within the yoga community to set professional standards for teacher training. In the late 1990s, Unity in Yoga, a conference organizer, merged with the Ad Hoc Yoga Alliance to create the Yoga Alliance, which two years earlier had begun working on creating minimum standards for yoga teachers. Despite opposition from within the yoga community, the new Yoga Alliance quickly gained traction among leading yoga media, schools, and teachers (although many never joined in and some continue to reject Yoga Alliance's self-anointed leadership role).

Yoga Alliance now sets forth widely recognized minimum standards for yoga teachers and teacher-training programs, including the minimum number of hours of training in each of five areas: (1) teaching methods, (2) techniques, (3) anatomy and physiology (including subtle energy), (4) philosophy and lifestyle, and (5) practice teaching. Schools whose curriculum meets or exceeds Yoga Alliance's minimum standards may apply to become a Registered Yoga School (RYS) at the two-hundred-hour or five-hundred-hour level, and teachers who graduate from an RYS are automatically eligible to register as a Registered Yoga Teacher (RYT) at the two-hundred-hour or five-hundred-hour level. In 2005, Yoga Alliance began recognizing and registering teachers with significant experience beyond basic training as Experienced Registered Yoga Teachers (E-RYT 200 or E-RYT 500). Registration with Yoga Alliance confers legitimacy as a yoga teacher and helps open the doors of the profession through easier access to liability insurance and professional teaching positions. Yoga Alliance promotes the following ethical code of conduct for all yoga teachers and schools:

1. Uphold the integrity of my vocation by conducting myself in a professional and conscientious manner.
2. Acknowledge the limitations of my skills and scope of practice and where appropriate, refer students to seek alternative instruction, advice, treatment, or direction.
3. Create and maintain a safe, clean, and comfortable environment for the practice of yoga.
4. Encourage diversity actively by respecting all students regardless of age, physical limitations, race, creed, gender, ethnicity, religion affiliation, or sexual orientation.
5. Respect the rights, dignity, and privacy of all students.
6. Avoid words and actions that constitute sexual harassment.
7. Adhere to the traditional yoga principles as written in the yamas and niyamas.
8. Follow all local government and national laws that pertain to my yoga teaching and business.

In 2009, several state finance directors, led by New Jersey, discovered Yoga Alliance's state-by-state registry of yoga schools and teachers and began a process to require state registration and licensing fees. This has resurrected the decade-old discussion and debate over the basic questions of regulation and oversight. While little is settled, Yoga Alliance, schools, and teachers continue navigating a professional path that is increasingly in the spotlight of the media, governments, and the ultimate beneficiaries of yoga—students. Along the path and certainly in the end what will most matter is how yoga teachers and schools choose to conduct themselves. In this, schools, teachers, and students are blessed by a richly interconnected community of mutual interest and support.

THE PATH OF THE TEACHER

Teaching yoga is an extension of practicing yoga. Whether you are just stepping onto the teaching path or have spent many years there maturing into a mentor teacher, as you practice so you discover anew the essence of yoga as a tool for self-transformation. Like in the practice, in teaching there are unlimited opportunities for seeing more clearly, feeling more fully, and living more happily. Teaching is also an extension of your larger life, for how you live is expressed in your teaching. Committing to this path will deepen your personal practice and bring yoga more into every aspect of your life.[2] Doing this consciously—making a considered and deliberate decision to teach yoga rather than casually assuming the role of a teacher—will make every part of your teaching practice a more natural expression of who you are as a person while allowing you to sustain yourself more simply in the teaching profession.

Your students will always be your best teachers. Listen to them, to what they say, and to what they don't say. Opening yourself with patience and compassion to how every student offers unique insights into the practice of doing and guiding yoga will help keep you grounded in the realities of your students. Your most challenging student may be your most relevant teacher. Honor, respect, and tap into these insights; they are the most essential foundation for being the best possible teacher.

Stay with your personal practice. Many yoga teachers become so consumed by teaching that their own practice fades. Not only is your practice a vital part of a balanced and healthy lifestyle, it is a bottomless well of experience for exploring and clarifying most of the questions that will arise in your teaching. Keep going back to that source. Beware of the common tendency among teachers to think you have done a practice by demonstrating asanas in the classes that you teach; it is not the same as when you are wholly focused in doing a yoga practice. Remembering Pattabhi Jois's oft-quoted statement that yoga is ninety-nine percent practice and one percent theory, do the practice, and the theory!

Everything in life has a rhythm. As you explore along the path of teaching, take time to pause and reflect on how you are feeling amid the shifting rhythms of your experience. Notice the changing terrain, whether it is new places, different students, or the evolution of your thinking and personal experience of the practice. Like pausing when empty of breath and sensing more clarity, occasionally take a break from teaching to gain deeper insight into how you are approaching the craft. Be as clear as you can in your motivation to teach. Allow the inevitable challenges that arise in teaching to be raw material for your personal development, always opening yourself to refining your teaching just as you help students to refine their practice of yoga.

Keep breathing. Namaste.

YOGA TEACHING RESOURCES

ONLINE RESOURCES

The Teaching Yoga Web site

www.markstephensyoga.com/teachingyoga.html

Developed in conjunction with this book, the Teaching Yoga Web site offers video vignettes showing hands-on adjustments, use of props, modifications, and variations for 108 asanas along with timely articles and a blog covering the art and science of teaching yoga.

Yoga Journal

www.yogajournal.com

The most comprehensive yoga Web site, its searchable database offers free access to articles from *Yoga Journal.* There is extensive information on all aspects of yoga, and a special section for teachers.

Human Anatomy

www.innerbody.com

Each topic has animations, hundreds of graphics, and thousands of descriptive links.

L.A. Yoga—Ayurveda and Health Magazine

www.layogamagazine.com

L.A. Yoga Magazine covers the practice and culture of yoga, ayurveda, and health.

Moving into Stillness

www.movingintostillness.com

Founded by Erich Schiffmann, this Web site offers online message boards with over three thousand registered users and nearly one hundred new messages posted each day.

Namarupa—Categories of Indian Thought Magazine

www.namarupa.org

Namarupa conveys the vast scope of sacred philosophical thought of India.

Pubmed

www.ncbi.nlm.nih.gov/pubmed

Searchable database for journal articles related to health, yoga, and related topics.

Yoga Directory

www.yogadirectory.com

Searchable database and links to yoga studios, teachers, events, and job opportunities.

Yoga Finder

www.yogafinder.com

Search engine geared towards finding numerous topics related to yoga, such as retreat centers, teacher training, and yoga opportunities. Post your yoga classified on this Web site.

Yoga Site

www.yogasite.com

Information on a wide-ranging areas relating to yoga; free teacher listings.

Yoga + Joyful Living Magazine

www.himalayaninstitute.org/yogaplus

Yoga + Joyful Living magazine delves deep into every aspect of conscious living, presenting time-honored practices and showing us how to apply them to our daily lives.

Yoga Tribe and Culture Films

www.ytcfims.com

The leading production company for innovative yoga, healing arts, and movement arts DVDs, YTC Films has produced over fifty original programs since 2006, including the best-selling Shiva Rea and Hemalaya Behl DVDs. An excellent media production resource for yoga teachers.

PROFESSIONAL ASSOCIATIONS

Most countries have independent yoga associations that vary quite widely in purpose, with some designed primarily for networking and others involved in setting standards for teacher training and certification.

British Wheel of Yoga

www.bwy.org.uk

> Founded in 1969, BWY is the United Kingdom's official governing body for yoga; it encourages and helps teachers to a greater knowledge and understanding of all aspects of yoga and its practice by provision of study, education, and training, sets standards for teacher training and certification, and maintains a regional networking and governance structure.

Iyengar Yoga National Association of the United States

www.iynaus.org

> Their mission is to disseminate and promote the art, science, and philosophy of yoga according to the teachings of B. K. S. Iyengar. The association oversees teacher training guidelines, holds annual certification assessments, and maintains a code of ethics for its teachers. IYNAUS also maintains an archive of Iyengar yoga materials and a national directory of certified teachers.

California Yoga Teachers Association

www.yogateachersassoc.org

> Founded in 1973 by a group of yoga teachers who wanted to connect and support each other through education and friendship, CYTA members later founded *Yoga Journal,* now a leading resource for the yoga community. Currently, CYTA functions as a not-for-profit foundation providing financial support for the Yoga Dana Foundation, a charitable institution described below.

Green Yoga Association

www.greenyoga.org

> The Green Yoga Association is dedicated to fostering ecological consciousness, reverence, and action in the yoga community through conferences and educational outreach.

International Association of Yoga Therapists

www.iayt.org

> IAYT supports research and education in yoga and serves as a professional organization for yoga teachers and yoga therapists worldwide. Its mission is to establish yoga as a recognized and respected therapy. IAYT also serves members, the media, and the general public as a source of information about contemporary yoga education, research, and statistics.

International Kundalini Yoga Teachers Association

www.kundaliniyoga.com

> IKYTA is a professional association to foster community, standards, and training for Kundalini yoga teachers.

Yoga Alliance

www.yogaalliance.org

> Yoga Alliance's mission is to lead the yoga community, set standards, foster integrity, provide resources, and uphold the teachings of yoga. It is the leading source for yoga teacher-training curriculum standards. They maintain a national Yoga Teachers Registry to recognize and promote teachers with training that meets Yoga Alliance standards. Teachers registered with Yoga Alliance are authorized to use the initials RYT (Registered Yoga Teacher) or the initials E-RYT (Experienced Registered Yoga Teacher) if they have significant teaching experience in addition to training. The registries are advertised and promoted to (a) the general public, (b) organizations that employ yoga teachers, and (c) organizations that review yoga teachers' credentials (hospitals, health insurance companies, governmental organizations, etc.).

Canadian Yoga Alliance

www.canadianyogicalliance.com

> A national alliance of yoga teachers and practitioners developed primarily for networking and sharing of professional resources.

INSTITUTES AND RESEARCH CENTERS

Esalen Institute

www.esalen.org

> Esalen is a place, as Thomas Wolfe said about America, where miracles not only happen, but where they happen all the time. And then there are the people—the people who live there and love the land, and the 300,000 more who have come from all over the world to participate in Esalen's forty-year-long Olympics of the body, mind, and spirit, committing themselves not so much to "stronger, faster, higher" as to deeper, richer, and more enduring.

Himalayan Institute

www.himalayaninstitute.org

> A leader in the field of yoga, meditation, spirituality, and holistic health, the Himalayan Institute was founded by Swami Rama. The mission of the Himalayan

Institute is to discover and embrace the sacred spirit of human heritage that unites East and West, spirituality and science, and ancient wisdom and modern technology.

Kripalu Center for Yoga and Health
www.kripalu.org

Kripalu is a nonprofit educational organization dedicated to promoting the art and science of yoga to produce thriving and healthy individuals and society. For more than thirty years, Kripalu has been teaching skills for optimal living through experiential education for the whole person: body, mind, and spirit. It is among the largest and most established retreat centers for yoga, health, and holistic living in North America.

Omega Institute for Holistic Studies
www.eomega.org

Omega Institute is among the nation's most trusted sources for wellness and personal growth. Omega offers diverse and innovative educational experiences that inspire an integrated approach to personal and social change. Located in Rhinebeck, New York, Omega welcomes more than 23,000 people to its workshops, conferences, and retreats in the Hudson Valley and at exceptional locations around the world.

White Lotus Foundation
www.whitelotus.org

White Lotus Foundation, created in 1967 by Ganga White, is one of the most established schools of yogic thought and practice today. Located in the mountains overlooking Santa Barbara, California, this renowned 40-acre retreat center is an oasis for yoga where Ganga and his wife, codirector, Tracey Rich, train teachers and students of all levels through a process of inquiry and self-expression that has nurtured many of the world's top teachers. Ganga is author of *Yoga Beyond Belief: Insights to Awaken and Deepen Your Practice.*

Yoga Research and Education Foundation
www.yref.org

Founded by Georg Feuerstein, YREF is a California nonprofit tax exempt 501(c)(3) educational corporation. YREF's primary objective is to conduct and promote research in any and all aspects of yoga.

YOGA STYLES AND TRADITIONS

Ananda Yoga
www.anandayoga.org

Anusara Yoga
www.anusara.com

Ashtanga Vinyasa Yoga
www.ashtanga.com

Bikram Yoga
www.bikramyoga.com

Integral Yoga
www.iyiva.com

Iyengar Yoga
www.iynaus.org

Kundalini Yoga
www.kundaliniyoga.com

Power Yoga
www.poweryoga.com
www.baronbaptiste.com

Sivananda Yoga
www.sivananda.org

Vinyasa Flow Yoga
www.markstephensyoga.com
www.seanecorn.com
www.shivarea.com

Yin Yoga
www.paulgrilley.com
www.sarahpowers.com

Yoga Therapy
www.iayt.org
www.kym.org
www.viniyoga.com

NONPROFIT YOGA SERVICE ORGANIZATIONS

Art of Yoga Project

www.theartofyogaproject.org

> The Art of Yoga Project leads teen girls in the juvenile justice system toward accountability to self, others, and community by providing practical tools to effect behavioral change.

Lineage Project

www.lineageproject.org

> The Lineage Project teaches at-risk and incarcerated New York City teenagers awareness-based practices to help consciously manage stress, increase self-awareness, and cultivate compassion and commitment to nonviolent engagement with their communities.

Off the Mat, Into the World

www.offthematintotheworld.org

> OTM is a program that aims to inspire and guide you to find and define your purpose and become active in your local or global community in an effective, sustainable, and joyful way. OTM is an educational, experiential, and motivational process for those interested in conscious activism and service.

Street Yoga

www.streetyoga.org

> Street Yoga teaches yoga, mindfulness, and compassionate communication to youth and families struggling with homelessness, poverty, abuse, addiction, trauma, and psychiatric issues.

The Yoga Group: Yoga for HIV/AIDS

www.yogagroup.org

> The Yoga Group provides free yoga classes to people living with HIV/AIDS and shares related information with yoga teachers and the poz community.

Yoga Dana Foundation

www.yogadanafoundation.org

> Yoga Dana Foundation was formed in 2007 as a not-for-profit charitable organization whose mission is to support yoga teachers who bring yoga to underserved communities. Yoga Dana Foundation is funded by grants from the California Yoga Teachers Association.

Yoga Ed.

www.yogaed.com

> Yoga Ed. develops and produces health and wellness programs, trainings, and products for teachers, parents, children, and health professionals that improve academic achievement, physical fitness, emotional intelligence, and stress management.

Yoga for the Special Child

www.specialyoga.com

> Yoga for the Special Child is a comprehensive program of yoga techniques designed to enhance the natural development of children with special needs.

GLOSSARY

a. "non-," as in ahimsa, nonviolence

abductor. muscle that draws a bone away from the midline of the body

adductor. muscle that draws a bone toward the midline of the body

adho. downward

adho mukha. downward facing

afflictions. the five forms of suffering (kleshas)

agni. fire

ahimsa. nonviolence; not hurting

ajna chakra. third-eye chakra

akarna. to the ear

anahata chakra. heart chakra

ananda. ecstasy; bliss; love

anjali mudra. the gesture of anjali, palms together at the heart

Anjaneya. the monkey god

antara. internal

antara kumbhaka. holding your breath after inhalation

anterior. forward, in front

anuloma. with the grain; refers to movement or breathing

apana. pelvis or lower abdomen

apanasana. pelvic floor poses

apana-vayu. the neurological force operating on the lower abdomen

aparigraha. freedom from hoarding or collecting

ardha. half

asana. to take one seat; a yoga pose; the third limb of ashtanga

Astavakra. an Indian sage and Sanskrit scholar; the asana Astavakrasana named for him

asteya. not stealing

atman. the true self; consciousness

aum. first described in the Upanishads as the originating and all-encompassing sound of the universe; alternately spelled *om*

avidya. ignorance

ayurveda. ancient Indian science; traditional form of Indian medicine

baddha. bound

bahya. external

bahya kumbhaka. suspension of the breath after complete exhalation

baka. crane

bandha. to bind; energetic engagement

bhadra. peaceful or auspicious

Bhagavad Gita. "Song of the Lord," a chapter in the epic Mahabharata and the most influential of all *shastras*

bhakti. the practice of devotion

Bharadvaj. an Indian sage

Bharirava. an aspect of Shiva

bhastrika. bellows used in a furnace; type of pranayama where air is forcibly drawn in and out through the nostrils

bhaya. fear

bheka. frog

bhuja. arm or shoulder

bhujanga. cobra

bhujapida. pressure on the arm or shoulder

Brahma. God; the supreme being; the creator; the first deity of the Hindu trinity

brahmacharya. celibacy or right use of sexual energy; one of the yamas

brahman. infinite consciousness

buddhi. intellect, seat of intelligence

cervical spine. the vertebrae of the neck

chakra. subtle energy center

chandra. moon

danda. staff or stick

dhanu. bow

dharana. mental concentration; the sixth limb of Patanjali's ashtanga yoga

dharma. virtuous duty

dhyana. meditation

dristi. gazing point

dukha. pain; sorrow; grief

dwi. two

eka. one

ekagrata. one-pointed mental focus

eka pada. one-legged or one-footed

extension. movement of a joint whereby one part of the body is moved away from another

flexion. bending movement that decreases the angle between two points

Galava. an Indian sage

garuda. eagle; name of the king of birds. Garuda is represented as a vehicle of
Vishnu and as having a white face, an aquiline beak, red wings, and a golden
body.

Gheranda. a sage, the author of the Gheranda Samhita, a classical work on
Hatha yoga

gomukha. cow head

guna. literally "rope," it refers to something that binds; in reference to yoga, it
refers to the three intertwined fundamental properties inherent in all
phenomena: sattva, rajas, tamas.

guru. gee, you are you; a spiritual preceptor, one who illuminates the spiritual
path

hala. plough

Hanuman. a monkey god, son of Anjaneya and Vayu

hasta. hand or arm

Hatha yoga. physical purification practices first described in written form in the
fourteenth century CE in the Hatha Yoga Pradipika

humerus. upper arm bone

hyperextension. extension of a joint beyond 180 degrees

ida. a nadi or channel of energy starting from the left nostril, moving to the
crown of the head, and descending to the base of the spine

insertion of muscles. end of the muscles that is distant from the center of the
body

Ishvara. the supreme being; brahman with form

isometric exercise. exercise in which the muscles do not get shortened

isotonic exercise. exercise that involves shortening of a muscle

jalandhara bandha. the chin lock where the chin is drawn toward the
collarbones

janu. knee

jathara. belly

jnana. sacred knowledge derived from meditation on higher truths of religion
and philosophy, which teaches people how to understand their own nature.

kapala. skull

kapalabhati. skull cleansing, a pranayama technique

kapha. one of the three ayurvedic humors

kapota. pigeon, dove

karma. action

karma yoga. the yoga of action

karna. ear

karnapida. ears squeezed

klesha. suffering through ignorance, egoism, desire, hatred, or fear

kona. angle

Koundinya. a sage

krama. sequence of moments; succession of moments

Krishna. a form of God

kriya. a purification process

krouncha. heron

kukkuta. rooster

kumbhaka. breath retention after a complete inhalation or exhalation

kundalini. pranic energy, symbolized as a coiled and sleeping serpent lying
    dormant in the lowest nerve center at the base of the spinal column; a form
    of Hatha yoga practice

kurma. turtle

kyphosis. forward curvature of the spine

laghu. simple; little; small; handsome

lateral. sideways; away from the midline of the body

lateral rotation. see external rotation

laya. to merge

lola. to swing or dangle

lordosis. backward curvature of the spine

lumbar spine. the vertebrae of the lower back

mahabandha. the great lock

Mahabharata. a major Sanskrit epic of ancient India; contains the Bhagavad Gita
    and major elements of Hindu mythology

maha mudra. the great seal

mala. garland, wreath

manos. the individual mind

mandala. spiritually significant concentric form used for meditation and rituals

manduka. frog

manipura chakra. navel chakra

mantra. sacred sound, thought, or prayer

Marichi. name of a sage who is one of the sons of Brahma

Matsyendra. lord of the fishes; a tantric adept

mayura. peacock

medial. toward the midline of the body

medial rotation. see *internal rotation*

moksha. liberation

mudra. seal; hand and finger positions or a specific combination of asana, pranayama, and bandha

mukha. face

mula. root, base

mula bandha. root lock; energetic engagement; sustained lifting of the perineum and levator ani

muladhara chakra. root chakra

nadi. literally "river"; energy channel

nadi sodhana. purification or cleansing of the nadis; pranayama technique for this purpose

nakra. crocodile

namaskara. salutation; greeting

nara. man

naravirala. sphinx

Nataraja. dancing Shiva

nauli. physical purification technique involving churning the belly

nava. boat

nidra. sleep

niyama. second limb Patanjali's eight-limbed path; consists of saucha, santosa, tapas, svadhyaya, and ishvarapranidhana

origin of a muscle. end of a muscle that is closer to the body center

pada. foot or leg

pada hasta. hand(s) to feet

padangustha. big toe

padma. lotus

parigha. gate

parigraha. hoarding

paripurna. full

parivrtta. crossed; with a twist

parsva. side; flank; lateral

paschimo. west; the backside of the body

phalaka. plank

pincha. chin; feather

pinda. fetus or embryo; body

pingala. a nadi or channel or energy starting from the right nostril, moving to the crown of the head and downward to the base of the spine

pitta. one of the three ayurvedic humors, sometimes translated as "bile" posterior. backward, opposite of anterior

prakriti. nature; the original source of the material world, consisting of sattva, rajas, and tamas

prana. life force; sometimes refers to the breath

pranayama. rhythmic yogic breathing; breath extension; the fourth limb of ashtanga

prasarana. sweeping movement of the arms

prasarita. spread out; stretched out

prasvasa. expiration

pratikriyasana. counterpose

pratiloma. against the hair; against the grain

pratyahara. independence of the mind from sensory stimulation; the fifth stage of ashtanga

prishta. back

puraka. inhalation

purna. complete

pursvo. east; the front of the body

pursvottana. the intense stretch of the front side of the body

raga. love, passion, anger

raja. king, ruler

rajakapota. king pigeon

rajas. impulsive or chaotic thought; the aspect of movement in nature; one of the three gunas

rechaka. exhalation, emptying of the lungs

sadhana. practice for achievement

sahasrara chakra. thousand-petaled lotus, located in the cerebral cavity

sahita. aided

sahita-kumbhaka. intentional suspension of breath

salabha. locust

salamba. with support

sama. equal; same

samadhana. mental peace

samadhi. bliss; meditative absorption

samasthihi. a state of balance

samskara. subconscious imprint

samyama. combined application of dharana, dhyana, and samadhi

santosa. contentment

sarvanga. the whole body

sattva. light/order; one of the three elements of prakriti

saucha. purity; cleanliness

sava. corpse

setu bandha. bridge

Shakti. life force, prana; consort of Shiva

shishula. dolphin

simha. lion

sirsa. head

sitali. a cooling form of pranayama

slumpasana. habitual collapse of the heart center associated with lackadaisical
slumping of the spine and torso

sukham. comfort; ease; pleasure

supta. supine; sleeping

surya. the sun

sushumna. central energy channel, located in the spinal column

svadhisthana chakra. seat of vital force, situated above the organs of generation

svana. dog

svasa. inspiration

Svatmarama. author of the Hatha Yoga Pradipika, the original book on Hatha
yoga

tada. mountain

tamas. dullness; inertia; ignorance; one of the three gunas

tantra. the practice of using all energies, including the mundane, for spiritual
awakening

tapa. austerity

tapas. heat; burning effort that involves purification, self-discipline, and
austerity

thoracic spine. the vertebrae of the rib cage

tibia. shinbone

tiriang mukha. backward-facing

tittibha. firefly

tola. balance; scales

tri. three

trikona. triangle

ubhaya. both

udana. a prana vayu

uddiyana. upward flying; a bandha

uddiyana bandha. drawing the lower abdominal core in and up

ujjayi. victorious

ujjayi pranayama. basic yogic breathing

Upanishads. to sit down by a guru to receive spiritual instruction; the core
teachings of Vedanta

upavista. seated with legs spread

urdhva. upward

ustra. camel

utkata. awkward; powerful; fierce

utpluti. lifting or pumping up

uttana. upright intense stretch

Uttanasana. forward bend

utthita. extended

vajra. thunderbolt

vakra. crooked

Vasistha. a Vedic sage

vata. one of the three ayurvedic humors, sometimes translated as "wind"

vayu. wind; vital air current

Vedanta. literally "end of the Vedas"; the dominant Hindu philosophical
tradition

Vedas. oldest sacred texts of humankind

vidya. knowledge; learning; lore; science

viloma. against the hair; against the order of things

vinyasa. to place in a special way; the conscious connection of breath and
movement

viparita. inverted; upside-down

vira. hero, brave

Virabhadra. a warrior

vishuddha chakra. pure; situated in the pharyngeal region

vrksa. tree

vrschika. scorpion

vyana. a prana vayu

yama. restraint; contain; the first of the eight limbs of ashtanga yoga

yoga. from the root *yuj,* meaning "to join," "to yoke," "to make whole"

yoga-robics. workout routines utilizing yoga asanas for purely physical exercise

LIST OF ASANAS

There is remarkable inconsistency in the names, pronunciation, physical forms, and descriptions of poses as described in the yoga literature. Different styles, traditions, lineages, teachers, books, and articles often give completely different names to the same physical form, or use the same name for different poses. Here we have drawn primarily from the most widely recognized sources, including *Yoga Journal*, B. K. S. Iyengar's *Light on Yoga*, and David Swenson's *Ashtanga Yoga*.

TABLE C—**Asanas**

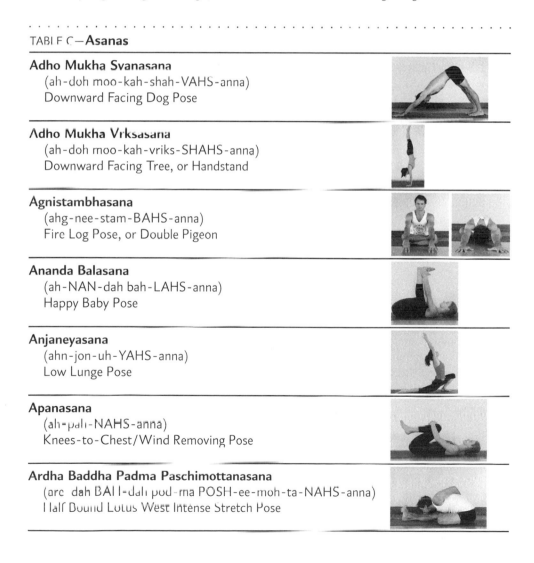

Adho Mukha Svanasana
  (ah-doh moo-kah-shah-VAHS-anna)
  Downward Facing Dog Pose

Adho Mukha Vrksasana
  (ah-doh moo-kah-vriks-SHAHS-anna)
  Downward Facing Tree, or Handstand

Agnistambhasana
  (ahg-nee-stam-BAHS-anna)
  Fire Log Pose, or Double Pigeon

Ananda Balasana
  (ah-NAN-dah bah-LAHS-anna)
  Happy Baby Pose

Anjaneyasana
  (ahn-jon-uh-YAHS-anna)
  Low Lunge Pose

Apanasana
  (ah-pah-NAHS-anna)
  Knees-to-Chest/Wind Removing Pose

Ardha Baddha Padma Paschimottanasana
  (are-dah BAH-dah pod-ma POSH-ee-moh-ta-NAHS-anna)
  Half Bound Lotus West Intense Stretch Pose

Ardha Baddha Padmottanasana
  (are-dah BAH-dah pod-mo-TAH-nahs-anna)
  Half-Bound Lotus Intense Stretch Pose

Ardha Chandrasana
  (are-dah chan-DRAHS-anna)
  Half Moon Pose

Ardha Matsyendrasana
  (are-dah MOT-see-en-DRAHS-anna
  Half Lord of the Fishes Pose

Ardha Uttanasana
  (are-dah OOT-tan-AHS-anna)
  Half Forward Fold

Ashta Chandrasana
  (ahsh-ta chan-DRAHS-anna)
  Eight Crescent Moon Pose

Ashtanga Pranam
  (ahsh-TAHN-gah pra-NAHM)
  Eight-Limbed Prostration

Astavakrasana
  (ah-stah-vah-KRAHS-anna)
  Eight-Angle Pose

Baddha Konasana
  (BAH-dah cone-AHS-anna)
  Bound Angle Pose

Baddha Padmasana
  (BAH-dah pod-MAHS-anna)
  Bound Lotus Pose

Bakasana
  (bahk-AHS-anna)
  Crane Pose

Balasana
  (bah-LAHS-anna)
  Child's Pose

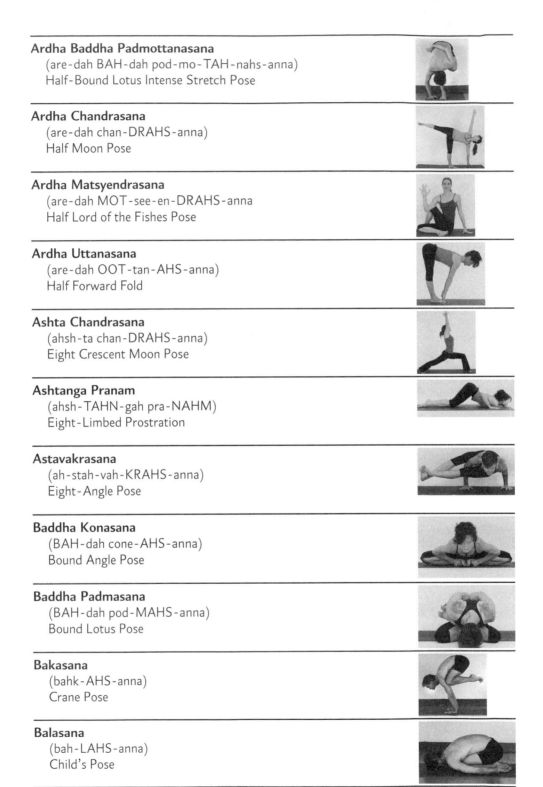

Bharadvajrasana
(bah-ROD-va-JAHS-anna)
Bharadvajra's Pose

Bhekasana
(beh-KAS-anna)
Frog Pose

Bhujangasana
(boo-jang-GAHS-anna)
Cobra Pose

Bhujapidasana
(boo-jah-pee-DAHS-anna)
Shoulder Pressing Pose

Chaturanga Dandasana
(chaht-ah-RON-gah don-DAHS-anna)
Four-Limbed Staff Pose

Dandasana
(don-DAHS-anna)
Staff Pose

Dhanurasana
(don-your-AHS-anna)
Bow Pose

Dwi Pada Koundinyasana
(DWEE pah-DAH koon-din-YAHS-anna)
Two Footed Koundinya's Pose

Eka Pada Koundinyasana
(eh-KAH pah-DAH koon-din-YAHS-anna)
One Footed Koundinya's Pose

Eka Pada Raj Kapotasana
(eh-KAH pah-DAH rahj cop-oh-TAHS-anna)
One Legged King Pigeon Pose

Eka Pada Sirsasana
(eh-KAH pah-DAH shear-SHAHS-anna)
One Foot Behind the Head Pose

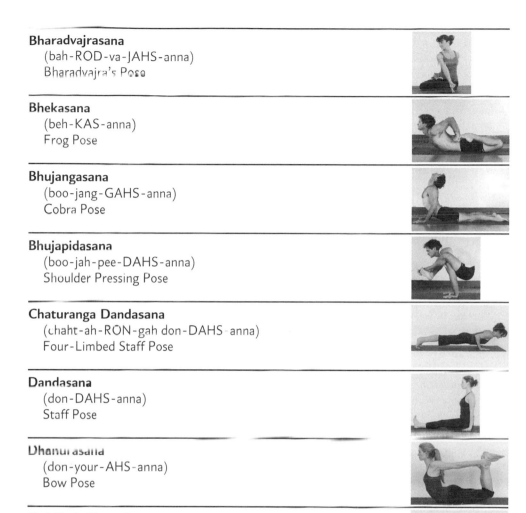

Eka Pada Viparita Dandasana
   (eh-KAH pah-DAH vee-pah-REE-tah don-DAHS-anna)
   One Foot Inverted Staff Pose

Galavasana
   (gah-LAH-vos-anna)
   Flying Crow Pose

Garudasana
   (gah-rue-DAHS-anna)
   Eagle Pose

Gomukhasana
   (go-moo-KAHS-anna)
   Cow Face Pose

Halasana
   (hah-LAHS-anna)
   Plow Pose

Hanumanasana
   (hah-new-mah-NAHS-anna)
   Monkey Pose

Janu Sirsasana
   (JAH-new shear-SHAHS-anna)
   Head to Knee Forward Bend Pose

Jathara Parivartanasana
   (JAT-hara par-var-tan-AHS-anna)
   Revolving Twist Pose

Kapotasana
   (cop-oh-TAHS-anna)
   Pigeon Pose

Karnapidasana
   (car-NAH-pee-DAHS-anna)
   Knees to Ears Pose

Krounchasana
   (crown-CHAHS-anna)
   Heron Pose

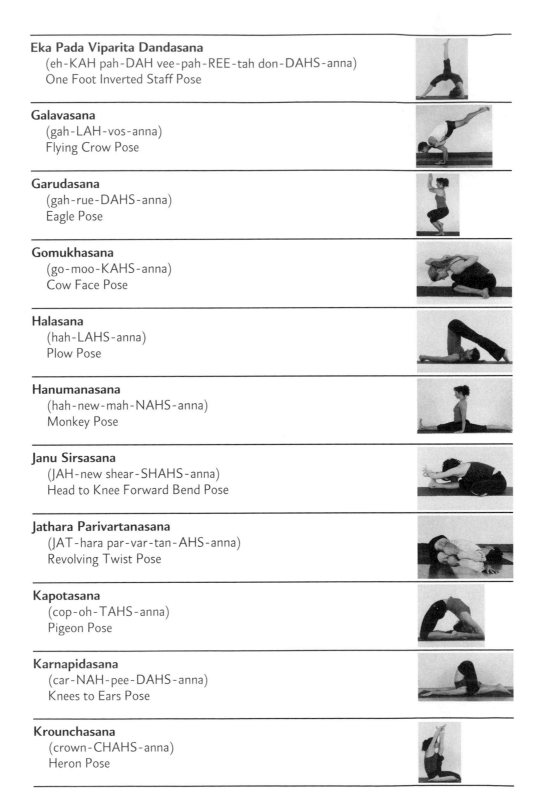

Kurmasana
(core-MAHS-anna)
Tortoise Pose

Laghu Vajrasana
(lah-gu VAJ rahs-anna)
Little Thunderbolt Pose

Lolasana
(lo-LAHS-anna)
Dangling Earring Pose

Marichyasana C
(mar-ee-chee-AHS-anna)
Marichi's Pose

Matsyasana
(mot-see-AHS-anna)
Fish Pose

Naraviralasana
(nah-VAHS-anna)
Sphinx Pose

Natarajasana
(nah-TAR-ah-JAHS-anna)
Dancer's Pose

Navasana
(nah-VAHS-anna)
Boat Pose

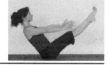

Padahasthasana
(PAH-dah haas-TAHS-anna)
Hands to Feet Pose

Padangusthasana
(PAH-da-goo-STAHS-anna)
Big Toe Pose

Padmasana
(pod MAHS anna)
Lotus Pose

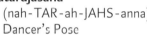

Parivrtta Ardha Chandrasana
   (par-ee-vri-tah ARE-dah chan-DRAHS-anna)
   Revolved Half Moon

Parivrtta Janu Sirsasana
   (par-ee-vri-tah JAH-new shear-SHAHS-anna)
   Revolved Head to Knee Pose

Parivrtta Parsvakonasana
   (par-ee-vri-tah pars-vah-ko-NAHS-anna)
   Revolved Side-Angle Pose

Parivrtta Trikonasana
   (par-ee-vri-tah tree-ko-NAHS-anna)
   Revolved Triangle Pose

Parsva Bakasana
   (pars-VAH bah-KAHS-anna)
   Side Crane Pose

Parsvottanasana
   (parsh-voh-tah-NAHS-anna)
   Intense Extended Side-Stretch Pose

Paschimottanasana
   (POSH-ee-moh-ta-NAHS-anna)
   Seated Forward Bend/West Stretching Pose

Phalakasana
   (pah-la-KAHS-anna)
   Plank Pose

Pincha Mayurasana
   (pin-cha my-yu-RAHS-anna)
   Feathered Peacock Pose

Pindasana
   (pin-DAHS-anna)
   Embryo Pose

Prasarita Padottanasana
   (pra-sa-REE-tah pah-doh-tah-NAHS-anna)
   Spread Leg Forward Fold

Pursvottanasana
(POOR-vo-ta-NAHS-anna
Upward Facing Plank/Eastern Intense Stretch Pose

Salabhasana A, B, C
(sha-la-BAHS-anna)
Locust Pose

Salamba Sarvangasana
(sha-LOM-bah sar-vahn-GAHS-anna)
Supported Shoulder Stand

Salamba Sirsasana I
(sha-LOM-bah shear-SHAHS-anna)
Supported Headstand I

Salamba Sirsasana II
(sha-LOM-bah shear-SHAHS-anna)
Supported Headstand II

Savasana
(shah-VAHS-anna)
Corpse Pose

Setu Bandhasana
(seh-too bahn-DAHS-anna)
Bound Bridge Pose, or Charlie Chaplin Pose

Setu Bandha Sarvangasana
(seh-too BAHN-dah sar-vahn-GAHS-anna)
Bridge Pose

Shishulasana
(SHE-shu-LAHS-anna)
Dolphin Pose

Supta Padangusthasana
(soup-TAH PAH-dahn-goo-STAHS-anna)
Reclining Big Toe Pose

Supta Parivartanasana
(soup-ta par-i-var-tan-AHS-anna)
Reclined Twist Pose

Supta Virasana
(soup-TAH veer-RAHS-anna)
Reclining Hero Pose

Tadasana
(tah-DAHS-anna)
Mountain Pose

Tiriang Mukha Eka Pada Paschimottanasana
(tear-ee-AHNG MOO-kah eh-KAH pah-dah
POSH-ee-moh-tahn-AHS-anna)
Three Limb Face One Foot Western Intense Stretch Pose

Tittibhasana
(tee-tee-BAHS-anna)
Firefly Pose

Tolasana
(toe-LAHS-anna)
Scales Pose

Upavista Konasana
(oo-pah-VEESH-tah ko-NAHS-anna)
Wide Angled Seated Forward Bend Pose

Urdhva Dhanurasana
(OORD-vah don-your-AHS-anna)
Upward Bow/Wheel Pose

Urdhva Kukkutasana
(OORD-vah koo-koo-TAHS-anna)
Upward Rooster Pose

Urdhva Mukha Svanasana
(URD-vah MOO-kah svah-NAHS-anna)
Upward Facing Dog

Urdhva Padmasana
(OORD-vah pod-MAHS-anna)
Upward Lotus Pose

Ustrasana
(oosh-TRAHS-anna)
Camel Pose

Utkatasana
(OOT-kah-TAHS-anna)
Awkward Pose, or Chair

Uttana Padasana
(OOT-anna pah-DAHS-anna)
Extended Leg Pose, or Flying Fish

Uttana Prasithasana
(OOT-annna pra-si-THAHS-anna)
Flying Lizard Pose

Uttanasana
(OOT-ta-NAHS-anna)
Standing Forward Bend

Utthita Hasta Padangusthasana
(oo-TEE-tah HAH-stah pah-dahn-goosh-TAHS-anna)
Extended Hand to Big Toe Pose

Utthita Parsvakonasana
(oo-TEE-tah pars-vah-ko-NAHS-anna)
Extended Side Angle Pose

Utthita Trikonasana
(oo-TEE-tah tree-ko-NAHS-anna)
Extended Triangle Pose

Vasisthasana
(vah-shish-TAHS-anna)
Side-Plank Pose

Viparita Dandasana
(vip-pah-ree-tah don-DAHS-anna)
Inverted Staff Pose

Viparita Karani
(vip-pah-ree-tah kuh-RAHN-ee)
Active Reversal, or Legs up the Wall

Virabhadrasana I
(veer-ah-bah-DRAHS-anna)
Warrior I Pose

Virabhadrasana II
   (veer-ah-bah-DRAHS-anna)
   Warrior II Pose

Virabhadrasana III
   (veer-ah-bah-DRAHS-anna)
   Warrior III Pose

Virasana
   (veer-RAHS-anna)
   Hero Pose

Vrksasana
   (vrik-SHAHS-anna)
   Tree Pose

ASANA ELEMENTS

TABLE D—**Sequencing Asanas**

ASANA	PREPARATION	INTEGRATION	EXPLORATION
Adho Mukha Svanasana	Anahatasana, Bidalasana, Phalakasana, Ardha Uttanasana, Uttanasana	Balasana, Apanasana, Supta Parivartanasana, Viparita Karani, Savasana	Use as a base for standing poses, to open the shoulders and chest for backbends and arm balances, and as preparation for full inversions.
Adho Mukha Vrksasana	Adho Mukha Svanasana, Tadasana, Phalakasana, Pincha Mayurasana, Supta Virasana, Garudasana arms, Gomukhasana arms	Uttanasana, Padahasth-asana, Balasana, wrist therapy (see Chapter 11)	Follow with Pincha Mayur-asana and Salamba Sirsasana I; release the feet overhead into Urdhva Dhanurasana; fold the legs into Padmasana and lower them to the shoulders into Urdhva Kukkutasana; scissor one leg forward and the other back and release into Hanumanasana.
Agnistambhasana	Gomukhasana, Eka Pada Raj Kapotasana Prep, Sukhasana, Baddha Konasana	Dandasana, Adho Mukha Svanasana, Virasana, Supta Virasana, Apanasana, Balasana	Follow with Eka Pada Raj Kapotasana A, B, C, Galavasana, Uttana Prasithasana, Padmasana, Urdhva Kukkutasana.
Ananda Balasana	Apanasana, Supta Padangusthasana	Apanasana, Viparita Karani	Extend the legs straight into a modified form of Supta Konasana.
Anjaneyasana	Adho Mukha Svanasana, Supta Padangusthasana, Apanasana, Ananda Balasana, Utkatasana, Prasarita Padottanasana, Virasana	Balasana, Adho Mukha Svanasana, Uttanasana	Use to open the hip flexors in preparation for backbends and arm balances in which the hips are extended; Ashta Chandrasana, Virabhadrasana I, Virabhadrasana III, Virasana, Supta Virasana, Hanumanasana.

ASANA	PREPARATION	INTEGRATION	EXPLORATION
Apanasana	Savasana, Virasana	Supta Baddha Konasana, Adho Mukha Svanasana	Ananda Balasana, Supta Padangusthasana
Ardha Baddha Padma Paschimottanasana	Dandasana, Paschimottanasana, Janu Sirsasana, Marichyasana A, Tiriang Mukha Eka Pada Paschimottanasana, Agnistambhasana, Padmasana	Balasana, Pursvottanasana, Setu Bandha Sarvangasana	Marichyasana B and D, Arkana Dandasana, Krounchasana, Eka Pada Raj Kapotasana, Eka Pada Sirsasana
Ardha Baddha Padmottanasana	Adho Mukha Svanasana, Uttanasana, Vrksasana, Garudasana, Padmasana	Tadasana, Urdhva Mukha Svanasana, Adho Mukha Svanasana	Keeping the foot in half-lotus, exhaling, float back to Chaturanga Dandasana and flow through to Adho Mukha Svanasana, hop to the front of the mat, and return to Tadasana before releasing the lotus foot.
Ardha Chandrasana	Utthita Trikonasana, Virabhadrasana II, Utthita Parsvakonasana, Vrksasana, Utthita Hasta Padangusthasana, Prasarita Padottanasana	Prasarita Padottanasana A, Malasana, Balasana; *do not* directly transition to Virabhadrasana III or Parivrtta Ardha Chandrasana	Keeping the top hip from rotating forward, bend the lifted leg to draw the foot back toward the upper hand, clasping the foot and either pulling it away from the hip or positioning the hand as in Bhekasana and pressing the heel to the hip. If easy, clasp with both hands.
Ardha Matsyendrasana	Supta Parivartanasana, Bharadvajrasana, Baddha Konasana, Janu Sirsasana, Virasana	Dandasana, Paschimottanasana, Apanasana, Ananda Balasana	Deeper twists, partial preparation for backbends and for twisting arm balances such as Parsva Bakasana.
Ardha Uttanasana	Dandasana, Supta Padangusthasana, Tadasana	Dandasana, Tadasana	Uttanasana
Arkana Dandasana	Dandasana, Marichyasana A	Apanasana, Adho Mukha Svanasana	Eka Pada Sirsasana series, Astavakrasana
Ashta Chandrasana	Anjaneyasana, Adho Mukha Svanasana, Supta Padangusthasana, Virasana, Utkatasana	Urdhva Mukha Svanasana, Adho Mukha Svanasana, Balasana	Use as base for transitioning into Virabhadrasana III, Parivrtta Ardha Chandrasana, Adho Mukha Vrksasana, and Parivrtta Parsvakonasana.

ASANA	PREPARATION	INTEGRATION	EXPLORATION
Astavakrasana	Dandasana, Jathara Parivartanasana, Arkana Dandasana, Chaturanga Dandasana, Marichyasana A, Paschimottanasana, Utthita Parsvakonasana, Bhujapidasana	Wrist therapy (see Chapter 11), Urdhva Mukha Svanasana, Adho Mukha Svanasana, Supta Baddha Konasana, Balasana	Use as base for transitioning through Eka Pada Koundinyasana I to Chaturanga Dandasana.
Baddha Konasana	Supta Padangusthasana, Ananda Balasana, Dandasana, Janu Sirsasana, Upavista Konasana, Paschimottanasana	Gomukhasana, Apanasana, Balasana, Adho Mukha Svanasana	Supta Baddha Konasana, Parivrtta Janu Sirsasana, Swastikasana, Marichyasana A, Arkana Dandasana, partial preparation for Eka Pada Sirsasana
Bakasana	Adho Mukha Svanasana, Phalakasana, Balasana, Baddha Konasana, abdominal core work, Virasana	Wrist therapy (see Chapter 11), Adho Mukha Svanasana, Balasana	Parsva Bakasana; Tittibhasana; explore as part of a Salamba Sirsasana II vinyasa (see Chapter 7); float to Chaturanga Dandasana; extend the torso, hips, and legs into Adho Mukha Vrksasana.
Balasana	Apanasana, Virasana	A deeply restorative pose in itself; Savasana	Extend the arms forward onto the floor. Transition to all fours and Adho Mukha Svanasana.
Bharadvajrasana A	Virasana, Gomukhasana, Baddha Konasana, Supta Padangusthasana, Supta Parivartanasana, Ardha Matsyendrasana	Dandasana, Paschimottanasana, Apanasana, Balasana	Bharadvajrasana B, Swastikasana.
Bharadvajrasana B	Bharadvajrasana A and its Prep poses; Janu Sirsasana A, Tiriang Mukha Eka Pada Paschimottanasana, Gomukhasana	Urdhva Mukha Svanasana, Adho Mukha Svanasana, Dandasana, Paschimottanasana, Apanasana, Balasana	Tiriang Mukha Eka Pada Paschimottanasana, Krounchasana
Bhekasana	Salabhasana B, Naraviralasana, Bhujangasana, Dhanurasana, Ustrasana, Prasarita Padottanasana C, Setu Bandha Sarvangasana	Balasana, Ardha Matsyendrasana, Adho Mukha Svanasana, Dandasana, Paschimottanasana	Eka Pada Raj Kapotasana, Urdhva Dhanurasana, Natarajasana
Bhujangasana	Salabhasana A, B, C, Naraviralasana, Dhanurasana, Urdhva Mukha Svanasana	Adho Mukha Svanasana, Balasana, simple twist, Apanasana, Supta Baddha Konasana	Urdhva Mukha Svanasana, Bhekasana

ASANA	PREPARATION	INTEGRATION	EXPLORATION
Bhujapidasana	Adho Mukha Svanasana, Prasarita Padottanasana A, Baddha Konasana, Malasana, Bakasana, Garudasana, Kurmasana	Adho Mukha Svanasana, Balasana with wrist therapy (see Chapter 11)	Tittibhasana, Bakasana, Eka Pada Bakasana, Astavakrasana
Bidalasana	Apanasana, Ananda Balasana, Balasana, Salabhasana A	Balasana, Svanasana	Anahatasana, Phalakasana, Adho Mukha Svanasana
Chakorasana	Krounchasana, Eka Pada Raj Kapotasana I and its Prep poses, Eka Pada Sirsasana A, B, C and their Prep poses	Setu Bandha Sarvangasana, Balasana, simple twists, wrist therapy (see Chapter 11)	Chaturanga Dandasana to Urdhva Mukha Svanasana to Adho Mukha Svanasana
Chaturanga Dandasana	Tadasana, Phalakasana, Adho Mukha Svanasana, Urdhva Mukha Svanasana	Adho Mukha Svanasana, Balasana with wrist therapy	Nakrasana
Dandasana	Supta Padangusthasana, Adho Mukha Svanasana, Ardha Uttanasana	Baddha Konasana, Supta Baddha Konasana, Viparita Karani, Svanasana	All seated forward bends, hip openers, and twists; Pursvottanasana to Tolasana to Lolasana to Chaturanga Dandasana
Dhanurasana	Salabhasana A, B, C, Urdhva Mukha Svanasana, Setu Bandha Sarvangasana, Anjaneyasana, Ashta Chandrasana, Virasana, Supta Virasana	Balasana, Apanasana, Ardha Matsyendrasana, Supta Parivartanasana	Parsva Dhanurasana, Bhekasana, Urdhva Mukha Svanasana, Ustrasana, Laghu Vajrasana
Dwi Pada Koundinyasana	Chaturanga Dandasana, Bakasana, Parsva Bakasana, Astavakrasana, Dandasana	Wrist therapy (see Chapter 11), Adho Mukha Svanasana, Balasana	Extend the upper leg back to Eka Pada Koundinyasana I, then float back to Chaturanga Dandasana; explore as part of a Salamba Sirsasana II vinyasa.
Eka Pada Koundinyasana I	Parivrtta Trikonasana, Parivrtta Parsvakonasana, Parsva Bakasana, Dwi Pada Koundinyasana, Parsvottan-asana, Chaturanga Dandasana, Marichyasana A	Wrist therapy (see Chapter 11), Adho Mukha Svanasana, Balasana	Float back to Chaturanga Dandasana; explore as part of a Salamba Sirsasana II vinyasa.

ASANA	PREPARATION	INTEGRATION	EXPLORATION
Eka Pada Koundinyasana II	Supta Padangusthasana, Utthita Hasta Padangusthasana, Chaturanga Dandasana, Anjaneyasana, Virabhadrasana II, Utthita Parsvakonasana	Wrist therapy (see Chapter 11), Adho Mukha Svanasana, Balasana	Float back to Chaturanga Dandasana; explore as part of a Salamba Sirsasana II vinyasa.
Eka Pada Raj Kapotasana I	Anjaneyasana, Virabhadrasana I, Baddha Konasana, Supta Baddha Konasana, Gomukhasana, Virasana, Supta Virasana	Chaturanga Dandasana to Urdhva Mukha Svanasana to Adho Mukha Svanasana, Balasana	Eka Pada Raj Kapotasana II, Eka Pada Sirsasana series
Eka Pada Raj Kapotasana II	Eka Pada Raj Kapotasana I and its Prep poses, Gomukhasana and Garudasana arms, Adho Mukha Svanasana, Shishulasana, Urdhva Dhanurasana, Viparita Dandasana	Chaturanga Dandasana to Urdhva Mukha Svanasana to Adho Mukha Svanasana, Balasana, simple twists	Natarajasana, Hanumanasana with backbend variation, Kapotasana, Raj Kapotasana
Eka Pada Sirsasana A, B, C	Eka Pada Raj Kapotasana I and its prep poses, Agnistambhasana, Tolasana, Lolasana	Chaturanga Dandasana to Urdhva Mukha Svanasana to Adho Mukha Svanasana, Balasana, simple twists	Chakorasana, Dwi Pada Sirsasana, Yogadrasana
Galavasana	Eka Pada Raj Kapotasana I, Utkatasana, Bakasana and its Prep poses	Chaturanga Dandasana to Urdhva Mukha Svanasana to Adho Mukha Svanasana, Balasana, wrist therapy (see Chapter 11)	Uttana Prasithasana, Eka Pada Bakasana
Garudasana	Tadasana, Utkatasana, Gomukhasana, Vrksasana	Tadasana, Uttanasana, Adho Mukha Svanasana, Baddha Konasana	Squeeze the elbows more firmly together while keeping them level with the shoulders.
Gomukhasana	Ardha Matsyendrasana, Virasana, Parivrtta Janu Sirsasana, Marichyasana C, Paschimottanasana	Dandasana, Baddha Konasana, Upavista Konasana, Adho Mukha Svanasana	Slide the heels forward until the lower legs are in a 180-degree plane, increasingly flexing the feet to protect the knees.
Halasana	Dandasana, Prasarita Padottanasana C, Setu Bandha Sarvangasana, Salamba Sarvangasana	Uttana Padasana, simple twists, Adho Mukha Svanasana, Viparita Karani, Savasana	Karnapidasana, Salamba Sarvangasana

ASANA	PREPARATION	INTEGRATION	EXPLORATION
Hanumanasana	Anjaneyasana, Virabha-drasana I, Supta Virasana, Supta Padangusthasana, Upavista Konasana, Janu Sirsasana	Balasana, Setu Bandha Sarvangasana	Eka Pada Raj Kapotasana I and II; explore the backbend variation or Hanumanasana.
Janu Sirsasana	Dandasana, Supta Padangusthasana, Baddha Konasana, Vrksasana, Paschimottanasana	Apanasana, Setu Bandha Sarvangasana, Gomukhasana	Upavista Konasana, Parivrtta Janu Sirsasana, Tiriang Mukha Eka Pada Paschimottanasana
Jathara Parivartanasana	Apanasana, Ardha Matsyen-drasana, Marichyasana C, Dandasana, yogic bicycles	Apanasana, Supta Baddha Konasana	Apply the awakened abdom-inals in twisting arm balances, including the Salamba Sirsasana II vinyasa.
Kapotasana	Ustrasana, Laghu Vajrasana, Supta Virasana, Urdhva Dhanurasana, Eka Pada Raj Kapotasana II, Gomukhasana	Simple twists followed by long-held seated forward bends	Eka Pada Raj Kapotasana II, then come to standing for Natarajasana.
Karnapidasana	Balasana, Dandasana, Paschimottanasana, Halasana	Uttana Padasana, simple twists, Adho Mukha Svanasana, Viparita Karani, Savasana	Explore long-held seated forward bends.
Krounchasana	Dandasana, Virasana, Paschimottanasana, Tiriang Mukha Eka Pada Paschimottanasana	Chaturanga Dandasana to Urdhva Mukha Svanasana to Adho Mukha Svanasana, Balasana	Pressing the hands onto the floor, pick up and float back to Chaturanga; follow with the Eka Pada Sirsasana to Chakorasana vinyasa.
Kukkutasana	Padmasana and its Prep poses	Dandasana, Paschimottanasana, Gomukhasana, Balasana	Urdhva Kukkutasana
Kurmasana	Dandasana, Paschimottan-asana, Baddha Konasana, Upavista Konasana	Simple twists, Setu Bandha Sarvangasana, Apanasana, Balasana	Apply the open hamstrings, hips, and torso in Tittibhasana.
Laghu Vajrasana	Ustrasana and its Prep poses, Virasana, Supta Virasana, abdominal core awakening	Balasana, simple twists, Supta Baddha Konasana, seated forward bends	Kapotasana, drop-backs from Tadasana to Urdhva Dhanurasana, Natarajasana.
Lolasana	Tolasana, Bakasana, abdom-inal core awakening	Apanasana, Ananda Balasana, Supta Baddha Konasana, Gomukhasana, Adho Mukha Svanasana	Slowly transition with continuous movement from Dandasana to Tolasana to Lolasana to Chaturanga Dandasana; transition into Bakasana and/or Adho Mukha Vrksasana.

ASANA	PREPARATION	INTEGRATION	EXPLORATION
Malasana	Baddha Konasana, Upavista Konasana, Marichyasana A, Virasana	Balasana, Paschimottan asana, Adho Mukha Svanasana, simple twists, Uttanasana	Arkana Dandasana, Bhujangasana, Bakasana, Tittibhasana
Marichyasana A	Dandasana, Paschimottan-asana, Ardha Baddha Padma Paschimottanasana, Anjaneyasana	Apanasana, Supta Baddha Konasana, Supta Parivartanasana	Ananda Balasana, Arkana Dandasana, Bhujangasana, Bakasana, Tittibhasana
Marichyasana C	Marichyasana A and its Prep poses, Ardha Matsyendrasana	Symmetrical forward bends, Baddha Konasana, Upavista Konasana, Supta Baddha Konasana	Ardha Matsyendrasana, Bharadvajrasana B, Parsva Bakasana, Eka Pada Koundinyasana II
Matsyasana	Padmasana and its Prep poses, Setu Bandha Sarvangasana, Uttana Padasana	Apanasana, Ananda Balasana, Svanasana	Transition into Uttana Padasana; after five breaths press the palms onto the floor by to the shoulders as if for Urdhva Dhanurasana, then exhaling draw the feet overhead to the floor while rolling over the head and landing in Chaturanga Dandasana.
Naraviralasana	Salabhasana A and B, Bhujangasana, Phalakasana	Balasana, simple twists, Supta Baddha Konasana, seated forward bends	Bhujangasana, Dhanurasana, Bhekasana
Natarajasana	Tadasana, Utthita Hasta Padangusthasana, Adho Mukha Svanasana, Shishul - asana, Gomukhasana, Anjaneyasana, Virabhadra-sana I, Supta Virasana, Virabhadrasana III, Urdhva Dhanurasana, Eka Pada Raj Kapotasana II	Ardha Uttanasana, Apanasana, Supta Parivartanasana, other simple twists and calming symmetrical forward bends, inversions, and Svanasana	Sit and tune-in inside.
Padahasthasana	Padangusthasana and its Prep poses	Tadasana, Adho Mukha Svanasana, Balasana, simple twists	Paschimottanasana, Upavista Konasana
Padangusthasana	Tadasana, Uttanasana	Tadasana, Adho Mukha Svanasana, Balasana, simple twists	Padahasthasana
Padmasana	Gomukhasana, Sukhasana, Dandasana, Eka Pada Raj Kapotasana I prep poses, Baddha Konasana, Virasana	Dandasana, Supta Padangusthasana, Adho Mukha Svanasana	Tolasana, Matsyasana, Urdhva Padmasana, Urdhva Kukkutasana

ASANA	PREPARATION	INTEGRATION	EXPLORATION
Parighasana	Supta Padangusthasana, Baddha Konasana, Janu Sirsasana, Upavista Konasana, Virasana, Utthita Trikonasana	Symmetrical forward bends, Adho Mukha Svanasana, Balasana	Parivrtta Janu Sirsasana, Utthita Trikonasana, Utthita Parsvakonasana
Paripurna Navasana	Adho Mukha Svanasana, Dandasana, Paschimottanasana	Apanasana, Supta Baddha Konasana, Adho Mukha Svanasana, Balasana, Ananda Balasana, Supta Konasana	Press up into Lolasana between each round; explore Ardha Navasana by bringing the lower back firmly onto the floor while lowering the legs and shoulders to about one foot off the floor, then with the palms in anjali mudra do several rounds of kapalabhati pranayama before lifting back up into Paripurna Navasana (repeat several times).
Parivrtta Ardha Chandrasana	Parivrtta Trikonasana and its Prep poses, Virabhadrasana III and its Prep poses	Uttanasana, Adho Mukha Svanasana, Balasana, Gomukhasana; *do not* directly transition to Ardha Chandrasana	Clasp the lifted foot with the lifted hand to explore a twisting backbend variation. Transition to Virabhadrasana III, then releasing the hands to the floor, float up into Adho Mukha Vrksasana and down to Chaturanga Dandasana.
Parivrtta Hasta Padangusthasana	Parivrtta Trikonasana and its Prep poses, Virabhadrasana III and its Prep poses, Utthita Hasta Padangusthasana and its Prep poses	Uttanasana, Adho Mukha Svanasana, Balasana, Gomukhasana	Transition to Virabhadrasana III, then release the hands to the floor, float up into Adho Mukha Vrksasana and down to Chaturanga Dandasana.
Parivrtta Janu Sirsasana	Utthita Parsvakonasana, Vrksasana, Baddha Konasana, Upavista Konasana, Janu Sirsasana	Symmetrical forward bends, Supta Baddha Konasana, Apanasana, Baddha Konasana	Upavista Konasana, Baddha Konasana, Kurmasana
Parivrtta Parsvakonasana	Anjaneyasana, Gomukhasana, Parivrtta Utkatasana, Ashta Chandrasana, Virabhadrasana I, Parivrtta Trikonasana	Urdhva Mukha Svanasana, Adho Mukha Svanasana, Balasana, Supta Baddha Konasana	Transition directly into Eka Pada Koundinyasana II, hold for five breaths, and then float back to Chaturanga Dandasana.

ASANA	PREPARATION	INTEGRATION	EXPLORATION
Parivrtta Trikonasana	Parsvottanasana, Prasarita Padottanasana, Utthita Trikonasana, Parivrtta Utkatasana, Parivrtta Ashta Chandrasana	Tadasana, Uttanasana, Urdhva Mukha Svanasana, Adho Mukha Svanasana, Balasana, Supta Baddha Konasana	Transition directly into Parivrtta Ardha Chandrasana.
Parsva Bakasana	Bakasana, Marichyasana A and C	Balasana with wrist therapy, Supta Baddha Konasana, Viparita Karani	Extend the legs into Dwi Pada Koundinyasana, scissor them into Eka Pada Koundinyasana I, then float to Chaturanga. Explore as part of a Salamba Sirsasana II vinyasa.
Parsvottanasana	Adho Mukha Svanasana, Ardha Uttanasana, Uttanasana, Gomukhasana, Utthita Trikonasana, Prasarita Padottanasana	Tadasana, Balasana, Apanasana, Supta Baddha Konasana, Supta Padangusthasana	Use as a base for transitioning into Parivrtta Trikonasana and Prep poses for Hanumanasana.
Paschimottanasana	Balasana, Supta Padangusthasana, Adho Mukha Svanasana, Dandasana, Janu Sirsasana	Simple seated and supine twists, Supta Baddha Konasana, Apanasana, Svanasana	Transition to Halasana and Karnapidasana; Upavista Konasana; Tiriang Mukha Eka Pada Paschimottan-asana, Krounchasana, Kurmasana.
Phalakasana	Adho Mukha Svanasana, Bidalasana, Ashtanga Pranam sequence	Adho Mukha Svanasana, Balasana, wrist therapy (see Chapter 11)	Lower to Chaturanga Dandasana; press back to Adho Mukha Svanasana; transition to Vasisthasana; lower to Shishula Phalak-asana and do several rounds of kapalabhati pranayama.
Pincha Mayurasana	Adho Mukha Vvanasana, Shishulasana, Gomukhasana (arms), Adho Mukha Vrksasana, Anjaneyasana, Virabhadrasana I, Supta Virasana	Balasana; sit in Virasana (or another other simple seated position) with Garudasana arms; simple supine or seated twists	Draw the toes to the forehead; draw the feet farther overhead to the floor, fully extending the legs into Viparita Dandasana.
Pindasana	Urdhva Padmasana and its Prep poses	Matsyasana, Uttana Padasana, Svanasana	Transition to Matsyasana, Uttana Padasana, then draw the legs over the head while pressing into the palms to land in Chaturanga Dandasana.

ASANA	PREPARATION	INTEGRATION	EXPLORATION
Prasarita Padottanasana A, B, C, D	Adho Mukha Svanasana, Supta Padangusthasana, Supta Baddha Konasana, Uttanasana, Utthita Trikonasana	Malasana, Garudasana, Uttanasana, Adho Mukha Svanasana, Balasana	From the B variation, transition directly into a Salamba Sirsasana II arm balance vinyasa; Uttanasana; Salamba Sirsasana I. The C variation opens the shoulders and chest for Setu Bandha Sarvangasana and Salamba Sarvangasana.
Pursvottanasana	Setu Bandha Sarvangasana, Ustrasana, Prasarita Padottanasana C, Anjaneyasana, Supta Virasana	Adho Mukha Svanasana, wrist therapy (see Chapter 11), Balasana, Supta Parivartanasana, seated forward bends	Extend one leg straight up into the Eka Pada variation.
Salabhasana A	Anjaneyasana, Ashta Chandrasana, Virabhadrasana I, Virasana, Gomukhasana, Bhujangasana, Naraviralasana	Balasana, simple twists, Supta Baddha Konasana, seated forward bends	Transition into the B and C variations, Dhanurasana, and Bhekasana.
Salabhasana B	Salabhasana A and its Prep poses, Setu Bandha Sarvangasana	Balasana, simple twists, Supta Baddha Konasana, seated forward bends	Transition into the C variation, Dhanurasana, and Bhekasana.
Salabhasana C	Salabhasana A and B and their Prep poses; Adho Mukha Svanasana	Balasana, simple twists, Supta Baddha Konasana, seated forward bends	Transition into Dhanurasana and Bhekasana.
Salamba Sarvangasana	Setu Bandha Sarvangasana, Prasarita Padottanasana C, Halasana, Viparita Karani, Virasana, Anjaneyasana	Halasana, Karnapidasana, Uttana Padasana, Supta Parivartanasana, Svanasana	Fold the legs into lotus position and balance with the knees resting in the hands in Urdhva Padmasana; alternately release the legs overhead into Setu Bandha Sarvangasana.
Salamba Sirsasana I	Adho Mukha Svanasana, Shishulasana, Uttanasana, core work, Salamba Sirsasana II	Balasana; explore neck therapy (see Chapter 11)	Twist; fold the legs into lotus position; lower the legs toward level with the floor and hold there for up to five breaths before extending them back up.
Salamba Sirsasana II	Prasarita Padottanasana B, Setu Bandha Sarvangasana, core work, Salamba Sirsasana I	Balasana, wrist therapy and neck therapy (see Chapter 11)	Use as a base for arm balance vinyasas; transition directly into Chaturanga Dandasana.

ASANA	PREPARATION	INTEGRATION	EXPLORATION
Samasthihi	Tadasana	Uttanasana, Adho Mukha Svanasana, Balasana	Maintain this quality of equanimity through whatever follows.
Savasana	For rest and integration following any other asanas	Allow at least five minutes in this asana	Slowly transition up to sitting.
Setu Bandha Sarvangasana	Anjaneyasana, Virasana, Supta Virasana, Salabhasana A and B, Dhanurasana	Apanasana, simple twists, Supta Baddha Konasana, Ananda Balasana, Balasana, seated forward bends	Use as a dynamic warm-up for deeper backbends, including Urdhva Dhanurasana; explore the Eka Pada variation.
Shishulasana	Adho Mukha Svanasana, Phalakasana, Gomukhasana and Garudasana arms	Balasana, simple twists, Supta Baddha Konasana, seated forward bends	Bhujangasana, Dhanurasana, Bhekasana, Ustrasana, Laghu Vajrasana
Supta Baddha Konasana	Baddha Konasana and its Prep poses, Supta Padangusthasana, Supta Virasana, Utthita Trikonasana, Virabhadrasana II	Apanasana, Supta Parivartanasana, Viparita Karani, Svanasana	Do the same asana with a block placed under the sacrum, with sandbags on the knees, and/or with a bolster under the back.
Supta Padangusthasana	Apanasana, Baddha Konasana, Adho Mukha Svanasana	Apanasana, Supta Parivartanasana, Viparita Karani, Svanasana	Supta Konasana, Upavista Konasana, Kurmasana
Supta Virasana	Anjaneyasana, Virasana, Setu Bandha Sarvangasana, Ustrasana	Bidalasana, Adho Mukha Svanasana, Balasana, Ananda Balasana, simple twists, Supta Baddha Konasana, seated forward bends	Apply the opening of the hip flexors and groins in exploring deeper backbends. From all fours, curl the toes under and again recline back, clasping the feet or knees as in Kapotasana; this is Prapada Paryankasana (Tiptoe Couch Pose).
Tadasana	Savasana, Bidalasana-Svanasana movements	Ardha Uttanasana, Uttanasana, Adho Mukha Svanasana, Balasana	Vrksasana and all other standing asanas
Tiriang Mukha Eka Pada Paschimottanasana	Dandasana, Paschimottanasana, Janu Sirsasana, Virasana	Urdhva Mukha Svanasana, Adho Mukha Svanasana, Apanasana, Ananda Balasana, Supta Parivartanasana	Krounchasana
Tittibhasana	Adho Mukha Svanasana, Utthita Trikonasana, Prasarita Padottanasana A, Baddha Konasana, Upavista Konasana, Bakasana, core work, Garudasana, Malasana, Bhujapidasana	Urdhva Mukha Svanasana, Adho Mukha Svanasana, Balasana, wrist therapy (see Chapter 11)	Flex the knees, drawing the heels back, up, and together into Bakasana, then float into Chaturanga Dandasana.

ASANA	PREPARATION	INTEGRATION	EXPLORATION
Tolasana	Padmasana and its Prep poses, core work	Dandasana, Pursvottan-asana, Urdhva Mukha Svanasana, Adho Mukha Svanasana, Balasana, wrist therapy (see Chapter 11)	Transition directly into Lolasana or Urdhva Kukkutasana.
Upavista Konasana	Supta Padangusthasana, Dandasana, Baddha Konasana, Prasarita Padottanasana A, Utthita Trikonasana	Dandasana, Marichyasana C, Virasana, Gomukhasana, Adho Mukha Svanasana, Balasana	Drawing the legs closer together, slide the arms out laterally under the legs, flex the knees, and extend the torso forward into Kurm-asana. Transition directly into Chaturanga Dandasana, or alternately into Bhujapid-asana and Tittibhasana.
Urdhva Dhanurasana	Adho Mukha Svanasana, Anjaneyasana, Virabhadrasana I, Virasana, Supta Virasana, Shishulasana, Bhujangasana, Setu Bandha Sarvangasana, Urdhva Mukha Svanasana, Viparita Dandasana	Apanasana, simple twists, Supta Baddha Konasana, Ananda Balasana, Balasana, seated forward bends	Brings the hands closer to the feet without compromising the parallel positioning of the feet; extend one leg straight up into the Eka Pada variation; draw up to standing in Tadasana and drop back into Urdhva Dhanurasana up to five times.
Urdhva Hastasana	Samasthihi, Tadasana, Anahatasana, Adho Mukha Svanasana	Tadasana, Uttanasana, Adho Mukha Svanasana, Balasana	Stretch to the side, first one way and then the other.
Urdhva Kukkutasana	Padmasana and its Prep poses, Bakasana, Salamba Sirsasana II	Urdhva Mukha Svanasana, Adho Mukha Svanasana, Balasana, Supta Baddha Konasana, wrist therapy (see Chapter 11)	Explore as part of a Salamba Sirsasana I vinyasa; from Adho Mukha Vrksasana, fold the legs into lotus and lower the lotus legs to the upper arms.
Urdhva Mukha Svanasana	Salabhasana A and B, Naraviralasana, Bhujangasana, Setu Bandha Sarvangasana, Phalakasana, Chaturanga Dandasana	Adho Mukha Svanasana, Ardha Matsyendrasana, Apanasana, Balasana	Transition to Bhujangasana, flex the knees and draw the toes toward the head.
Urdhva Padmasana	Padmasana and its Prep poses, Baddha Konasana, Padmasana, Salamba Sarvangasana	Matsyasana, Uttana Padasana, Supta Parivartanasana, Svanasana	Transition to Pindasana; alternately, place the hands under the sacrum and extend the lotus legs up and forward; add a slight twist, placing just one hand under the sacrum.

ASANA	PREPARATION	INTEGRATION	EXPLORATION
Ustrasana	Anjaneyasana, Virabhadra-sana I, Virasana, Supta Virasana, Salabhasana, Setu Bandha Sarvangasana	Balasana, simple twists, Supta Baddha Konasana, Ananda Balasana, seated forward bends	Transition to Laghu Vajrasana and Kapotasana.
Utkatasana	Tadasana, Adho Mukha Svanasana, Salabhasana B, Virasana	Uttanasana, Adho Mukha Svanasana, Balasana	Add a twist with Parivrtta Utkatasana, keeping the knees even with each other so the hips are even and the sacrum more open.
Uttana Padasana	Dandasana, Paripurna Navasana, Virasana, Setu Bandha Sarvangasana	Apanasana, simple twists, Svanasana	Use this asana to help strengthen the neck musculature in preparation for Setu Bandhasana ("Charlie Chaplin Pose").
Uttana Prasithasana	Marichyasana A and C, Eka Pada Raj Kapotasana Prep poses, Arkana Dandasana, Bakasana, Galavasana, Astavakrasana	Upavista Konasana, Supta Baddha Konasana, Apan-asana, Balasana, wrist therapy (see Chapter 11)	Float lightly into Chaturanga Dandasana.
Uttanasana	Supta Padangusthasana, Adho Mukha Svanasana, Tadasana, Ardha Uttanasana	Malasana, Supta Baddha Konasana, Apanasana, Balasana, Svanasana	Transition into Padangusth-asana and Padahasthasana; alternately extend one leg back and up into Eka Pada Adho Mukha Vrksasana ("Standing Splits").
Utthita Hasta Padangusthasana	Supta Padangusthasana, Tadasana, Vrksasana, Utthita Trikonasana, Utthita Parsvakonasana	Tadasana, Garudasana, Urdhva Mukha Svanasana, Adho Mukha Svanasana, Balasana	Draw the straight lifted leg higher up toward the shoulder without bending the standing leg, losing pelvic neutrality, or flexing the spine.
Utthita Parsvakonasana	Supta Padangusthasana, Tadasana, Malasana, Urdhva Hastasana, Vrksasana, Utthita Trikonasana, Virabhadrasana II	Urdhva Mukha Svanasana, Adho Mukha Svanasana, Prasarita Padottanasana C, Apanasana, Balasana	Draw the upper arm around behind the back and the lower arm under the front leg to clasp the wrist of the straight upper arm, transitioning into either Eka Pada Koundinyasana A or Svarga Dvidasana (Bird of Paradise Pose).

ASANA	PREPARATION	INTEGRATION	EXPLORATION
Utthita Trikonasana	Supta Padangusthasana, Tadasana, Vrksasana, Adho Mukha Svanasana, Virabhadrasana II	Tadasana, Adho Mukha Svanasana, Garudasana, Gomukhasana, Balasana	Transition into Ardha Chandrasana while keeping the standing foot in place and the upper hip rotated on top of the lower hip.
Vasisthasana	Adho Mukha Svanasana, Utthita Trikonasana, Vrksasana, Utthita Hasta Padangusthasana, Ardha Chandrasana, Phalakasana, Prasarita Padottanasana B and D, Supta Padangusthasana	Urdhva Mukha Svanasana, Adho Mukha Svanasana, Gomukhasana, Balasana, wrist therapy (see Chapter 11)	Transition into Vishvamitrasana or Eka Pada Koundinyasana A.
Viparita Dandasana	Adho Mukha Svanasana, Anjaneyasana, Virabhadra-sana I, Shishulasana, Supta Virasana, Pursvottanasana, Gomukhasana, Setu Bandha Sarvangasana, Urdhva Dhanurasana	Apanasana, simple twists, Supta Baddha Konasana, Ananda Balasana, Balasana, seated forward bends	Explore extending one leg straight up into the Eka Pada variation; alternately, walk the feet closer to the elbows and spring up into Pincha Mayurasana.
Viparita Karani	A deeply restorative asana that can be practiced on its own or after any other asana	Apanasana, Supta Baddha Konasana, Savasana	Place a strap around the thighs and a sandbag on the feet to stabilize the position and deepen its restorative effects.
Virabhadrasana I	Tadasana, Adho Mukha Svanasana, Anjaneyasana, Ashta Chandrasana, Gomukhasana, Virasana, Virabhadrasana II	Urdhva Mukha Svanasana, Adho Mukha Svanasana, Supta Padangusthasana, Supta Baddha Konasana, Apanasana, Ananda Balasana, Balasana	Use as base for Dancing Warrior or for transitioning into other standing asanas; alternately, fold the arms into Garudasana or Gomukhasana position to prepare the shoulders for easier flexion in Urdhva Dhanurasana, Adho Mukha Svanasana, or Adho Mukha Vrksasana.
Virabhadrasana II	Tadasana, Anjaneyasana, Ashta Chandrasana, Baddha Konasana, Supta Padangusthasana, Utthita Trikonasana, Vrksasana	Urdhva Mukha Svanasana, Adho Mukha Svanasana, Gomukhasana, Paschimottanasana, Balasana	Use as a base for exploring Utthita Parsvakonasana, Utthita Trikonasana, Ardha Chandrasana, Svarga Dvidasana, and other externally rotated hip standing asanas.

ASANA	PREPARATION	INTEGRATION	EXPLORATION
Virabhadrasana III	Tadasana, Anjaneyasana, Ashta Chandrasana, Supta Padangusthasana, Vrksasana, Uttanasana, Virabhadrasana I	Malasana, Garudasana, Supta Baddha Konasana, Balasana; *do not* directly transition to Ardha Chandrasana	Use as base for Parivrtta Ardha Chandrasana, Parivrtta Hasta Padangusthasana, Natarajasana and Adho Mukha Vrksasana.
Virasana	Apanasana, Balasana, Baddha Konasana, Gomukhasana	Phalakasana, Adho Mukha Svanasana	Recline back into Supta Virasana.
Vrksasana	Supta Padangusthasana, Baddha Konasana, Tadasana, Utthita Trikonasana, Virabhadrasana II	Tadasana, Ardha Uttanasana, Uttanasana, Garudasana, Balasana	Use as a base for transitioning into Utthita Hasta Padangusthasana; alternately, explore staying balanced with the eyes closed.
Yogic bicycles	Jathara Parivartanasana, Paripurna Navasana, Ardha Matsyendrasana, Marichyasana C	Apanasana, Supta Parivartanasana, Ananda Balasana, Supta Baddha Konasana	Explore in conjunction with core abdominal movements, including Paripurna to Ardha Navasana and Jathara Parivartanasana.

NOTES

CHAPTER ONE—ANCIENT ROOTS OF MODERN YOGA

1. Pattabhi Jois elaborates on this, writing that in order to achieve *brahmacharya* one must avoid "mixing with vulgar people, going to crowded areas for recreation, reading vulgar books that disturb the mind, going to theaters and restaurants, and conversing secretly with strangers of the opposite sex" (Jois 2002, 8).

2. See Muktananda (1997).

CHAPTER TWO—MODERN HATHA YOGA

1. In more recent years, the yoga movement has taken off more globally, particularly in Asia. See Ferretti (2008).

2. Even many of Vivekananda's biographers recognize the earlier development of yoga in the United States under the influence of the transcendentalist movement in New England. See www.ramakrishavivekenanda.info for an online biography.

3. See D. G. White's (2009, 243–248) discussion of the extension of yoga to the West.

4. The yoga–body sculpting extreme was met in 2001 with the Warner Home Video production of *Yoga: Buns of Steel,* starring Rolf Junghans and Tracey Bradford.

5. This version is implicitly called into question in Sjoman's *The Yoga Tradition of the Mysore Palace* (1996), which makes a compelling case for Krishnamacharya and his protégés as creative forces in the conscious evolution of yoga, with Ashtanga Vinyasa an original synthesis of traditional Indian martial arts forms, British calisthenics, and earlier Hatha yoga.

6. The most thorough description of Ashtanga Vinyasa is found in Maehle (2006). David Swenson's classic *Ashtanga Yoga: The Practice Manual* (1999) has fallen out of favor with more purist ashtangis, who consider his suggested use of props and modifications a dilution of Jois's teachings.

7. Dr. Robert Gotlin, director of orthopedic and sports rehabilitation at Beth Israel Medical Center in New York City, says that he sees up to five Bikram-related injuries a week (A. Stephens 2005).

8. Desikachar's translation of this same sutra gives us "When cleanliness is developed it reveals what needs to be constantly maintained and what is eternally clean," while Bouanchaud translates the same passage as "Purity protects one's body and brings nonphysical relationships with others" (Desikachar 1995, 178).

9. The newsreel was published on YouTube: http://www.youtube.com/watch?v=lmOUZQi_6Tw (accessed May 12, 2006).

10. See, in particular, B. K. S. Iyengar's *The Tree of Yoga* (1988), *Light on the Yoga Sutras of Patanjali* (1993), *Yoga* (2001), and *Light on Life* (2005).

11. Note that this version of Ashtanga Vinyasa history stands in stark contrast to the story given by Pattabhi Jois, contributing to the mystification noted earlier.

12. For further exploration, see Shannahoff-Khalsa (2004) and Sovatsky (1998).

CHAPTER THREE—SUBTLE ENERGY

1. It is worth reflecting on the etymology of the term *individual*, derived from the Latin *individuum*, meaning "inseparable from." In a curious shift of meaning that coincided with the rise of capitalism in the West, our essential inseparability gave way to the idea of an isolated being. To explore this further, see Williams (1985).

2. Finger (2005) gives specific physical locations and attributes for each chakra. As noted earlier, many others, including Johari (1987), dispute this specific association of chakras with physical elements.

CHAPTER FOUR—BODY STRUCTURE AND MOVEMENT

1. Calais-Germain (1991, 62) and Thomas Myers (1998, 82) offer two contrasting views of this source of balance.

2. Weak biceps exacerbate elbow hyperextension, a condition exacerbated by the nature of asana practice, in which the biceps are never concentrically contracted against significant resistance. There is an interesting spiritual/philosophical element to this: In most asana practice, most effort pushes out away from the body and only rarely draws in toward the body.

CHAPTER FIVE—CREATING SPACE FOR SELF-TRANSFORMATION

1. The Yoga Sutras of Patanjali describe this condition as one of the kleshas. For an excellent discussion of the psychological aspects of this separation and how yoga can heal the consequent suffering, see Cope (1999). We explore this later in this chapter.

2. As noted in Chapter Two, there is significant emerging evidence showing that exercise in extreme heat can cause serious injuries. See note 7 in Chapter Two for further exploration.

3. To get an idea of the possibilities, see B. K. S. Iyengar (2001) for numerous examples of the use of chairs and other props.

4. For a strong argument in favor of this position, see Farhi (2006, 81–82).

5. The question of what is spiritual—*and what is not spiritual*—is succinctly and beautifully discussed by Remen in her article.

6. This point is emphasized by Farhi (1999), who stresses that "each asana acts as a container for subtle and dynamic inner movement."

7. The practice of mindfulness is found in a variety of spiritual disciplines, most notably in Zen Buddhism; see Hanh (1975). For an eclectic resource on cultivating being present in the moment, see Watts (1980). More recently, Eckhart Tolle has helped popularized the practice of being in the moment through his writings and talks, including *The Power of Now* (1999); and Sarah Powers, (2008) explores mindfulness and asana practice.

8. *Aum* is mentioned in all of the Upanishads, where it is set forth as a profound object or spiritual meditation, its sound equated with Brahma. It is discussed extensively in the Chandogya Upanishad, Taittiriya Upanishad, and Mandukya Upanishad. See the Katha Upanishad (1.2.15) for a simple definition of *aum* as "the highest" syllable, the "aim of all human desire," which in knowing the support of this sound, its meaning, makes one "adored in the world of Brahma."

9. On time and spirit, see Medina (1996); on the day-night cycle and human behavior, see Thompson and Harsha (1984).

10. In the past few years we have seen the development of "yin" and "yang" yoga, and sometimes "yin-yang" yoga, the Chinese terms for the same essential polarities that can be seen together as the archetypal parents, the "first bifurcation of the primal, cosmogenic reality, now united in productive harmony" (Zimmer 1972, 127). In other traditions they are called "Father Heaven and Mother Earth," "Zeus and Hera," "Uranos and Gaia," "T'ien and Ti," etc. Where yoga classes use these epithets to describe their approach, it can signify that other traditions are being incorporated into the practice, such as Sarah Powers's activation of Chinese meridians through specific asana sequences in her approach to yin yoga. To explore, see Campbell's (1949, 97–171) discussion of "Initiation" as well as Zimmer (1972). On yin yoga, originally developed by Pauli Zink, see Grilley (2002).

11. Jody Greene (personal communication, 2009) has rightly suggested that we problematize and retire the self-limiting and archaic typologies that cast energetic qualities as male-female polarities. Why should we accept that to be "expansive" is somehow more masculine than feminine, or that to be "integrative" is more feminine than masculine? While there may be heuristic value in offering conceptual polarities, associating them with gender, which is relatively fluid and unfolding in human development, only reinforces misconceptions about the qualities of maleness and femaleness that take us further away from a sense of wholeness.

12. There are hundreds of sources on Ganesha. Courtright (1985) provides a scholarly treatment of Ganesha that many purist Hindus have assiduously sought to have removed from circulation; Getty's *Ganesa* (1936) is among the earliest introductions to Ganesha in the English language; Swami Chinmayananda (1987) offers a traditionalist interpretation that may have motivated Courtright's work; a delightful rendition is found in Kapur's *Ganesha Goes to Lunch* (2007).

13. Blitz, a follower of Krishnamurti and student of Desikachar (he first brought Desikachar to Europe in the early 1960s), founded Club Méditerranée with his father in 1950, offering luxury vacation retreats with yoga classes, prefiguring a trend of the 1990s and 2000s.

14. Expanding on this idea, Desikachar (1998) relates that the revered scriptures of ancient India "prepare definitions, classification, and methods appropriate to each individual. Taken into account are personal interests, vocation, age, sex, family, social position, and cultural setting. There are detailed descriptions of proper attitudes toward the self and others: of when to act and when not; when to speak, when to be silent."

15. See the Yoga Sutras of Patanjali, especially II.27-31.

16. Dean Ornish (1998, 211), a medical doctor, asked Swami Satchidananda, "What is the root of healing?" Satchidananda replied, "Contentment. Contentment comes by quieting down the mind and body enough—whether through meditation, yoga, or prayer—to experience an inner sense of joy and well-being...."

17. See Cope (2006), especially pages 231-262.

CHAPTER SIX—TECHNIQUES AND TOOLS FOR TEACHING

1. The "normal force" itself is derived from Newton's Second Law, the Law of Resultant Force. For discussion, see Shabana (1999); Espinoza (2005, 141); or the original Newton (1999).

2. For a discussion of grounding and elongation through the spine, see Scaravelli (1991).

3. Schiffmann devotes a chapter of his *Yoga* (1996) to elaborating on Kramer's lines of energy approach, offering a useful set of techniques that students can apply in developing this aspect of their practice.

4. This relationship between drawing muscular energy to the core of the body while radiating out from the core to the periphery is found in many styles of Hatha yoga, albeit with different terminology and slightly different emphasis.

5. While most Hatha yoga styles recognize these polarities, the few that explicitly address them in asana instruction emphasize somewhat different oppositions and energetic actions. Cf. B. K. S. Iyengar (2001); Devereux (1998); Schiffmann (1996); Holleman (1999, 27); and Rea (2005, 75-76).

6. The ubiquitous sequence of Plank–Chaturanga–Up Dog–Down Dog should be demonstrated on a fairly regular basis. See Chapter Seven for the instructions.

7. The terms *passive* and *active* are often used in different ways depending on the context of the discussion. See Ganga White's (2007, 119-121) discussion of active and passive holding.

8. There is considerable debate in the medical and scientific communities about stretching. For an overview, see Shrier and Gossal (2000). Several studies on duration of static stretching show no increase in flexibility after thirty seconds. See Bandy and Irion (1994) for a study showing

duration longer than thirty seconds having no acute effect on hamstring flexibility. In one study of passive stretching versus active movement, the application of "awareness through movement" was shown to result in significantly more muscle length than passive stretching, indicating that muscle length can be increased through a process of active movement that does not involve stretching; see J. Stephens (2006).

9. The value of dynamic practice for beginners is emphasized by Desikachar (1995, 29–31).

10. The concept of yoga chikitsa is recognition that yoga is a process for healing that involves transforming the conditioned patterns that influence every aspect of one's life. It is also the name given to the primary series of Ashtanga Vinyasa yoga, one of the overarching aspects of the Viniyoga approach and at the center of Iyengar's practice and teachings.

11. See Farhi (2006, 89–91) for an insightful discussion of touching.

12. There is a wide range of views on sexual relations between teachers and students. At one extreme is an insistence on celibacy, particularly in the more renunciate lineages, which settles the matter. At the other extreme we find near-complete license given to teachers in acting on sexual attraction to students, as in John Friend's (2006, 92) statement: "When a sexual attraction occurs between you and a student, wait some weeks before acting on the attraction."

13. Some styles of yoga, particularly Ashtanga Vinyasa, are inclined toward very strong physical adjustments. In the hands of an ill-informed or insensitive teacher, this can be dangerous.

14. The "one size fits all" approach in which teachers insist that all students do all asanas in the same form and without props will likely fade into obscurity as more and more students come to appreciate that they can experience yoga with a greater sense of safety and freedom, and thus as a source of deeper self-transformation, when they modify asanas and use props.

CHAPTER SEVEN—TEACHING ASANAS

1. As discussed in Chapter Two, Indra Devi, B. K. S. Iyengar, Pattabhi Jois, and T. V. K. Desikachar brought this tradition to the West. Their students have subsequently given us various hybrid forms of asana practice that include Vinyasa Flow, Power yoga, Anusara, Prana Vinyasa, and a variety of other approaches and brands.

2. There are hundreds of books on asanas. The following are especially insightful: B. K. S. Iyengar (1966), B. K. S. Iyengar (2001), Schiffmann (1996), Holleman (1999), Devereux (1998), Maehle (2006), Lasater (1995), Desikachar (1995), and Mohan (1993). *Yoga Journal* magazine has hundreds of outstanding articles on asanas, including many written for teachers.

3. For details on the anatomy of pada bandha, see the discussion of the feet in Chapter Four. For more on balance in the feet, see Holleman (1999) and Little (2001).

4. For more details on the functions of and benefits to muscles and joints used in twists, read Gudmestad (2003) and Cole (2005).

5. See Schatz (2002) for the position that inversion will not cause endometriosis. Many others still argue against inversion during menstruation: Geeta Iyengar (1995, 77) writes that "During the monthly period, 48–72 hours complete rest is advisable. Asanas should not be practiced." Clennell (2007, 18), drawing from Geeta Iyengar, goes even farther, advising against "poses in which your head is lower than your torso, hips, and legs."

CHAPTER EIGHT—TEACHING PRANAYAMA

1. Many traditional spiritual perspectives give primacy to "being present," yet some also appreciate the natural human capacity for reflection and imagination, sensing context, and thinking of alternative possibilities. While opening ourselves to what Eckhart Tolle describes as the "power of now" as part of conscious awareness, we need not limit ourselves to a belief or sense of the "now" being all there is. For further exploration, see Kramer and Alstad (2009).

2. Differing definitions are found in the Vedas, Upanishads, Yoga Sutras of Patanjali, tantric literature, and the classical Hatha yoga literature from the fourteenth to seventeenth centuries. See Chapter Three for a discussion of prana. To explore more recent interpretations, see Rosen (2002), Rosen (2006), and B. K. S. Iyengar (1985).

3. Various translations use the terms *perfected, accomplished,* or *mastery.* There is wide debate over when and under what conditions pranayama can be safely practiced. While B. K. S. Iyengar states that asanas must first be perfected, in other commentary regarding inhalation, exhalation, and retention, he states that "all are to be performed, prolonged, and refined according to the capacity of the aspirant" (B. K. S. Iyengar 1993, 165).

4. The Chinese had earlier developed a partly philosophical, partly physiological concept of breathing, *lien chi,* meaning transmuting the breath into the soul substance or the vital essence from the air; see Morse (1934).

5. See Farhi (1996, 74–90) on breathing patterns.

6. These exercises are adapted from the detailed anatomical practices discussed in Calais-Germain (2005, 176–203). See Netter (1997, plate 183) for muscles of inspiration and expiration.

7. See Ganga White (2007, 66–67) for a succinct discussion of this debate.

8. Breath retention practice is found in the Yoga Sutras, where the cessation of breath is associated with chitta vritti nirodaha, calming the fluctuations of the mind (Yoga Sutras II.49–52). The term *kumbhaka* appears in the Hatha Yoga Pradipika (II.43–46) along with a more elaborate description of its practice. Here we focus on forms of *sahita-kumbhakas,* those that concern the threefold practices of inhalation, exhalation, and retention. A fourth form, *kevala-kumbhaka,* spontaneously arises from these practices and transcends the phases of breathing; beyond technique, in kevala-kumbhaka the body-breath-mind are in effortless suspension. According to the Hatha Yoga Pradipika, there are eight kumbhaka practices (all sahita): *surya-bheda, ujjayi, seetkari, sitali, bhastrika, bhramari, morchha,* and *plavini.*

9. Beyond inhalation, exhalation, and retention.

10. Regarding both kapalabhati and bastrika, Iyengar (1985, 180) tells us, "if people perform them because they believe that they awaken the kundalini, disaster to body, nerves, and brain may result." Yet the Hatha Yoga Pradipika, Iyengar's primary source, says that this pranayama "quickly arouses kundalini. It is pleasant and beneficial, and removes obstruction due to excess mucus accumulated at the entrance to brahma nadi" (Hatha Yoga Pradipika II.66).

11. Also see Powell (1996).

12. The approach here draws primarily from the Hatha Yoga Pradipika (II.7–9) and from Bailey's (2003) lucid insights into the balancing of prana.

CHAPTER NINE—TEACHING MEDITATION

1. For a practical modern-day treatment, see Cope (1999).

2. There is a tendency for many spiritual practices to offer promised outcomes in exchange for commitment to a particular practice, guru, or religion. It is no different in much of yoga. For a fascinating discussion, see Kramer and Alstad (2009).

3. For a discussion of how dharana can be experienced amid a variety of activities, see Cope (2006, 68–71).

4. See Eliade's (1958, 69–73) discussion.

5. See Fischer-Schreiber et al. (1994).

6. There are infinite mudra possibilities. For guidance, see Hirschi (2000).

7. See Kempton (2002) for a variety of approaches to using the breath in meditation.

8. There are infinite mantra meditations. For a guided audio meditation practice, try Stryker (2005).

9. This is a modified version of the counting meditation technique I learned from Erich Schiffmann in 1993. For more on his approach, see Schiffmann (1996).

10. This perspective blends the author's separate conversations with Sally Kempton and Daniel Odier. For more on Odier's approach and his translation of the Vijnana Bhairava, see Odier (2004).

CHAPTER TEN—SEQUENCING AND PLANNING CLASSES

1. For a broad overview of vinyasa krama, see Mohan (1993, 125–158) and Desikachar (1995, 25–43).

2. See Hardy et al. (1983).

3. See Schiffmann (1996, 89–94) for detailed guidance.

4. In some yoga styles and traditions, including Ashtanga Vinyasa and Bikram, the sequence of asanas is preset. Yet even with set sequences, you can help students ease or deepen their practice with variations that draw from the same sequencing principles applied in creatively sequenced classes.

5. The classic source is Geeta S. Iyengar (1995). Clennell (2007) expands on Iyengar's thinking. For a contrasting perspective, see Benagh (2003).

6. Finger (2005) offers a variety of chakra-oriented sequences.

CHAPTER ELEVEN—SPECIALIZED TEACHING

1. This section is designed for yoga teachers working with common student injuries. For guidance on how yoga can promote healing of a wide variety of ailments, see McCall (2007) and the *Journal of the International Association of Yoga Therapists.*

2. For more detailed guidance on methods for developing alignment and addressing pain in students with scoliosis, see E. B. Miller (2003).

3. Allison Woolery (2004) and her associates at UCLA have conducted the most compelling research. For more extensive reading on yoga for depression, see Weintraub (2004).

4. To explore this line of thinking about depression, see Keedwell (2008) as well as Neese and Williams (1994).

5. This is Patricia Walden's interpretation as presented by McCall (2007, 267–268).

6. These suggestions draw from a variety of sources, of which one of the most insightful and succinct is Ferretti (2006).

7. For fascinating stories of how fear can limit a woman's cervical dilation in labor, see Gaskin (2003, 133–142).

8. For specific modifications of asanas in working with these two classes of students, there are excellent pre/postnatal books that closely correspond to the two groups: for more basic pre/post classes, see Balaskas (1994); for regular yoga classes and experienced students, see Freedman (2004).

9. For specific exercises, see Calais-Germain (2003); this book should be required reading for all pre/postnatal yoga teachers.

CHAPTER TWELVE—THE YOGA PROFESSION

1. For more on marketing yourself as a yoga teacher, see Payne (2000).

2. Farhi (2006) examines these larger life relationships in her book on ethics in teaching yoga.

REFERENCES

Aboy, Adriana. 2002. Indra Devi's legacy. *Hinduism Today* 24.

Aiyar, K. N., trans. 1914. *Thirty minor Upanishads, including the Yoga Upanishads.* Madras, India: Vasanta.

Aldous, Susi Hately. 2004. *Anatomy and asana: Preventing yoga injuries.* Calgary: Functional Synergy.

Alstad, Diana. 1979. Exploring relationships: Interpersonal yoga. *Yoga Journal* (March 1979).

Alter, Michael J. 1996. *Science of flexibility* 2nd ed. Champaign, IL: Human Kinetics.

Ashtanga Yoga. 2006. Video, http://www.youtube.com/watch?v=lmOUZQi_6Tw.

Avalon, Arthur. 1974. *The serpent power: Being the Sat-Cakra-Nirupana and Paduka-Pancaka.* New York: Dover.

Avari, Burjor. 2007. *India: The ancient past.* Abingdon, UK: Routledge.

Ayyanga, T. R. S. 1952. *The Yoga Upanishads.* Adyar, India: Adyar Library.

Bailey, James. 2003. Balancing act. *Yoga Journal* 176 (September/October 2003), http://www.yogajournal.com/wisdom/927.

————. 2006. *Living ayurveda reader.* Santa Monica, CA: self-published.

Balaskas, Janet. 1994. *Preparing for birth with yoga.* Boston: Element.

Bandy, William D., and Jean M. Irion. 1994. The effect of time on static stretch on the flexibility of the hamstring muscles. *Physical Therapy* 74(9): 845–50.

Baptiste, Baron. 2003. *Journey into power: How to sculpt your ideal body, free your true self, and transform your life with yoga.* New York: Fireside.

Benagh, Barbara. 2003. Inversions and menstruation. *Yoga Journal*, http://yogajournal.com/practice/546_1.cfm.

Bhajan, Yogi. Kundalini Research Institute, http://www.kriteachings.org/teachertraining.htm.

Birch, Beryl Bender. 1995. *Power yoga: The total strength and flexibility workout.* New York: Fireside.

————. 2000. *Beyond Power yoga: 8 levels of practice for body and soul.* New York: Fireside.

Bouanchaud, Bernard. 1999. *The essence of yoga: Reflections on the Yoga Sutras of Patanjali.* New York: Sterling.

Briggs, Tony. 2001. The gift of assisting. *Yoga Journal*, http://www.yogajournal.com/for_teachers/1024.

Calais-Germain, Blandine. 1991. *Anatomy of movement.* Seattle: Eastland.

————. 2003. *The female pelvis: Anatomy and exercises.* Seattle: Eastland.

————. 2005. *Anatomy of breathing.* Seattle: Eastland.

Campbell, Joseph. 1949. *The hero with a thousand faces.* New York: Pantheon.

Chaudburi, Haridas. 1965. *Integral yoga.* London: Allen & Unwin.

Chinmayananda, Swami. 1987. *Glory of Ganesha.* Bombay: Central Chinmaya Mission Trust.

Chödrön, Pema. 2007. *Always maintain a joyful mind, and other Lojong teachings on awakening compassion and fearlessness.* Boston: Shambhala.

Choudhury, Bikram. 2000. *Bikram's beginning yoga class.* New York: Penguin Putnam.

Clennell, Bobby. 2007. *The woman's yoga book: Asana and pranayama for all phases of the menstrual cycle.* Berkeley, CA: Rodmell.

Cole, Roger. 2005. With a twist. *Yoga Journal* (November 2005).

_____. Protect the knees in lotus and related postures. *Yoga Journal,* http://www.yogajournal. com/for_teachers/978.

Cope, Stephen. 1999. *Yoga and the quest for the true self.* New York: Bantam.

_____. 2006. *The wisdom of yoga: A seeker's guide to extraordinary living.* New York: Bantam-Bell.

Courtright, Paul B. 1985. *Ganesa: Lord of obstacles, lord of beginnings.* New York: Oxford University Press.

Davidson, Ronald M. 2003. *Indian esoteric Buddhism: A social history of the tantric movement.* New York: Columbia University Press.

_____. 2005. *Tibetan renaissance: Tantric Buddhism in the rebirth of Tibetan culture.* New York: Columbia University Press.

Desikachar, T. K. V. 1995. *The heart of yoga: Developing a personal practice.* Rochester, VT: Inner Traditions.

_____. 1998. *Health, healing, and beyond: Yoga and the living tradition of Krishnamacharya.* New York: Aperture.

Devereux, Godfrey. 1998. *Dynamic yoga: The ultimate workout that chills your mind as it charges your body.* New York: Thorsons.

Dharma, Krishna. 1999. *Mahabharata: The greatest spiritual epic of all time.* Badger, CA: Torchlight.

Easwaran, Eknath, trans. 1987. *The Upanishads.* Tomales, CA: Nilgiri.

Eliade, Mircea. 1958. *Yoga: Immortality and freedom.* New York: Pantheon.

Espinoza, Fernando. 2005. An analysis of the historical development of ideas about motion and its implications for teaching. *Physical Education* 40(2).

Farhi, Donna. 1996. *The breathing book: Good health and vitality through essential breath work.* New York: Henry Holt.

_____. 1999. Asana column: Supta Padangusthasana. *Yoga Journal* (May/June 1999).

_____. 2006. *Teaching yoga: Exploring the teacher-student relationship.* Berkeley, CA: Rodmell.

Ferretti, Andrea. 2006. Feel happier. *Yoga Journal,* http://www.yogajournal.com/lifestyle/2562.

_____. 2008. Yoga metropolis. *Yoga Journal,* http://www.yogajournal.com/lifestyle/2686.

Feuerstein, Georg. 1998. *Tantra: The path of ecstasy.* Boston: Shambhala.

_____. 2001. *The yoga tradition: Its history, literature, philosophy and practice.* Prescott, AZ: Hohm.

Finger, Alan. 2005. *Chakra yoga: Balancing energy for physical, spiritual, and mental well-being.* Boston: Shambhala.

Fischer-Schreiber, Ingrid, Stephan Schuhmacher, and Gert Woerner. 1994. *The encyclopedia of Eastern philosophy and religion.* Boston: Shambhala.

Flood, Gavin D. 1996. *An introduction to Hinduism.* Cambridge: Cambridge University Press.

Flynn, Kimberly. 2003. FAQ, http://www.ashtangayogashala.com.

Folan, Lilias. 1976. *Lilias yoga and you.* New York: Bantam.

Frawley, David. 1999. *Yoga and ayurveda: Self-healing and self-realization.* Twin Lakes, WI: Lotus.

Freedman, Françoise Barbira. 2004. *Yoga for pregnancy, birth and beyond.* New York: Dorling Kindersley.

French, Roger Kenneth. 2003. *Medicine before science: The rational and learned doctor from the Middle Ages to the Enlightenment.* Cambridge: Cambridge University Press.

Friend, John. 2006. *Anusara yoga teacher training manual* 9th ed. The Woodlands, TX: Anusara.

Gambhirananda, Swami. 1989. *Taittiriya Upanishad.* Calcutta: Advaita Ashram.

Gannon, Sharon, and David Life. 2002. *Jivamukti yoga: Practices for liberating body and soul.* New York: Ballantine.

Gardner, Howard. 1993. *Frames of mind: The theory of multiple intelligences.* New York: Basic.

Gaskin, Ina May. 2003. *Ina May's guide to childbirth.* New York: Bantam.

Getty, Alice. 1936. *Ganesa: A monograph on the elephant-faced god.* Repr., Oxford: Clarendon, 1992.

Ghosh, Aurobindo Akroyd. 1914. *The synthesis of yoga.* Pondicherry, India: SABDA.

Grilley, Paul. 2002. *Yin yoga: Outline of a quiet practice.* Ashland, OR: White Cloud.

Gudmestad, Julie. 2003. Let's twist again. *Yoga Journal* (January/February 2003)

Hackett, Paul G. forthcoming. *The life and works of Theos Bernard,* http://c250.columbia.edu/ c250_celebrates/remarkable_columbians/theos_bernard_scholar.html.

Hanh, Thich Nhat. 1975. *The miracle of mindfulness: A manual on meditation.* Boston: Beacon.

Hardy, L., R. Lye, and A. Heathcote. 1983. Active versus passive warm up regimes and flexibility. *Research Papers in Physical Education* 1(5): 23–30.

Hirschi, Gertrud. 2000. *Mudras: Yoga in your hands.* Boston: Weiser

Hittleman, Richard. 1982. *Richard Hittleman's yoga: 28 day exercise plan.* New York: Bantam.

Hoff, Benjamin. 1982. *The Tao of Pooh.* New York: Dutton.

Holleman, Dona, and Orit Sen-Guppta. 1999. *Dancing the body light: The future of yoga.* Amsterdam: Pandion.

Huxley, Aldous. 1962. *Island.* New York: Harper and Row.

Iyengar, B. K. S. 1966. *Light on yoga.* New York: Schockten.

———. 1985. *Light on pranayama: The yogic art of breathing.* New York: Crossroad.

———. 1988. *The tree of yoga.* Boston: Shambhala.

———. 1993. *Light on the Yoga Sutras of Patanjali.* Columbia, MO: South Asia.

———. 2001. *Yoga: The path to holistic health.* London: Dorling Kindersley.

———. 2005. *Light on life: The yoga journey to wholeness, inner peace, and ultimate freedom.* New York: Rodale.

Iyengar, Geeta S. 1995. *Yoga: A gem for women.* Spokane: Timeless.

Johari, Harish. 1987. *Chakras: Energy centers of transformation.* Rochester, VT: Destiny.

Jois, Sri K. Pattabhi. 2002. *Yoga mala.* New York: North Point.

Jung, Carl. 1953. Yoga and the West. *The collected works of Carl Jung Vol. 1.,* ed. Sir Herbert Read, Michael Fordham, and Gerard Adler. New York and Princeton, NJ: Bollingen.

Kapur, Kamla K. 2007. *Ganesha goes to lunch: Classics from mystic India.* San Rafael, CA: Mandala.

Keedwell, Paul. 2008. *How sadness survived: The evolutionary basis of depression.* Oxford: Radcliffe.

Keele, Kenneth D. 1952. *Leonardo da Vinci on movement of the heart and blood.* London: Lippencott.

Kempton, Sally. 2002. *The heart of meditation: Pathways to a deeper experience.* South Fallsburg, NY: SYDA Foundation.

Kest, Bryan. 2007. Bryan Kest's Power yoga, http://www.poweryoga.com (accessed 2007).

Khalsa, Gurmukh Kaur. 2000. *The 8 human talents.* New York: HarperCollins.

Kornfield, Jack. 1993. *A path with heart: A guide through the perils and promises of spiritual life.* New York: Bantam.

Kramer, Joel. 1977. A new look at yoga: Playing the edge of mind and body. *Yoga Journal* (January 1977).

———. 1980. Yoga as self-transformation. *Yoga Journal* (May/June 1980).

Kramer, Joel, and Diana Alstad. 1993. *The guru papers: Masks of authoritarian power.* Berkeley, CA: North Atlantic.

———. 2009. *The passionate mind revisited: Expanding personal and social awareness.* Berkeley, CA: North Atlantic.

Kriyananda, Swami (J. Donald Walters). 1967. *Ananda Yoga for Higher Awareness.* Nevada City, NV: Crystal Clarity.

Kriyananda, Swami. 2008. What is yoga?, http://www.expandinglight.org/yoga/what-is.htm.

Lad, Vasant. 1984. *Ayurveda: The science of self-healing.* Twin Lakes, WI: Lotus.

Lasater, Judith. 1995. *Relax and renew: Restful yoga for stressful times.* Berkeley, CA: Rodmell.

Levine, Stephen. 1979. *A gradual awakening.* Garden City, NJ: Anchor.

Little, Tias. 2001. From the ground up. *Yoga Journal* (November 2001).

Lutyens, Mary. 1975. *Krishnamurti: The years of awakening.* Repr., Boston: Shambhala, 1997.

MacShane, Frank. 1964. Walden and yoga. *New England Quarterly* 37:322–42.

Maehle, Gregor. 2006. *Ashtanga yoga: Practice and philosophy.* Novato, CA: New World Library.

Mallinson, James, trans. 2004. *The Gheranda Samhita.* Woodstock, NY: YogaVidya.com.

Manchester, Frederick. 2002. *The Upanishads: Breath of the eternal.* New York: Signet Classics.

McCall, Timothy, 2007. *Yoga as medicine: The yogic prescription for health and healing.* New York: Bantam Dell.

Medina, John J. 1996. *The clock of ages.* Cambridge: Cambridge University Press.

Menon, Ramesh. 2003. *The Ramayana.* New Delhi: HarperCollins.

Michaels, Axel. 2004. *Hinduism: Past and present.* Princeton, NJ: Princeton University Press.

Miller, Barbara Stoler. 1986. Why did Henry David Thoreau take the Bhagavad-Gita to Walden Pond? *Parabola* 12.1 (Spring 1986): 58–63.

Miller, Elise Browning. 2003. *Yoga for scoliosis.* Menlo Park, CA: self-published.

Mittelmark, Raul Artal, Robert A. Wiswell, and Barbara L. Drinkwater, eds. 1991. *Exercise in pregnancy, 2nd ed.* Baltimore: Williams & Wilkins.

Mohan, A. G. 1993. *Yoga for body, breath, and mind: A guide to personal reintegration.* Portland, OR: Rudra.

Mohan, A. G., and Indra Mohan. 2004. *Yoga therapy: A guide to the therapeutic use of yoga and ayurveda for health and fitness.* Boston: Shambhala.

Moore, Keith L., and Arthur F. Dalley. 1999. *Clinically oriented anatomy, 4th ed.* Baltimore: Lippincott Williams & Wilkins.

Moore, Thomas. 1994. Care of the soul: A guide for cultivating depth and sacredness in everyday life. New York: HarperCollins.

Morrison, Judith. 1995. *The book of ayurveda.* London: Gaia.

Morse, William R. 1934. *Chinese medicine.* New York: Hoeber.

Muktananda, Swami. 1997. *Nothing exists that is not Siva: Commentaries on the Siva Sutra, Vijnanabhairava, Gurugita, and other sacred texts.* South Fallsburg, NY: Siddha Yoga Publications.

Muktibodhananda, Swami, trans. 1993. *Hatha Yoga Pradipika: Light on yoga.* Munger, India: Bihar School of Yoga.

Myers, Esther. 2002. *Hands-on assisting: A guide for yoga teachers.* Toronto: Explorations in Yoga.

Myers, Thomas. 1998. Poise: Psoas-pirifomis balance. *Massage Magazine* (March/April 1998): 72–83.

———. *Body cubed: A therapist's anatomy reader.* Self-published.

Narayanananda, Swami. 1979. *The primal power in man, or the Kundalini Shakti,* 6th rev. ed. Gylling, Denmark: Narayanananda Universal Yoga Trust.

Neese, Randolph M., and George C. Williams. 1994. *Why we get sick: The new science of Darwinian medicine.* New York: Vintage.

Netter, Frank H. 1997. *Atlas of human anatomy, 2nd ed.* East Hanover, NJ: Novartis.

Newton, Isaac. 1999. *The principia: Mathematical principles of natural philosophy.* Trans. I. Bernard Cohen and Anne Whitman. Berkeley, CA: University of California Press.

Nikhilananda, Swami, trans. 2008. *Chandogya Upanishad,* http://www.bharatadesam.com/spiritual/upanishads/chandogya_upanishad.php.

Odier, Daniel. 2004. *Yoga Spandakarika: The sacred texts at the origins of tantra.* Rochester, VT: Inner Traditions.

Ornish, Dean. 1998. *Love and survival: 8 pathways to intimacy and health.* New York: HarperCollins.

Pattanaik, Devdutt. 2003. *Indian mythology: Tales, symbols, and rituals from the heart of the subcontinent.* Rochester, VT: Inner Traditions.

Payne, Larry. 2000. *The business of teaching yoga.* Los Angeles: Samata.

Pizer, Ann, interviewer. 2007. Yoga guide, http://www.about.com (accessed May 18, 2007).

Postacchini, F., and M. Massobrio. 1983. Idiopathic coccygodynia: Analysis of fifty-one operative cases and a radiographic study of the normal coccyx. *Journal of Bone and Joint Surgery* 65(8): 1116–24.

Powell, Barbara. 1996. *Windows into the infinite: A guide to the Hindu scriptures.* Fremont, CA: Jain Publishing.

Powers, Sarah. 2008. *Insight yoga.* Boston: Shambhala.

Prabhavananda, Swami, and Christopher Isherwood, trans. 1944. *Bhagavad-Gita.* Los Angeles: The Vedanta Society.

Ramaswami, Srivatsa. 2000. *Yoga for the three stages of life: Developing your practice as an art form, a physical therapy, and a guiding philosophy.* Rochester, VT: Inner Traditions.

———. 2005. *The complete book of vinyasa yoga.* New York: Marlowe.

Rea, Shiva. 1997. *Hatha yoga as a practice of embodiment.* Masters thesis, Univ. of California, Los Angeles, Dance Department.

———. 2002. You are here. *Yoga Journal,* http://www.yogajournal.com/wisdom/460.

———. 2005. *Embodying the flow teacher training manual.* Unpublished.

———. 2007. Namaskaram. In *Iyengar: The yoga master,* ed. Kofi Busia. Boston: Shambhala.

Remen, Rachel Naomi. 1993. On defining spirit. *Noetic Sciences Review* 27 (Autumn 1993).

Rosen, Richard. 2002. *The yoga of breath: A step-by-step guide to pranayama.* Boston: Shambhala.

———. 2003. Here comes the sun. *Yoga Journal* 176 (September/October 2003).

———. 2006. *Pranayama beyond the fundamentals: An in-depth guide to yogic breathing.* Boston: Shambhala.

Ross, Steve. 2003. *Happy yoga: 7 reasons why there's nothing to worry about.* New York: HarperCollins.

Satchidananda, Swami. 1970. *Integral Hatha yoga.* Austin, TX: Holt, Rinehart and Winston.

———, trans. 1978. *The Yoga Sutras of Patanjali.* Buckingham, VA: Integral Yoga.

Satprem. 1968. *Sri Aurobindo, or the adventure of consciousness.* Pondicherry: Sri Aurobindo Ashram Press.

Satyadharma, Swami. 2003. *Yoga Chudamani Upanishad: Crown jewel of yoga.* New Delhi: Yoga Publications Trust.

Scaravelli, Vanda. 1991. *Awakening the spine: The stress-free new yoga that works with the body to restore health, vitality and energy.* New York: HarperCollins.

Schatz, Mary Pullig. 2002. A woman's balance: Inversions and menstruation, http://www.iyengar-ch/Deutsch/text_menstruation.htm.

Schiffmann, Erich. 1996. *Yoga: The spirit and practice of moving into stillness.* New York: Pocket.

———. 2007. A Tribute. In *Iyengar: The yoga master,* ed. Kofi Busia. Boston: Shambhala.

Shabana, Ahmed A. 1999. *Dynamics of multibody systems,* 3rd ed. Cambridge: Cambridge University Press.

Shamdasani, Sonu, ed. 1996. *The psychology of Kundalini yoga: Notes of the seminar given in 1932 by C. G. Jung.* Princeton: Princeton University Press.

Shannahoff-Khalsa, David S. 2004. An introduction to Kundalini yoga meditation techniques that are specific for the treatment of psychiatric disorders. *Journal of Alternative and Complementary Medicine* 10(1): 90–1.

Shrier, Ian, and Kav Gossal. 2000. The myths and truths of stretching: Individualized recommendations for healthy muscles. *Physician and Sportsmedicine* 28(8).

Singer, Charles A. 1957. *A short history of anatomy and physiology from the Greeks to Harvey.* New York: Dover.

Sivananda Yoga Center. 1983. *The Sivananada companion to yoga.* Repr., New York: Fireside, 2000.

Sjoman, N. E. 1996. *The yoga tradition of the Mysore palace.* New Delhi: Abhinav.

Sovatsky, Stuart. 1998. *Words from the soul: Time, East/West spirituality, and psychotherapeutic narrative.* New York: State University of New York Press.

Sparrowe, Linda. 2003. *Yoga.* New York: Universe.

Stein, W. B. 1965. Thoreau's first book, a spoor of yoga: The Orient in a week. *Emerson Society Quarterly* 41:3–25.

Stenhouse, Janita. 2001. *Sun yoga: The book of Surya Namaskar.* St.-Christophe, France: Innerspace.

Stephens, Anastasia. 2005. Health: The Bikram backlash. London: *The Independent,* January 25.

Stephens, J. et al. 2006. Lengthening the hamstring muscles without stretching using "awareness through movement." *Physical Therapy* 86(12): 1641–50.

Strom, Max. 1995. Stiff white male. *Yoga Journal* (June 1995).

Stryker, Rod. 2005. *Meditations for life.* Los Angeles: Para Yoga.

Svoboda, Robert. 1988. *Prakriti: Your ayurvedic constitution.* Bellingham, WA: Sadhana.

Svoboda, Robert, and Arnie Lade. 1995. *Tao and dharma: Chinese medicine and ayurveda.* Twin Lakes, WI: Lotus.

Swatmarama, Swami. 2004. *Hatha Yoga Pradipika.* Woodstock, NY: YogaVidya.com.

Swenson, David. 1999. *Ashtanga yoga: The practice manual.* Austin, TX: Ashtanga Yoga Productions.

Taylor, F. Sherwood. 1949. *A short history of science and scientific thought.* New York: Norton.

Thompson, Marcia, and David Harsha. 1984. Our rhythms still follow the African sun. *Psychology Today* 12 (January 1984): 50–4.

Tigunait, Pandit Rajmani. 1999. *Tantra unveiled: Seducing the forces of matter and spirit.* Honesdale, PA: Himalayan Institute Press.

Tirtha, Swami Sada Shiva. 2006. *The ayurvedic encyclopedia.* Coconut Creek, FL: Educa.

Todd, Mabel. 1937. *The thinking body.* Repr., New York: Dance Horizons, 1972.

Tolle, Eckhart. 1999. *The power of now: A guide to spiritual enlightenment.* Novato: New World Library.

Troels, B. 1973. Achilles heel rupture. *Acta Orthopaedica Scandinavica.* 152(suppl.): 1–126.

Van Vrekhem, Georges. 1999. *Beyond man: The life and work of Sri Aurobindo and the mother.* New Delhi: HarperCollins.

Vasu, Rai B. Chandra, trans. 2004. *The Siva Samhita.* New Delhi: Munshiram Manoharial.

Vaughan, Kathleen. 1951. *Exercises before childbirth.* London: Faber.

Vishnudevananda, Swami. 1960. *The complete illustrated book of yoga.* New York: Julian.

Watts, Alan. 1980. *Om: Creative meditations.* Berkeley, CA: Crystal Arts.

Weintraub, Amy. 2004. *Yoga for depression: A compassionate guide to relieve suffering through yoga.* New York: Broadway.

White, David Gordon. 1996. *The alchemical body: Siddha traditions in medieval India.* Chicago: University of Chicago Press.

———, ed. 2000. *Tantra in practice.* Princeton, NJ: Princeton University Press

———. 2003. *Kiss of the yogini: "Tantric sex" in its South Asian contexts.* Chicago: University of Chicago Press.

———. 2009. *Sinister yogis.* Chicago: University of Chicago Press.

White, Ganga. 2007. *Yoga beyond belief: Insights to awaken and deepen your practice.* Berkeley, CA: North Atlantic.

Williams, Raymond. 1985. *Keywords: A vocabulary of culture and society.* New York: Oxford University Press.

Witzel, Michael, ed. 1997. *Inside the texts, beyond the texts: New approaches to the study of the Vedas.* Cambridge, MA: Harvard University Press.

Woolery, Allison, et al. 2004. A yoga intervention for young adults with elevated symptoms of depression. *Alternative Therapies in Health and Medicine* 10(2): 60–3.

Yeats, W. B., and S. P. Swami. 1937. That is perfect. In *The ten principal Upanishads.* New York: Macmillan.

Yesudian, Selvarajan, and Elisabeth Haich. 1958. *Sport and yoga.* Paris: Albin Michel.

Yogananda, Paramahansa. 1946. *Autobiography of a yogi.* Los Angeles: Self-Realization Fellowship.

Zimmer, Heinrich. 1972. *Myths and symbols in Indian art and civilization.* New York: Bollingen Foundation.

INDEX

ABOUT THE AUTHOR

An esteemed yoga instructor who has trained over seven hundred yoga teachers, Mark Stephens conducts classes, workshops, teacher trainings, and retreats worldwide. He is also the author of *Yoga Sequencing: Designing Transformative Yoga Classes* (North Atlantic Books, 2012). Practicing yoga since 1991 and teaching since 1996, Mark has sought out complementary approaches along his path as student and teacher, studying Ashtanga Vinyasa, Iyengar, 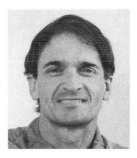 Vinyasa Flow, Tantra, yoga therapy, traditional yoga philosophy, and modern philosophies of being and consciousness. He has taught yoga at conferences (Yoga Journal, IDEA), in traditional studios (Yoga Works, L.A. Yoga Center, Santa Cruz Yoga), and in alternative settings (inner-city schools, juvenile institutions, treatment centers, prisons, and mental hospitals). He received *Yoga Journal*'s first annual Karma Yoga Award for his nonprofit work with Yoga Inside Foundation in 2000. In 2002 Stephens opened L.A. Yoga Center, an eclectic yoga studio offering Ashtanga Vinyasa, Iyengar, Vinyasa Flow, Anusara, Kundalini, and other forms of Hatha yoga. He currently lives and teaches in Santa Cruz, California, and is the founder and director of teacher training at Santa Cruz Yoga.